Clinical Decision Making in the Diagnosis and Treatment of Fluency Disorders

Delmar Publishers' Online Services
To access Delmar on the World Wide Web, point your
browser to:
http://www.delmar.com/delmar.html
To access through Gopher: gopher://gopher.delmar.com
(Delmar Online is part of "thomson.com", an internet site with
information on more than 30 publishers of the International
Thomson Publishing organization.)
For information on our products and services
email: info@delmar.com
or call 800-347-7707

Clinical Decision Making in the Diagnosis and Treatment of Fluency Disorders

Walter H. Manning, Ph.D.
The University of Memphis

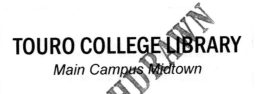

Delmar Publishers

I⊤P An International Thomson Publishing Company

Albany • Bonn • Boston • Cincinnati • Detroit • London • Madrid • Melbourne
Mexico City • New York • Pacific Grove • Paris • San Francisco • Singapore • Tokyo
Toronto • Washington

TO THE READER

Publisher does not warrant or guarantee any of the products described herein or perform any independent analysis in connection with any of the product information contained herein. Publisher does not assume, and expressly disclaims, any obligation to obtain and include information other than that provided to it by the manufacturer.

The reader is expressly warned to consider and adopt all safety precautions that might be indicated by the activities described herein and to avoid all potential hazards. By following the instructions contained herein, the reader willingly assumes all risks in connection with such instructions.

The publisher makes no representations or warranties of any kind, including but not limited to, the warranties of fitness for particular purpose or merchantability, nor are any such representations implied with respect to the material set forth herein, and the publisher takes no responsibility with respect to such material. The publisher shall not be liable for any special, consequential, or exemplary damages resulting, in whole or in part, from the reader's uses of, or reliance upon, this material.

Cover Design: Sergio Sericolo
Delmar Staff:
Acquisitions Editor: Kimberly A. Davies
Marketing Manager: Dawn Gerrain
Developmental Editor: Debra Flis
Project Editor: Coreen Rogers
Production Coordinator: John Mickelbank
Art and Design Coordinator: Vincent S. Berger
Editorial Assistant: Donna L. Leto

COPYRIGHT © 1996
By Delmar Publishers
A division of International Thomson Publishing Inc.
The ITP logo is a trademark under license
Printed in the United States of America
For more information, contact:

Delmar Publishers
3 Columbia Circle, Box 15015
Albany, New York 12212-5015

International Thomson Publishing Europe
Berkshire House 168-173
High Holborn
London, WC1V7AA
England

Thomas Nelson Australia
102 Dodds Street
South Melbourne, 3205
Victoria, Australia

Nelson Canada
1120 Birchmount Road
Scarborough, Ontario
Canada M1K 5GA

International Thomson Editores
Campos Eliseos 385, Piso 7
Col Polanco
11560 Mexico D F Mexico

International Thomson Publishing GmbH
Königswinterer Strasse 418
53227 Bonn
Germany

International Thomson Publishing Asia
221 Henderson Road
#05-10 Henderson Building
Singapore 0315

International Thomson Publishing - Japan
Hirakawacho Kyowa Building, 3F
2-2-1 Hirakawacho
Chiyoda-ku, Tokyo 102
Japan

Dedication

This book is dedicated to Sallie Starr Hillard. Sallie was a friend, a colleague, and a counselor. She was a grand clinician, in part, because she was a person with marvelous wisdom and grace. She was there at the beginning of this book. I believe that she is able to know its completion.

Contents

Preface

The primary goal of this book is to convey to students, as well as professional clinicians, the enthusiasm and excitement of working, and growing with, people who have disorders of fluency. During the formulation and development of the profession of speech pathology in this country, particularly during the decades from the late 1920s through the 1960s, the area of fluency disorders was a major focus of the research and writing in our journals and texts. A review of the early issues of the *Journal of Speech Disorders* (published from 1936 through 1946) or the initial volumes of the *Journal of Speech and Hearing Disorders* confirms that a large proportion of the articles addressed stuttering diagnosis and treatment. As the scope of practice continued to expand in the field of communication disorders, fluency disorders became but one of many areas that students were presented with during their academic and clinical program. Today, students and professionals are exposed to areas of study that were not even acknowledged in the field only a few years ago. At the present time, speech-language pathologists are asked to become generalists across the wide range of human communication disorders, as the scope of practice for the field has expanded dramatically during the past two decades.

The depth of the field is also changing. Because clinicians are asked to become knowledgeable about so many different communication disorders and related areas, there is concern that the qualifications of professionals for serving any one disorder are being compromised. As a result, during the next few years, many professional clinicians will have the opportunity to become certified as specialists in specific disorder areas. Specialty recognition will require the demonstration of additional academic and clinical experience beyond the basic graduate degree. Moreover, continued recognition will require continued education. Specialty recognition is being driven both by evident professional needs and by a consumer demand for better services. There is no doubt that these certification requirements will result in a higher level of professional help for clients with fluency disorders.

As the field of communication disorders continues to evolve, the critical mass of information will continue to rapidly expand. Even within a single area of study such as fluency disorders, the literature is extensive and additional material is continually becoming available via computer and electronic networks. The single most difficult choice in preparing a text is not what to include, for there are many informative and intriguing manuscripts available. Rather, the most difficult decision is what portion of the ongoing flow of new information by many diligent authors to omit. In preparing a text, there is also the desire to pay homage to those who have gone before and to acknowledge the colleagues you feel privileged to be working alongside, in, as Charles Van Riper often said, the vineyard of fluency disorders.

Reading the volumes of literature can be intimidating, even for someone who has been a clinician and researcher in the field for many years. As Conture (1990) has pointed out, it is easy to feel as though you are drowning in a sea of information, especially when some of it is conflicting. One wonders, as other authors have, what there is to say that is new. So much about stuttering and stutterers has been said before—in some cases, probably more times than it needs to be. One of the reasons for writing this book is to find out what I know and what I need to know about fluency disorders. This work is based on knowledge gained from a variety of texts, an extensive review of representative descriptive and experimental research, and twenty-five years of research and clinical work with individuals who have fluency disorders. It is also based on a successful experience of self-management of my own stuttering.

There are discussions in this text that have not appeared in past literature (e.g., humor as both a clinician and treatment variable, signs of progress during and following treatment) or, in some cases, very little (e.g., characteristics of older stutterers, characteristics of effective clinicians, rationale and procedures for eliciting fluency breaks in young children). Other information has appeared only in recent years (the problems of maintaining long-term progress and the serious issue of relapse following treatment). We have attempted to introduce new ideas and to take a slightly different approach to some of the old ones.

The intervention philosophy in this text is comprehensive. That is, I believe that successful treatment involves many levels of change. Fluency problems are multidimensional, involving, at the very least, behavioral, attitudinal, and cognitive features. For most people, counseling is an important component of long-term success. For a successful treatment outcome, each of these levels needs to be addressed. We need to change speech behavior, to be sure, but we also need to change ways of interpreting what is occurring during our attempts at human communication. Our goal is to change, not only the nature of a fluency disorder, but, more importantly to help the *person* who comes to us with the problem. While we are interested in decreasing the frequency and changing the form of the stuttering, we are even more interested in reducing the handicap that this problem creates for the speaker.

No one should expect anyone who has recently completed a graduate program to be perfect in their work, including speech-language pathologists. One or more classes, a text, and the initial years of experience with clients provide only a beginning to a lifelong career of learning about how to help people. How, then, can we expect our clients to swiftly master their speech and all of the fearful communication situations that are available to them? However, if we do the job well, it is reasonable to expect our clients to be able to independently assess the situation, make decisions that are informed and truthful, use appropriate techniques for conceptualizing the situation and self-managing their speech, and create a new interpretation of their internal control as it relates to their speech. If they can do these things most of the time, our clients will be better able to cope with their speech and their lives. Moreover, they will not be nearly as handicapped as they have been in the past, which, after all, is the true measure of successful intervention.

This book is not intended to provide comprehensive coverage for courses in fluency disorders. With the current base of information concerning this communication disorder, no single book can serve that purpose. There are sources that have been especially helpful in obtaining information for this text. The series of editions of Bloodstein's *Handbook on Stuttering* (1987) provides an ongoing review of the past and current literature. Van Riper's texts on the treatment (1973) and nature of stuttering (1982) also provide exhaustive sources embedded with wonderful clinical intuition. Starkweather (1987) provides a critical review of the characteristics of normal fluency with insightful comments that explain the contrast between normal and abnormal fluency breaks. Silverman (1996) provides a brilliant explanation of the historical development of the major views of stuttering etiology. Peters and Guitar (1991) give the reader a lucid and detailed explanation of the major intervention strategies for fluency disorders as well as detailed descriptions of specific treatment techniques. In addition, Conture (1990) presents the student with a thoughtful and highly readable explanation of specific treatment techniques for both children and adults.

The fundamental objectives that have guided the preparation of this text are:

1. to generate an enthusiasm in clinicians, especially graduate students, for working with children and adults who stutter,

2. to discuss clinical decision making from the perspective of individual client needs,

3. to provide the clinician with choices of treatment strategies and associated techniques,

4. to discuss aspects of diagnosis and treatment that have been discussed very little or not at all in the literature,

5. to suggest questions for clinical investigation in the general area of fluency disorders.

It is fitting at the outset to comment on some of the terms used in this book. Throughout the chapters, the clinician or speech-language pathologist is referred to by using feminine pronouns and clients are referred to by using masculine pronouns. Obviously, there are both male and female clients and clinicians, but since it reflects the most common clinical situation, this description will be used to enhance the consistency of the reading. An even more important issue is what to call the person who is doing the stuttering. In var-

ious clinical contexts, he or she is referred to as client, patient, or even consumer. For consistency, the term most often used in this book is *client*.

During the past few years, there has been discussion concerning the appropriateness of using the term *stutterer*. Some argue that the term is too all-
encompassing and serves as a label that can negatively influence and limit how
we define the problem as well as the person. Clearly, a person who happens
to stutter also takes on many other roles. Some have suggested using the term
"person who stutters" or PWS. While such terms are generally seen as being
more descriptive, they can be extremely cumbersome and often result in an
awkward writing style that is difficult to read and understand. Recently, a friend
with a background in psycholinguistics pointed out that the suffix *-er* means
someone or something that performs the action of the root verb: someone who
does, not someone who *is*. Thus, the term *stutterer* would refer to someone
who stutters, and not someone whose life is defined by stuttering. As we shall
see, the variability of stuttering behavior also contributes to the problem of
what to call people who happen to sometimes stutter. That is, the terminology is complicated because, unlike someone who is blind or deaf or has lost
a limb, the person who stutters is often fluent. Indeed, many people who
stutter have no difficulty calling themselves stutterers and even show pride
in using the term, particularly if they are fluent much of the time.

The approach I have chosen for this book is to use *person who stutters* whenever possible. However, I will also use the term *stutterer* when it facilitates
the clarity of the writing. In any case, I want to state at the outset the earnest
belief that, indeed, terms do not define the person. Clearly, each client is vastly
more than someone who stutters. Such a view is at the heart of any comprehensive and humanistic approach to the problem. Just as the clinician makes
decisions based on the needs of the client throughout the intervention process,
a choice can be made about what terms are best in each case. If the client, at
the outset of treatment, attaches a stigma to the term *stutterer* and would
feel more comfortable using something such as *a person who stutters* or *PWS*,
then, for the time being, these are likely to be the best terms. In any case, the
terminology should not become part of the problem.

The treatment of fluency disorders should be exciting and fun. It ought to
be exciting, for to the degree that we as clinicians enter the process, model
the behavior we want to change, take risks with our clients, and even experience setbacks with them, we grow as well. Thus, much of the process of fluency treatment is a shared psychotherapeutic experience and, typically, a good
one. Welcome to the vineyard! If you stay awhile, it won't be long before you
find that there is a wealth of knowledge, goodwill, and support to be found
among your colleagues.

Acknowledgments

I greatly appreciate the many students and colleagues at the University of Memphis who provided critical evaluations of this manuscript. Genuine thanks is given to my good friend of many years, Terry Beachy, whose clinical and editorial insight for choosing the best words is greatly valued. Her belief in this project was a large part of my incentive. Acknowledgment is also given to my mentors and friends—people like Gene Cooper, Dan Beasley, and Anne Manning—whose support will always be valued. Thank you also to three wonderful children, Tracy, Jody, and Matt. Lastly, I want to note my appreciation of the clients who continue to show me the many facets of fluency disorders, including the courage essential for change and growth.

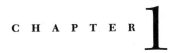

Clinician Characteristics

INTRODUCTION

To begin a book on fluency disorders by discussing the characteristics of the clinician is unusual. Often, the first chapter instead includes a description of the symptoms or presents historical views of the problem. However, because the emphasis of this text is on the clinician's clinical decision making and the choices that must be made by the one who will conduct the diagnosis and treatment, it seems an ideal place to begin. Not everyone—not even all clinicians— are equally effective when trying to assist children and adults who have fluency disorders. Experienced clinicians and even some clients have suggested that some clinician characteristics are more desirable than others. If this is the reader's first exposure to the field of fluency disorders, this initial chapter may help you to determine whether or not helping people with such problems is likely to be satisfying, both for you and the client.

The purpose of this chapter is twofold. First, we will examine some characteristics of the clinicians who have been identified as being especially effective in working with children and adults who stutter. We will discuss the attitudes as well as the personal and professional attributes that are most desirable for the clinician who effectively guides a client through the treatment process. In the second half of the chapter, we will introduce an attribute of the clinician-client relationship that reflects the essential properties of the therapeutic process—humor.

THE IMPORTANCE OF THE CLINICIAN

There is no exclusive set of attributes that define the model clinician. Even if this were the case, no clinician could be expected to possess all the desirable attributes that are discussed in this chapter. Each client comes to us with different needs and requires, at various points during the treatment process, different attributes and different roles of the clinician. Moreover, the professional and personal attributes of the clinician will interact with the characteristics of the client, resulting in a unique combination during each therapeutic relationship. After many years of observing both student and professional clinicians as well as asking clients about their perceptions of their clinicians, it is clear that some clinicians are considerably better than others at motivating and guiding their clients. The attitudes and abilities these clinicians possess distinguish them from the clinicians who are less effective. It is the effective clinicians who are able to discover appropriate therapeutic strategies and design associated techniques. Perhaps more than any other quality, the best clinicians are uncommonly effective in motivating and supporting their clients along the often arduous path of treatment.

In contrast to the numerous investigations of children and adults who stutter, relatively few questions have been asked about the attributes of the clinicians who provide the treatment. Those authors who have considered this side of the treatment process, specifically in the area of fluency disorders (Cooper & Cooper, 1985c; Van Riper, 1975) provide convincing arguments that the clinician is not only a, but *the* critical part of the process. Regardless of the treatment strategy or specific techniques, Cooper and Cooper maintain that the person who is administering the treatment is the most important variable in the process of change.

The importance of the clinician is perhaps more apparent when a counseling-based treatment is used. Murphy and Fitzsimons (1960) contend that during counseling, the "most important single variable affecting the success in the treatment of stutterers is—the clinician" (p. 27). However, as Cooper and Cooper (1985b) state, even if treatment takes the form of an archetypal program of behavioral modification, "It does matter who is doing the conditioning" (p. 21). Regardless of the overall treatment strategy, the clinician plays a critical role in orchestrating a successful treatment program. For that matter, the clinician often is a major factor in determining whether the client even stays in treatment long enough for meaningful change to take place. Just as in teaching, parenting, and coaching, in the treatment of fluency disorders, it makes a real difference who is serving as a guide and mentor.

Clinician Attitudes About Stuttering and Stutterers

Our attitude about those who come to us for help and our understanding of their communication problems have a fundamental influence on how we approach them as people during both assessment and treatment. What the clinician has been told and what she has been able to observe about stuttering and the people who stutter will determine whether she will even have the desire to work with such clients. There are clinicians who choose to, or at least would like to, avoid working with children and adults who stutter (Ainsworth, 1992; Cooper, 1975c, 1985; St. Louis & Durrenberger, 1992; Van Riper, 1992; Wingate, 1971). Clinicians who do not find it enjoyable and rewarding to work with people who stutter should not do so, as their lack of enjoyment will show. Obviously, at the outset of training, it is natural for anyone to be anxious. However, if a clinician has received a quality education and continues to be apprehensive about working with people who stutter, this is one indication that he or she is not yet qualified. People who stutter will not get the best possible treatment unless they can find a clinician who is not merely competent, but enthusiastic about the process of change.

The disturbing results of several investigations indicate that some professional clinicians have opinions of stuttering, and particularly of the people who stutter, that are not accurate. The findings of these investigations are consistent with each other and have included large numbers of both student and professional clinicians from many states throughout the country (Cooper and Cooper, 1985a; Curlee, 1985; Lass, Ruscello, Pannbaker, Schmitt, & Everly-Myers, 1989; Mallard, Gardner, & Downey, 1988; Matkin, Ringle, & Snope, 1983; St. Louis & Lass, 1981). Sommers and Caruso (1995) noted that directors of university training programs and public school supervisors found both preservice clinical experience and postgraduate in-service training to be lacking in the area of fluency disorders. University program directors reported that clinical clock hours for master's degree students in the area of fluency disorders were considerably less (average, 20.2 hours, standard deviation, 18.7) than for language disorders (average, 104.2 hours, standard deviation, 52.8) or articulation-phonology disorders (average, 77.4 hours, standard deviation, 56.3).

A survey of 597 certified professional clinicians done by Matkin, Ringle, and Snope (1983) indicated that these clinicians rated themselves as being much less competent with fluency disorders than with other communication disorders. Curlee (1985) found that 40 percent of the respondents from accredited programs did not believe that their students were being adequately prepared to serve clients with fluency disorders. A review of clinician attitudes toward stuttering done by Cooper and Cooper (1992) provides the most recent example of these opinions. These authors determined the attitudes of 1,872 speech-language pathologists from twenty-one states. Seventy-five percent of the subjects held a graduate degree in education. The subjects completed the Clinician Attitudes Toward Stuttering Inventory (CATS) (Cooper, 1975a). Clinicians responded to fifty attitudinal statements by circling words on a five-point strength-of-agreement scale. The results of the 1991 survey were contrasted to an identical survey of 674 clinicians conducted between 1973 and 1983.

The results of the 1991 survey indicated that, as a group, the clinicians showed attitude changes over the years that indicated the development of a more enlightened view of stuttering and people who stutter. For example, in comparison to the earlier results, the 1991 data indicated that a smaller percentage of the professional clinicians held the view that most stutterers have psychological problems (35.7% versus 41.9%). The view that parents are the primary factor causing stuttering in their children became less frequently expressed (10.6% versus 17.9%). Moreover, a larger proportion of clinicians now held the view that early intervention with young children is likely to yield success (63.4% versus 49.5%).

However, the results from the 1991 survey also indicated that there continued to be large percentages of clinicians who held the following views:

- 12.6 percent of the subjects agreed that most speech clinicians are adept in treating stuttering (75.5% disagreed).

- 2.1 percent of the clinicians agreed that they felt more comfortable in working with individuals who stutter than working with articulatory defective individuals (93.2% disagreed).

- 57.8 percent of the clinicians agreed that there are some personality traits that are characteristic of stutterers (18.4% disagreed).

The view of stuttering that clinicians will have is profoundly influenced by the nature of the academic and clinical instruction they receive during their degree programs. At this writing the national accrediting association in the field, the American Speech-Language-Hearing Association (ASHA), has failed to mandate that students must obtain even a minimum number of hours in diagnosing and treating children and adults with fluency disorders. In addition, the association does not require that a student take even a single course in fluency disorders. Thus, depending on the academic and clinical preparation provided by specific graduate programs, the view clinicians have about stuttering and stutterers may be a narrow one. Hopefully, the recent efforts toward specialty certification through ASHA will help to elevate the level of training received by many clinicians.

If stuttering is presented as a mysterious disorder, an enigma, clinicians will naturally be wary about treating these clients. Stuttering may indeed be an enigma, for the syndrome is complex and much of the problem lies under the surface. Van Riper (1982), responding to the suggestion that stuttering is like a riddle, stated that "[It] is more than a riddle. It is at least a complicated, multidimensional jigsaw puzzle, with many pieces still missing" (p. 1). Sheehan frequently argued the case that stuttering was like an iceberg, with only small portions of the problem visible to those who were unwilling to look below the surface (Sheehan, 1970). Years later, Sheehan (1980) offered the pointed comment that "defining stuttering as [only] a fluency problem borders on professional irresponsibility. It ignores the person. It ignores his feelings about himself" (p. 392).

However, stuttering is a problem that is not significantly more complex than many other human behavioral problems (Ham, 1993). It is true that there is much to learn about the many aspects of this handicap to communication. On the other hand, clinicians also need to appreciate that much of stuttering behavior is rule governed. Many of the factors that precipitate and maintain stuttering are understood, and many children and adults achieve extraordinary success in modifying both their speech and their handicap as a result of treatment. As students have the opportunity to observe clinicians who are unafraid of stuttering and have had success with several people, they will be more likely to be enthusiastic about the assessment and treatment of fluency disorders. These experienced clinicians know what success looks and sounds like, changes that can be shown to the new clinician.

One of the substantial problems faced by students taking part in any clinical experience is that they are not likely to see a long view of progress. They are not able to follow clients throughout the continuum of change. It is all too rare, even for the professional clinician, to follow a client for more than a few months or years following dismissal from treatment. Most students lack the chance to observe a client even during the range of formal treatment—the time during which the client pays a professional for services—let alone informal treatment—the much longer period when the client gradually assumes the role of clinician and develops the "response-ability" required for self-treatment. The window available to student clinicians in graduate programs is a small one. When the overall picture of behavioral, affective, and cognitive change is unavailable, it is understandable that the treatment process will appear enigmatic. However, if student clinicians know what to look for and can be shown progress during treatment (both in the behavioral changes and in attitudinal and cognitive changes of the person who stutters), then helping these speakers will be more likely to be viewed as a positive rather than an aversive, experience. A central principle is indicated in the comments of Daly (1988), who noted that the better clinicians tend to be those who hold a belief that their clients have the capacity for success as a result of treatment. Such conviction by the clinician is essential according to Van Riper (1973), who stated the belief that "out of the therapist's faith can come the stutterer's hope" (p. 230).

CLINICIAN PERSONALITY ATTRIBUTES

The therapeutic relationship has been studied extensively in the fields of counseling and clinical psychology. The results of these investigations began finding their way into the literature in speech-language pathology during the 1960s. Although the clinician-client relationship is clearly important in all aspects of clinical intervention in communication disorders, it is especially critical in the area of fluency disorders because of the strong interactive therapeutic component. Research in the fields of counseling and psychology has provided consistent evidence that therapeutic exchanges are more likely to facilitate optimum change or gain if the clinician is able to communicate messages of empathy, positive regard, genuineness, and concreteness (Berenson & Carkhuff, 1967; Carkhuff & Berenson, 1967; Truax & Carkhuff, 1966).

Van Riper (1975) provided the first comprehensive description of the desirable attributes of a stutterer's clinician. He described personality characteristics such as *empathy*, an authentic sensitivity for the client; *warmth*, a respect or positive regard for the client; *genuineness*, an openness and the ability to disclose oneself as a real person; and *charisma*, an ability to arouse hope, appearing confident yet humble, frank yet tactful. As Van Riper (1973) stated: "Like fishermen, good therapists are optimists. Most of them have come to have profound respect for the latent potential for self-healing that exists in all troubled souls" (p. 230).

Undoubtedly, such characteristics would be desirable for any clinician working with a person for any reason. They would be valuable characteristics to have in a friend or colleague. Moreover, just as it is possible to be successful as a friend or colleague without all of these attributes, it is possible to be a successful clinician without possessing enormous amounts of each. However, clinicians that possess such characteristics not only make the treatment process more effective, they also make it more enjoyable.

Cooper and Cooper (1985b) also provided a description of several desirable attributes of the effective clinician. Many of the attributes described by these authors coincide with their view of fluency treatment as an interpersonal communication experience. The effective clinician brings to this interpersonal experience certain desirable attitudes and personality attributes. The Coopers suggested that, especially during the early stages of treatment, the client-clinician relationship should be a major focus of discussion. They stated that the clinician should be able to *openly express* both negative as well as positive feelings to the client. However, as the clinician is expressing these feelings, it is important that the clinician also *indicate a belief in the worth and potential* of the client. As treatment becomes challenging and the client is asked to make behavioral, attitudinal, and cognitive changes, the clinician should be *continually honest* in reinforcing the client's feelings of self-worth. This, the Coopers prudently note, is much easier to do when the clinician enjoys working with the client, which may not always be the case. They warn that clinicians need to resist the urge to tell clients how they should feel. Instead, they should foster an expression of client feelings. The clinician may, however, indicate that although she understands a client's feelings, she does not share them or at least does not necessarily agree that they are warranted by the situation. Moreover, of course, experienced clinicians are able to indicate the difference between disapproval of feelings expressed by the client and the client's worth.

Cooper and Cooper (1985b) state that the clinician should be "*devoid of dogma*" and have the ability to adapt the therapeutic approach to the client's uniqueness and needs. This is another way of saying that good clinicians are client directed rather than treatment directed. The clinician must be able to recognize subtle client responses that provide cues for direction and indicate progress. Experienced clinicians are not slowed down by a client's negative response to the demands and challenges. They are, in short, able to be a constant ally and to persevere along with the client when the process becomes difficult. Experienced clinicians *inform the client* by providing information about the latter's status and progress in treatment. Cooper and Cooper submit that clients, at any point in treatment and regardless of age or mental abilities, should be able to describe just where they are in treatment in both behavioral and attitudinal terms. Finally, effective clinicians are able to attend to the details of record keeping and report writing.

Most people come to the professional field of speech-language pathology with many of these basic personality attributes, attitudes, and abilities. It is not clear whether some or all of these basic characteristics can be created or enhanced as a function of academic and clinical experience. What is clear, however, is that given these basic personality characteristics, clinicians can achieve proficiency in several intervention skills that increase their effectiveness.

CLINICIAN INTERVENTION SKILLS

This section will discuss, given the aforementioned attitudes and personality attributes, some of the intervention abilities that I believe can be acquired and developed during the student's education. There is, of course, considerable overlap across each of these abilities.

Becoming Less Inhibited

Becoming desensitized to stuttering is an important first step in understanding the behavior and the person we are treating. Only after the clinician is able to become uninhibited about stuttering in general, and about herself in particular, will treatment proceed (Van Riper, 1982).

The clinician needs to become less inhibited about many aspects of stuttering. First of all, clinicians often need to overcome a concern about doing something "wrong" in therapy that will hurt the stutterer and make him worse. This common perspective is likely related to the notion that there is something psychologically amiss or unstable about the person who stutters and that such clients are especially susceptible to emotional trauma. In part, this attitude may be a result of the diagnosogenic view of stuttering etiology advocated during the period from the 1950s through the late 1960s, which stated that stuttering was created by inappropriate listener reactions to the fluency breaks of young children. Alternately, such a cautious approach may be related to the idea that any increase in the frequency of stuttering is necessarily bad. As we will discuss in later chapters, stuttering is highly variable and changes in the frequency of the overt behaviors can be attributable to many factors, only one of which is the clinician.

In extreme instances, it may be possible to make the stuttering, or even the stutterer, in some sense worse. If, for example, the clinician is truly an unqualified, uncaring, and insensitive person, the client and, conceivably, the stuttering could become worse. However, a qualified clinician who is inhibited about saying or doing something during treatment for fear of somehow injuring a client possesses a naive view of the person doing the stuttering. On the contrary, most people who stutter are stable and highly durable, especially those who have the courage to ask for help and initiate treatment. Clinicians, if they have enough training and experience, should have no more fear about doing the "wrong" thing during the treatment of a child or adult who stutters than they would have with a client with any other communication disorder.

The relationship between clinician and client is an important aspect of the process of change during treatment. There is no question, especially with adults who stutter, that there is a strong counseling or psychotherapeutic component at the center. There are aspects of this process of the nature of change and growth that impact on the clinician as well as the client. It is rare that only one person grows during good, interactive treatment. Indeed, such growth is often experienced most clearly during the mixture of personalities and perceptions that take place in group treatment activities. Students have often commented after completing their clinical experiences in fluency disorders that they miss the exciting and challenging experiences of group treatment.

Nevertheless, because the process of change and growth is a dynamic one, it is not necessarily something that all clinicians are initially comfortable about entering. One alluring aspect of the early behavior modification programs in fluency disorders in the late 1950s, 1960s, and 1970s was the belief that the role of the clinician was limited to the identification and modification of overt stuttering behaviors. The behaviors that were audible and variable on the surface were the major focus of treatment. It is not that the clinicians were not making decisions. Frequency counts were made, contingencies were agreed upon, and rewards and punishments were dispensed based on the client's performance. The treatment process was clear, goals were explicit, and fluency was charted and changed. The approach was relatively easy to teach to students as well as to clients. Some clients did well, as they do in all treatment approaches. Some even stayed well. However, the point is not whether behavior modification approaches are effective. A particular treatment strategy can only be evaluated based on the needs and response of the client. The point is that in any treatment, including current behavioral modification programs (which tend to include a more broad-based approach that focuses on more than the speaker's surface behaviors), the clinician needs to be unafraid. She needs to be uninhibited about stuttering and the people doing the stuttering if she expects the client, parents, teacher, or spouse to also adopt this attitude.

Obtaining experience with clients in any clinical area is difficult—frightening, even. At the outset, the clinician will be overloaded. Even if she has a sense of the overall direction of treatment and knows about a variety of treatment techniques, at best she has seen only a portion of the total treatment sequence.

Although there may have been the opportunity to observe clients on video-tape in the clinic, *she* has not been the one who has made the process happen.

One of the best aspects of the treatment videotapes produced by the Stuttering Foundation of America is that the clinician, Charles Van Riper, demonstrates an uninhibited and assertive interactive style with the young adult, male client. He models attributes of empathy, genuineness, warmth, charisma, and particularly frankness, as he works through the treatment process with his young adult client. Van Riper is obviously unafraid of stuttering. He moves forward in treatment with a distinct sense of direction and an uninhibited attitude.

Another beneficial aspect of these videotapes is that the student can see an enlarged window of change as the client progresses through treatment. There is some indication that students can increase their level of self-efficacy about clinical performance with fluency clients as a function of (only) academic training (Rudolf, Manning, and Sewell, 1983). There is, of course, no substitute for a successful clinical experience.

Opening Your Focus

One of the characteristics of someone who is learning a new activity is the amount of attention given to the techniques. When first learning a sport such as soccer, for example, it is necessary to learn such techniques as passing, receiving, and shooting the ball. Later, with more experience, one moves beyond the techniques. The accomplished player has a broader, less technical view of the game. With experience, the view includes the strategies of the event, and particularly an analysis of the other team's strengths and weaknesses. The participant's focus begins to open up. Although the techniques remain essential to the accomplishment of the overall strategy, the most important aspect of the process is not what to do or how, but when to do it and why. Similar to inexperienced players or coaches, new clinicians tend to focus on techniques of the moment rather than the overall, long-term strategies. Even more to the point, new clinicians are more likely to focus on the techniques rather than the person they are trying to help. They are apt to think to themselves, "What do I *do* in therapy today?" rather than, "What does my client need from me now, and how does that fit with the long-term goal of treatment?"

We are not suggesting that specific treatment techniques are unimportant. They are, of course, every bit as essential as knowing how to pass and handle the ball is to playing soccer. You cannot play the game if you are not able to handle the ball—and you cannot treat people who stutter if you are not able to identify specific accessory behaviors, tabulate the percentage of syllables stuttered, and demonstrate specific stuttering or fluency modification techniques. Techniques are unquestionably important, the professional clinician must know many of them, and know them well. However, they are not the most important aspect of the process. The ability to look beyond the techniques—even beyond the treatment program—and see the client is something that distinguishes the experienced clinician from the novice, the technician from the professional.

Just as the new instructor is less likely to vary the prepared text or stray more than a few steps away from the podium, the less experienced player is more likely to have a rigid, preplanned attack. A preplanned strategy may work for a time, particularly if the opponent is easy. However, it will not work indefinitely, especially if the opponent is challenging. The accomplished participant is flexible; he or she can see what is occurring on the field in a broader sense. The accomplished athlete (or coach) is more likely to be aware of, and willing to change, strategy, based on circumstances and the competition. The clinician's decisions and actions are primarily dictated by the other players. They most certainly are not dictated by a textbook or by dogma. Table 1–1 suggests several continuums that serve to distinguish the technician from the professional.

Table 1-1. Continuums that distinguish clinical decision making by a technician and by an experienced professional.

Technician	⟷	Professional
technique directed	⟷	client directed
preplanned procedures	⟷	flexible procedures
dogmatic treatment	⟷	treatment alternatives
narrow focus, on problem	⟷	open focus, on person

For decades, Van Riper stated that "the client is the guide," not the clinician, and certainly not the text or the treatment techniques. There is no one dogmatic path up the mountain. Rather, the path is likely to be different for each client. We must know what the client needs and when. This seems rather complicated—and it is. However, before we throw up our hands at the challenge facing us with each new client, it is important to realize that much of what most clients need is similar; we can expect to see certain patterns of attitude and behavior. Moreover there are basic clinician as well as client skills that will contribute to the process of change.

Calibrating to the Client

At the outset of the first several treatment sessions, we clinicians find ourselves overloaded with information presented by the client. Not only are we introduced to expected surface behaviors that we have seen before, but we will also be presented with some new behaviors that are unique to this person. Some of these behaviors may be obvious and explicit in the form of struggle behavior (see Chapters 3 and 4). Other behaviors may occur rarely or not at all during the initial sessions. Some of the behaviors that were learned long ago and have become part of this person's response to stuttering may only surface during more stressful speaking situations. These behaviors may be observed only rarely, if at all, during treatment sessions. We may be able to observe these surface behaviors only if we accompany the person into speaking situations they enter daily, for example, at school or at work. Alternately, we may note these behaviors if we call clients unexpectedly at home or by chance meet them in some location outside the formal clinical setting. In any case, there are apt to be many surface behaviors, several of them unique to one person, and it will take a while to become calibrated to them.

In addition to tuning in to the stuttering behaviors, it will also take a while to become calibrated to the way the new client speaks when not stuttering. In order to specify the nature of the client's stuttered speech, it is essential to specify the quality of the person's nonstuttered speech. What is it about the surface behaviors of this person's speech that indicates to us that they are not stuttering? Is the client able to produce truly fluent speech that, as Stark-weather (1987) indicates, is characterized by an easy, smooth, relatively effortless flow? On the other hand, is their speech characterized by something less than a smooth, effortless quality? Is the client achieving fluency or just "not stuttering"? Is the speech fluent in a technical sense but characterized by a degree of instability? An essential step in calibrating yourself to the client is being able to differentiate and contrast at least three levels of fluency: stuttered speech, unstable speech, and fluent speech.

One procedure that aids in the calibration process, especially during the first several meetings, is to pantomime the client's speech (Van Riper, 1973). That is, the clinician follows the client's speech by shadowing what he is saying. In this way the clinician is able to get a feel for how the client may, for example, slightly slow his speech before a feared word. The clinician can begin to sense how the client scans ahead and "pretastes" words while considering whether to try moving through them. Using audio- or videotapes early in treatment can assist clinicians in tuning in to their new client. The clinician can become calibrated to the client's speech patterns by pantomiming the tapes at the office, at home, or while driving in the car. Although on the surface, the client may appear to be fluent, with time the clinician will be able to detect instances when the client is speaking carefully and making a concerted effort not to stutter. The speech is unstable and the clinician will get the sensation that the client is "talking on thin ice"; the client is not stuttering in a technical sense yet seems as though he may fall through at any moment.

As we become calibrated to the new client, we will begin to notice how the client's speech looks as well as how it sounds. We can begin to tune in, not only to the surface structure, but, and perhaps even more important, to the deep structure of the person. What are the cues signaling that this speaker may feel some loss of control, some helplessness, as he approaches, and even goes through, a feared word? Although the speaker may not have overtly stuttered on a word, he may not have felt completely in control of his speech. It is as though the stuttering were just under the surface. Until we become calibrated to that person, we are not likely to detect such occurrences.

In observing the surface and deep structure of the client's speech, experienced clinicians are apt to minimize talk and maximize observation. One way to tune in to someone is to stop talking. More experienced clinicians use silence and are not intimidated by it. They use it as a time for reflecting on what the client has said. Interpersonal communication is not stopped during silence. Body language, eye contact, and facial expressions tell much about the status of what has been said—and left unsaid. Silence on the part of the clinician may even be thought of as providing the client with a degree of independence. Van Riper (1975) suggested that when the clinician finds herself uttering more than four or five sentences in a row, "warning lights should go off." This is especially true, he suggested, if the sentences contain many *I*'s and *We*'s.

Taking Risks

Clinicians must be prepared to lead the way in treatment. We must be able to demonstrate our willingness to take risks if we are asking our client to do so. Sheehan (1970) made the insightful comment that "the Achilles heel of most normal speaking therapists who try to work with stutterers is simply that they are not willing to do what they ask their stutterers to do" (p. 283). If we are afraid of stuttering and the tasks that await our client on the road to change, how can we expect him to follow our recommendations and to move forward? We do not have to do so often, but we will occasionally be called upon to demonstrate our willingness to take risks and to lead the way into speaking situations. Each situation is an opportunity to demonstrate that it is possible to be reasonably calm in the midst of stuttering; it is possible to openly stutter and not completely lose control. Alternately, depending on how difficult this experience is for you as the clinician, it is a chance to demonstrate that, despite your obvious anxiety, you are committed to helping the client. You are willing to enter the field of play (Manning, 1991). You will, for example, voluntarily stutter to a stranger on the street as your client observes. You will openly stutter on the question, "Pardon me, do you have the ta . . . ta . . . ta . . ." until the listener gives you the time of day. You can tell the client that you are committed to helping him, which is fine, but showing him is far better.

It is easy to talk about the tasks, about what needs to be done to change the behaviors and attitudes associated with the problem. However, it is quite another thing to enter into the hard, often grueling, tasks that must be done. As Peck (1978) suggested, the cornerstone of any clinical relationship is the commitment on the part of the clinician, who must be willing to join in the struggle rather than sitting back and playing a professional role. There will be times during successful treatment where the clinician will be asked to take the field and join in the struggle, not to talk about commitment, but to demonstrate it. If the clinician is able to do so and to show that she is a stable and understanding ally, the client will be much more likely to go beyond his previously established boundaries.

There are times during treatment—especially if it is conducted outside of the safe environment of the clinic room or building—that you as the clinician will need to "step up to the plate" and lead the way. If clients know that you are willing, they will come to know that you understand the dynamics of stuttering and what it is to be a person who stutters. Moreover, they will know that you are committed to the treatment process. Take your turn at stuttering with a stranger on the street, in a store, on the telephone. Don't talk about it—just do it! Do not tell, but rather *show* the client that it is possible to change both stuttering itself and ways of thinking about it.

The clinician may model risk-taking behavior in speech and nonspeech activities. Just as the client is asked to venture outside his previously established speech boundaries, the clinician can model behavior that includes presentations to colleagues or social groups. Alternately, the clinician can take on athletic challenges, such as walking, running, or swimming, or professional challenges, such as coordinating a social event or writing an article, pamphlet, or book. By taking risks yourself, it is possible to model new boundaries for the client; to extend a little beyond your previous endeavors.

Challenging the Client

Assuming that we are able to provide the security of a committed clinical relationship and a strategy for change with the client, we then must begin pushing the person forward. However, change is difficult even when the motivation exists. Changing the surface structure and, especially, the deep structure of stuttering is difficult. If it were easy, anyone could do it and there would be far fewer people handicapped by the problem of stuttering. However, it is difficult to alter the equilibrium that has been established in one's psyche and in the roles that the stutterer and his listeners have played for many years. Change involves work; it is time-consuming, and it is usually expensive. At the very least, it is an inconvenience.

Because of the difficulties involved in change, it is not apt to occur without some force. The current ways of speaking and thinking about speaking must be moved off-center. There will be times during treatment when the clinician will have to push hard, and demand that specific, concrete tasks be accomplished. Moreover, on more than a few of those occasions, even the most motivated of our clients will not comply. They may not comply because they do not understand the task, because we move too fast and the task is too difficult, or simply because they do not want to do what needs to be done. Nonetheless, pushing the client—just as in parenting, teaching, or coaching—beyond his previous levels of performance also shows respect for his potential.

If clinicians, including myself, are to be faulted for any one thing, we are most likely guilty of not pushing our adult clients hard enough. Most adult clients come to us knowing that the task is difficult. They often want us to push them harder, but we are fearful of eliciting a negative reaction. There is some evidence that greater progress in fluency treatment is made when the client is pushed to the point of eliciting negative feelings toward the clinician (Cooper & Cooper, 1965; Manning & Cooper, 1969). As Cooper and his associates have suggested, the dynamic process of change is not likely to yield an all-positive client-clinician relationship. Just as change is a function of a teacher-student, parent-child, or coach-player relationship, there will be times when progress is especially hard and the mentor must do what is necessary, and not what the client would prefer to do. Thus, there will be times during treatment when the effective clinician will say and demand things that the client does not want to hear. Moreover, there will be periods when, based on our clinical experience and our long range view of the treatment process, we will have to stand firm in our clinical decisions. However, being the "bad guy" can sometimes be good, especially when it promotes the long-term progress of our clients.

HUMOR AND THE CLINICIANS

We turn now to a final but sensitive indicator of successful clinicians, the ability to use humor during the clinical process. The focus of our discussion of humor in this chapter concerns clinician attributes. However, our discussion of these attributes and the rationale behind the use of humor will also provide the basis for information found in subsequent chapters on assessment and intervention.

A Historical Perspective

Humor may seem like a funny thing to discuss in relation to clinician attributes. Kuhlman (1984) reported that during the first two decades of behavior therapy (1950–1970) there was not a single reference to humor in the literature. This lack of interest in the therapeutic value of humor was clearly the case in the area of fluency disorders. Van Riper (1973) commented briefly about the significance of humor for the person who stutters, describing it in terms of an antiexpectancy device used to lessen the severity of stuttering. He also referred to Bryngelson (1935), as well as Luper and Mulder (1964), who recommended that stutterers learn to joke about their stuttering in order to help others feel more at ease and to themselves develop more optimistic attitudes about their problem.

However, since the early 1970s there has been a substantial and progressive increase in the therapeutic use of humor, particularly in the professional fields of clinical psychology, counseling and allied health. During the last twenty-five years, the value of humor began to be recognized as a legitimate part of the human healing process, a way to maintain both physical and psychological health (McGhee & Goldstein, 1977).

The interest in humor in the clinical setting during the 1970s may have occurred, at least in part, because of an increased interest in the humanistic tradition and a renewed appreciation of the cognitive aspects of behavioral intervention in psychology, counseling, and related fields. The research on humor in general and especially as applied to various forms of treatment for human physical and behavioral problems, began to blossom in the mid-1970s. Perhaps more than any single event, the publishing of Norman Cousins' book, *Anatomy of an Illness,* in 1979 (describing his recovery from the life-threatening disease of ankylosing spondylitis) provided a major impetus for the appreciation of the therapeutic potential of humor by the general public as well as researchers in many areas of human development. Writing and research on humor increased dramatically. Formal and informal networks of professionals interested in the potential of humor in human growth and adjustment were formed (Robinson, 1991). The need to understand the uses and benefits of humor was becoming obvious to researchers throughout the world. Subsequent years have seen the formation of many groups with associated newsletters and meetings, all with an interest in promoting the benefits of humor in various aspects of personal and professional life. Although it is evident that empirical support is needed for much of what is discussed in the literature, the benefits are often striking and the therapeutic potential is obvious.

Beginning in the 1970s the field of psychotherapy saw an increased call for clinicians who were empathic, spontaneous, flexible, and creative (Kuhlman, 1984). It was reasoned that selecting such a person was the best way to increase the likelihood of creating an effective professional through the academic and clinical training processes. Most of us would choose as a colleague someone who possessed these characteristics—and most clients would be likely to choose such a clinician.

The characteristics proposed by Kuhlman are closely related to another personality characteristic: the ability to appreciate and use humor with yourself and with others. Morreall (1982) noted that a person with a sense of humor is more likely to interact well with others than a person lacking humor. Individuals with a sense of humor tend to be more imaginative and flexible and correspondingly less likely to become obsessed with a particular issue or approach to a problem. In addition, a person with a sense of humor is more likely to be open to suggestions from others and more approachable (Morreall, 1982).

Alport (1937, 1961), Maslow (1968), Rogers (1951, 1961), and Combs and Snygg (1959) all identified humor as an essential attribute of a healthy and fully functioning person. It is only recently, however, that this attribute has been acknowledged as a vital characteristic of clinicians. Burton (1972) stated the issue clearly: "One thing every therapist must have is a feeling for the comic. This balances his feeling for the tragic. I am suspicious of any therapist who never laughs." (p. 93). In a similar vein, Rosenheim (1974) commented on the therapeutic potential of humor by saying:

> The unique value and potency of humor in psychotherapy derives mainly from its intrinsic attributes of intimacy, directness and humaneness.

Thus, it draws patient and therapist into a closer alliance than is often possible through a more formal, purely rational modality. Laughing with a patient . . . puts to the test and strengthens the accurate perception of both internal and interpersonal realities. (p. 591)

What's So Funny?

Kuhlman (1984) suggested that trying to define and understand humor is like trying to do so for the concept of "learning." When theories of humor are contrasted, there is little agreement on many of the most fundamental points (Davis & Farina, 1970). However, a review of even a portion of the literature on humor, especially in the area of "therapeutic humor," clearly indicates that there are some valuable concepts for the speech-language pathologist. The fact that humor has been positively correlated with such personality characteristics as enthusiasm, playfulness, hopefulness, excitement, and vigorousness and negatively correlated with fear, depression, anger, indifference, and aloofness (McGhee & Goldstein, 1977) should alert the clinician to the importance of humor during both the assessment and intervention aspects of treatment.

Attempts to understand the essence of humor and its therapeutic potential have evolved through at least three stages of research. The initial stage of research on humor has been defined by Goldstein (1976) as the *pretheoretical* stage. This stage began during the early part of the twentieth century and continued until about 1940. Published manuscripts during this period consisted largely of correlational and observational studies of laughter and smiling—when and how people responded to humor-producing stimuli. There were relatively few attempts to develop or test a particular theory. Goldstein termed the next stage of humor research the *psychoanalytic* phase. Beginning in the 1940s and continuing until the 1970s, this phase was concerned almost exclusively with Freudian theory of wit and humor. Sigmund Freud viewed humor as a potential reducer of stress and placed it alongside the neurotic and psychotic disorders as a basic mechanism of adaptation to human suffering. The essential difference was that humor was thought of as a nonpathological adaptation. In addition, Freud (1928, 1961) asserted that perceived humorousness is related to the degree with which one is able to empathize and assume the role of the person who is the focus of humor.

The third and current stage of research on humor began during the 1970s and stressed the *cognitive* foundations of humor; what it is that causes a person to interpret a particular event as humorous. The change from a Freudian view of humor to a cognitive approach corresponded to the loss of interest in the psychoanalytic view of human behavior and a corresponding increase in Jean Piaget's cognitive-structural view of humor development and behavior.

Two similar views of humor provide a good beginning for appreciating the possibilities for intervention with individuals who stutter. Morreall (1982) suggested that laughter is the natural expression of the feeling of amusement in response to a *sudden conceptual shift*. He suggested that the essence of humor is found in the enjoyment of incongruity. Associated with incongruity is a conceptual shift (not necessarily an emotional one) in the way we consider an event. This conceptual shift must be *immediate*, and the change in the conceptual states be relatively large. When the shift is predictable or anticipated, the degree of humor decreases accordingly. Davis and Farina (1970) advance a similar explanation for a humorous event. They include as basic features of humor, *contradiction* or *incongruity*, as well as the *integration* of contradictory ideas or concepts, which take place *suddenly*. These authors also emphasize a sudden shift that results in new *insight* about the relationship of ideas or concepts. Furthermore, this new insight results in an objective, in contrast to an emotional, experience of the concepts. "We may say that on the cognitive side, laughter results from the sudden insightful integration of contradictory or incongruous ideas, attitudes, or sentiments which are experienced objectively" (Davis & Farina, 1970, p. 307).

Humor in Psychotherapy

Psychotherapists and counselors have differing views on the efficacy and worth of humor during the treatment process. To some clinicians, treatment is "serious business" and not a place where humorous things are likely to take place. On the other hand, there are clinicians who argue that a humorous view of the circumstances presented to us by life could be considered an appropriate issue for the process of treatment (Schimel, 1978). Because of the inherent difficulty of persuading clinicians to consider the possibilities of humor during treatment, some authors have attempted to relate humor to prevailing theoretical approaches. This, of course, is one way of assigning some importance to an aspect of treatment that is likely to have little credibility for some clinicians. One can imagine this group reacting to the suggestion of using humor in the treatment of a handicapping problem by saying "Be serious! Change is difficult, even painful. How can you possibly imply that there is something humorous about such an overwhelming problem." Not surprisingly, clients also may have this initial response to the appropriateness of humor during treatment.

USING HUMOR IN TREATMENT

It is important to consider the way we think about humor in a treatment sense. The semantics of the phrase, "using humor," suggests that humor is a device that the clinician brings to the treatment session in the same way as a questionnaire or treatment technique. To think in terms of *using* humor gives the impression that a clinician will arrive at the treatment session with a well-rehearsed series of jokes (Kuhlman, 1984).

Rather than thinking of using humor in this sense, Kuhlman (1984) proposed that humor is more appropriately viewed as an integral part of the *interactional* aspects of treatment. Rather than a device or tool, humor is related to the client-clinician relationship and to the sense of timing therein. He suggested that spontaneity is the essence of all effective humor, and certainly of humor occurring during treatment. Accordingly, until the clinician is calibrated to the client and until some level of intimacy has been established in the therapeutic relationship, humor is not likely to serve a beneficial purpose.

The fact is, humor and laughter frequently take place during successful treatment, including treatment for fluency disorders. Until recently though, it has not been discussed in the literature (Manning & Beachy, 1994). There is, during effective treatment, the enthusiasm and excitement of exploration. The resulting change in insight often leads to an expression of humor, and conversely, humor can lead to insight. E. B. White (1954/1960) wrote that "humor at its best is a kind of heightened truth—a super truth." Most behavioral strategies seek to expand the client's awareness of the problem that brought him to treatment. Alport (1961) demonstrated the close relationship between insight and humor, finding a positive correlation of .88 between the two. He further noted that insight and humor were related to an individual's capacity for self-objectification and the ability to construe oneself as both subject and object (Kuhlman, 1984). That is, humor reflects a person's ability to step away and *distance* himself from his situation in order to gain a degree of insight. The distance provides for a degree of objectivity that allows us to see ourselves from a new angle or with a "god's eye" view. The new view that we are able to provide through humor is the first of three basic qualities (conceptual shift, distancing, and mastery) that make humor an effective force for the clinician.

The Conceptual Shift

The conceptual shift that is an integral part of humor and permits a more objective view is not likely to be part of the treatment process early in the therapeutic relationship. The initial treatment sessions often are spent gathering information such as acquiring baseline performance, obtaining demographic data, developing procedural guidelines, and becoming calibrated to the client. During and following these initial stages, the clinician begins to become attuned to the client. Once the therapeutic relationship becomes stable, humor is more likely to become part of the relationship. As the sessions continue, an interactional environment will begin to be established in which spontaneity and the expression of something other than the preliminary aspects of the relationship can occur.

As more intimacy is established in the clinician-client relationship, the limits of appropriate humor can expand, as can the number and severity of the taboos that may be violated in safety (Kuhlman, 1984). Humor creates a relaxed atmosphere and encourages communication, particularly on sensitive matters (McGhee & Goldstein, 1977). Although humor is not the only force in the process of promoting a client's conceptual shift about himself and his problem, it can play an important role in the process of change during treatment (Kuhlman, 1984).

As humor facilitates a new insight about an old problem, the client may respond with pleasure or laughter. A kind of catharsis may take place, and for the first time, a new way of looking at the problem may result. According to Kuhlman (1984), the client's laughter, if spontaneous and genuine, can be taken as a sign of validation of a change in insight. On occasion, a client's initial reaction to a new view of the problem or the situation may be one of anger. He may not like the view that the new insight provides, especially if the old view is comforting. Consequently, the appropriateness of a humorous interpretation of an event must be judged within the context of the therapeutic relationship *at that particular moment*. To be appropriate as well as effective, the timing must be both accurate and spontaneous.

It has often been suggested that an integral part of a comprehensive behavioral treatment strategy involves the client's development of a new belief system—a paradigm shift—about himself and the problem (Cooper, 1993; Covey, 1989; Kuhlman, 1984; Hayhow & Levy, 1989, Peck, 1978; Van Riper, 1973). During that process, the client tends to, more or less effectively, ward off the clinician's views and perspective on the problem. As Kuhlman (1984) suggested, although people seek treatment in order to feel better, they are often less than enthusiastic about the behavioral and cognitive changes necessary to achieve the goals of treatment. The client is apt to cling to established perspectives and belief patterns because they are familiar, comfortable, and self-protective (Hayhow & Levy, 1989). The client is often too close to the situation, especially a threatening or emotionally laden one, to see it any other way. Alternately, he has viewed the situation for so long from a particular angle that no other view seems possible. Humor can assist both the clinician and the client in viewing the situation from other angles, other perspectives. As Kuhlman (1984) stated, before a client is able to adopt a new belief system, he must acknowledge and dismiss the old one as being in error in some way. Although humor does not have to be a part of the process, it is often an effective and pleasurable way to facilitate and share the changing view.

Distancing with Humor

In order to facilitate the development of a new cognitive perspective and begin to form a new belief system about both oneself and the problem, it is necessary to step away from the situation somewhat (Kuhlman, 1984). It is not necessary to step back a great distance, but only far enough to see its paradoxical aspects. Until the person is able to move back somewhat, especially from a threatening experience or a problem that creates anxiety, the paradoxical aspects of the situation will not be readily apparent. However, as the client, with the clinician's assistance, is able to achieve greater distance, it will be possible to gradually gain objectivity by viewing the problem with the third eye of humor. Rather than endlessly reliving earlier experiences with the old view, new interpretations will become possible. Humor promotes the possibility that the client will begin to play with the possibilities and have fun considering a variety of new interpretations of the experience.

Morreall (1982) also discussed the role of distancing in humor. He suggested that humor has a liberating effect. Something is funny because it violates what is supposed to be sacrosanct, it goes against the rational or, certainly, the accepted order of things. Morreall (1982) made the observation that humor enables us to achieve some distance and perspective, not only in situations where we are failing, but also in situations where we are succeeding; humor can prevent us from overrating our achievements. The more developed a person's sense of humor, the wider the range of situations in which the clinician can achieve the distance required to laugh. For the clinician, and certainly for the client, it is important to appreciate that to the extent that we can achieve this distance from the practical aspects of a situation, we will be free from being dominated by it. Moreover, to the degree that a person can appreciate the humor in his or her own personal situation, that person will be liberated from the dominance of emotions and more likely to have an objective view.

Mastery and Humor

Lefcourt and Martin (1989) found that the expression of humor is also related to a feeling of mastery of a task or situation. Their interpretation of this relationship relates to the view of humor as a reducer of stress. As Kuhlman (1984) pointed out, the relationship between mastery and humor is readily observed in children as they face problem-solving situations. Laughter is often a by-product of children's shift from one cognitive stage to another as they master a new problem. Problem solving, especially when the experience is a new one, is exhilarating (Levine, 1977). The client's subsequent behavior change suggests that some reorganization of internal reality (insight) has been achieved, which allowed the problem to be solved.

This perspective of humor and mastery also coincides with the view of humor suggested by Freud (1928). That is, the humor process includes a cognitive reorientation in the face of stress (Martin & Lefcourt, 1983; Nezu, Nezu, & Blissett, 1988). The ability to appreciate as well as use humor has been shown to be related to a person's internal locus of control, which provides an indication of how much he or she perceives events as a consequence of his or her own behavior (Craig, Franklin, & Andrews, 1984). Subjects who hold an internal locus of control were found to smile and laugh more in the face of stress (Lefcourt, Sordoni, & Sordoni, 1974). Martin and Lefcourt (1984) found that people with better locus of control scores demonstrate greater ability to take multiple perspectives when problem solving as well as to resist the effects of persuasion. Persons whose locus of control is more internally based are more able to consider alternative constructions for their experiences. Though having multiple perspectives regarding an issue does not necessarily lead to humor, the experience of humor is believed to require a person's ability to view a situation or event from multiple perspectives (Lefcourt & Martin, 1989).

Lefcourt and Martin (1989) suggested that in order to have a greater ability to entertain alternative interpretations for experiences, one must perceive oneself as an actor, a determiner of one's fate, and an active maker of choices. Only by making choices among available options can one be free. In the absence of choice, one is more likely to feel controlled and constrained. Thus, in the exercise of choice and the ability to consider alternative interpretations, there is a connection between a sense of mastery and the potential for humor (Lefcourt & Martin, 1989).

CONCLUSIONS

We have addressed in this chapter the most important component of the treatment process for people who stutter: the clinician. We have considered the impact of the clinician's attitudes and intervention skills on the treatment process. We have also introduced the variable of humor, as both a clinician characteristic as well as an indication of client change and progress during treatment. As we will see in the chapters to follow, many variables influence the likelihood of success, both during and following treatment. However, the one constant is the person guiding the process. It takes energy and optimism on the part of the clinician, and it is demanding work. Each client provides a challenge that tests us repeatedly, and it is necessary and appropriate that we ask ourselves if we are up to the task. It can be hard to prevent burnout. However, if being a clinician is thought of as a continual process of learning and growth we can renew ourselves with continuing education opportunities and other avenues of personal enrichment. Much of our growth comes from the people we are trying so hard to help. The best clinicians know that clients have much to teach us and that we often benefit nearly as much from the treatment process as they do. Although we have been down this path before, the territory and timing of the steps will be new for our companion, to whom we must attend closely and with both determination and esteem.

RECOMMENDED READINGS

Cousins, N. (1979). *Anatomy of an illness*, New York: Norton.
Robinson, V. M. (1991). *Humor and the health professions*. Throrfare, NJ: Slack, Inc. (See the chapters in the section titled, "Humor in Health and Illness").

Van Riper, C. (1975). The stutterer's clinician. In Jon Eisenson (Ed.), *Stuttering, A Second Symposium* (pp. 453–492).

Van Riper, C. (1979). *A career in speech pathology.* Englewood Cliffs, NJ: Prentice Hall Inc. (See chapters titled, "The Clinician's Skill," pp. 103–114, and "The Rewards of Therapy," pp. 115–138.)

Etiology, Onset, and Development

INTRODUCTION

Perhaps no other disorder of human communication has been described in so many different ways. Stuttering has been called, among other things, a mystery, an enigma, a puzzle, and a riddle (Blumel, 1957). Because stuttering can look and feel very different depending on how one approaches it, Wendell Johnson used the analogy of a group of blind men examining an elephant. Because no examiner was able to see the entire concept, each came to a very different conclusion about the nature of the animal they were investigating. Similarly, because the large majority of the syndrome of stuttering lies beneath the surface, stuttering also has been equated to an iceberg (Sheehan, 1970). These different characterizations, each in their own way, can be descriptive and informative. However, they also indicate the confusion that the syndrome holds for even the most experienced researcher and clinician in the field. While there appears to be gradually increasing agreement about the most appropriate possibilities for intervention, there continues to be great uncertainty, and therefore mystery, about how the problem of stuttering arises in the first place.

This uncertainty is such that it could be argued that one sign of the competent clinician is that she does not easily provide an answer to the question of etiology. As we shall see, glib answers about such a complex syndrome may be one sign of a less knowledgeable professional. However, even though clinicians and researchers may not yet have a complete answer about the etiology of the problem, it is important for the clinician to have an opinion. The clinician should have, if not a complete answer, at least a reasonable response to the question of causation, and she should be able to demonstrate her awareness of the etiological possibilities for the clients whom she will see.

One of the first and most frequent questions the clinician will be asked by clients, parents, and other professionals is, "What causes stuttering?" The clinician's response to this question will frequently be her first opportunity to demonstrate her competence and understanding concerning the syndrome. The response will also set the stage for the client's interpretation of himself and his speech. Telling someone that the stuttering is a symptom of a psychological conflict resulting from a pregenital conversion neurosis is considerably different than saying that his stuttering may be the result of a combination of physiological predisposing factors and learned adaptive behaviors. In addition, as many current tests demonstrate, the clinician's understanding about the possible etiologies of the problem will have an influence on the clinician's treatment decisions (Bloodstein, 1995; Conture, 1990; Culatta and Goldberg, 1995; Ham, 1990; Peters & Guitar, 1991; Silverman, 1996; Starkweather, Gottwald, & Halfond, 1990). If the clinician believes that fluency failure can result from communication demands that exceed a child's limited capacity for speech and language production, some treatment decisions will undoubtedly be more appropriate than others. Finally, the clinician's explanation of etiology will influence the parents' response to their situation, including how they deal with any guilt they may have about their child's speech and how they react when their child produces either fluent or stuttered speech.

Although stuttering is often an aversive phenomenon, it nevertheless holds a fascination for most people. Stuttering characters appear with some frequency in movies and books, and no doubt much of this appeal centers on the mystery of the etiology, and students of the field only have to mention to one or more people that they are taking a course in stuttering in order to elicit a flood of queries about the disorder. The initial questions will usually center on etiology, the psychological components of the problem, and the nature of treatment.

Many writers have proposed relatively simple solutions concerning the etiology of stuttering. To be sure, there have always been beguiling leads that result in a wave of furious investigation. Although there are some etiological models that appear to explain much of what is known about the onset and development of the problem, there are many exceptions, speakers whose development and behavior fail to follow the proposed models.

Undoubtedly, the problem of stuttering is complex. In a few select cases we are able to identify, with reasonable certainty, a likely cause. For example, there are instances of sudden onset, such as in neurogenic or psychogenic stuttering, where it is possible to identify specific events that appear to have precipitated the problem (see Chapter 4). Given our current understanding, however, the precise reasons for the large majority of *developmental* stuttering are unknown. At least in most cases, the syndrome appears to arise from a combination of several factors that come together within a requisite time interval. In addition, the cause or causes of stuttering may well be novel for different individuals. *Fortunately, in most cases, it is not necessary for the clinician to know the precise cause of the problem in order to provide the speaker with substantial help.*

Silverman (1996) makes the barbed, but accurate, comment that should any so-called authority propose that he or she understands the cause, let alone a cure for this disorder, all but the most naive clinicians will tend to be highly suspicious of anything else the person may utter. A student of the field does not have to travel far before coming face-to-face with such claims. Conture (1990) reflects the understanding of those who have worked for years in the field when he says that no one has developed a program that provides an answer to all people who stutter. He provides a forthright view when he says:

> I don't know what causes stuttering. I also don't know the best way to treat it. I don't even know if there is *one* way. I'm not sure if anyone else does either. Of one thing I am sure, however: The history of stuttering reflects a multidimensional problem that has repeatedly and successfully defied unidimensional solutions. (p. 1)

So, despite claims to the contrary, it is good to suspect *anyone* who appears to have all the answers and to claim high levels of success with those who stutter. The problem, especially for adolescents and adults, is plainly not that simple. If there were a single or obvious reason why people stutter, the answer would have been found long ago. Many intelligent and dedicated people have spent lifetimes (see Van Riper, 1990) searching for a cause. It may be, of course, that there is no one answer but, rather, many. Moreover, though explanations about etiology vary across researchers and clinicians, there are probably seeds of truth in many.

What clinicians and clients believe about the etiology of stuttering also influences the many stereotypes on the part of the general public about the people who are doing the stuttering (Bloodstein, 1987; Silverman, 1992; Van Riper, 1982). Nearly all the stereotypes pertaining to people who stutter tend to be negative (Bloodstein, 1995; Doopdy, Kalinowski, & Armonson, 1993; Lass et al., 1992) and the information the clinician is able to provide to other professionals as well as the general public should illuminate the problem rather than obscure it.

If the reader has doubts concerning the attitudes and reactions of listeners to someone who stutters, give yourself the following challenge. Pose as a person with a moderate-to-severe stuttering problem in a variety of social, educational, and vocational situations. With a partner to help record your behavior as well as that of the listeners, make a series of telephone calls and enter into a series of face-to-face speaking situations. Determine your level of anxiety in each situation. Keep a record of the verbal and nonverbal reactions of your listeners. It is advisable to enter several (more than ten) speaking situations during one session, for it will take many encounters to begin to become desensitized to the experience. There will be occasions during treatment sessions when it will be appropriate for you, the clinician, to take this role—to do what you are asking your client to do. As you challenge yourself to this experience you will gradually become desensitized and appreciate the dynamics of the situation. You will also find that many listeners will react to you as though you are, at the very least, unintelligent. Listeners may speak slowly, using excessively simple vocabulary and syntax. Although many listeners also will demonstrate a surprising amount of empathy, the experience is apt to reveal the stereotypes that many people have about stuttering. What the clinician communicates to the general public about the etiology of the problem can do much to shed light on the stereotypes people tend to have about stuttering and the people who are speaking that way. There is much to learn about fluency disorders, and it is the clinician's responsibility to enlighten all those who are interested enough to listen.

DEFINITIONS OF RELATED TERMS

Before discussing etiological models of stuttering, we will define some related terms. The term *stammering* can be found in some early literature in this country, where it tended to be used interchangeably with stuttering. While currently the term *stuttering* is used in the United States, *stammering* is often used to mean essentially the same thing in Europe. A major self-help group in Great Britain, for example, is called the British Stammering Association.

The term *disfluent* is often used in the literature to indicate the fluency breaks of normal speakers, while the term *dysfluent* is used to describe the abnormal fluency breaks of people who stutter. According to a variety of medical dictionaries, the prefix *dis* means reversal, separation, or duplication. The prefix *dys*, on the other hand, means difficult, impaired, painful, bad, or disordered. However, because there is considerable overlap in the nature of the fluency breaks of normal and stuttering speakers, there have been ambiguous findings. The speech of people who stutter contains many "normal" fluency breaks, and it is not always clear which surface behaviors differentiate disfluent from dysfluent speech. It is, of course, a matter of degree. The fact that the two words are pronounced the same can lead to additional confusion. As we will see later, normal speakers have many fluency breaks, with some of them characterized by tension and struggle behavior, features that are associated with stuttered speech. In part, because of this overlap along the continuum of what is generally considered normal and what is considered to be abnormal speech, Peters and Guitar (1991) use the term *disfluent* speech when referring to normal as well as abnormal fluency breaks. As we will discuss in Chapter 3, fluent speech is characterized by ease of production.

Fluent speech is also distinguished by the flow of information. That is, the listener is able to attend to the content of the speech rather than the manner of production.

It is important to point out that the following discussion concerns the development of stuttering in young children. Although the onset of developmental stuttering may begin (or at least is diagnosed) as late as the early years of adolescence (ages eight through eleven), the vast majority of people who stutter begin doing so during the early childhood years, ages two through six (Andrews & Harris, 1964).

Primary stuttering (Bluemel, 1932) describes a transient phenomenon in which a child's fluency breaks are easy and he is generally unaware of his problem. The child displays no special effort or tension during speaking. The motoric behaviors taking place in the speech production mechanism at the outset of the behavior are referred to as *core* (Van Riper, 1982) or *Alpha* (Conture, Rothenberg, & Molitor, 1986) behaviors. These primary, or initial, behaviors are differentiated from the *secondary* or *accessory* behaviors that gradually develop around the core of the small breaks or pauses in speech. The secondary behaviors, it is generally agreed, are learned responses or attempts to cope with the initial break in the flow. For whatever reason, it is the core behaviors that form the initial temporal breaks in the flow of the child's speech. As we will discuss, these core breaks in the timing of speech may indicate the incipient stages of stuttering in young children. These breaks, at their most basic level, take the form of easy repetitions and prolongations. However, as awareness increases and struggle behavior develops, there may be blockages or disruptions in airflow, phonation, or even respiration. The essential question that theories of etiology attempt to explain is why these core behaviors take place and why they occur in some children and not in others.

SOME DEFINITIONS OF STUTTERING

The variety of definitions for stuttering that have been offered over the years gives the reader an indication of the many ways to view the problem. Many definitions do not actually define the problem but merely reflect the author's view of the etiology. Johnson's 1946 definition, for example, reflected his view of etiology when he argued that stuttering was what the stutterer does to avoid nonfluency. During the 1940s and 1950s he came to define stuttering as an anticipatory, apprehensive, hypertonic avoidance reaction. Johnson's view was that stuttering was a learned response to environmental events and something that the person (a) does, not something that happens to him; (b) expects to (anticipates will) occur; (c) is fearful (apprehensive) about doing; (d) is tense (hypertonic) about; and (e) tries to keep from happening (avoidance). Today, most would agree that this was a reasonably restrictive definition and that stuttering can occur in the absence of some or even most of these attributes.

One definition of stuttering is offered by the World Health Organization (1977). This definition points out that, in contrast to the view of many non-professionals, people who stutter know what it is they want to say. For someone to tell a person who stutters to stop and think what he wants to say indicates a lack of understanding about what is occurring. The person who stutters knows precisely what he wants to say. He is unable, however, to move through the sounds or make the transitions from one sound to another so that it can be said. The World Health Organization states that stuttering includes "disorders in the rhythm of speech in which the individual knows precisely what he wishes to say, but at the time is unable to say it because of an involuntary, repetitive prolongation or cessation of a sound" (1977, p. 202).

Taking a similar approach, Van Riper (1982) and Perkins (1983) suggest that a fluency break is more likely to be *normal* if it is the result of "linguistic uncertainty." That is, the speaker is hesitating because he needs the time to conceive what it is he wants to say: this is a formulative break. Stuttering is more likely if there is a closure or constriction of the vocal tract—a motoric break.

Views of stuttering as a classical and operant conditioned behavior are reflected in Brutten and Shoemaker's 1967 definition that "stuttering is that form of fluency failure that results from conditioned negative emotion" (p. 61). For those who view stuttering as a type of primary neurosis, a symptom of a basic emotional or psychological conflict, there is the trend to define stuttering by citing the presumed source of the conflict rather than describing the stuttering behavior (symptoms). Coriat (1943), for example, describes stuttering as a psychoneurosis characterized by the persistence of early, pregenital oral nursing, oral sadistic, and anal sadistic elements. In 1958 Glauber described stuttering as "a symptom in a psychopathological condition classified as a pregenital conversion neurosis" (p. 78). Perhaps the most memorable explanation of this type was offered by Fenichel in 1945 who stated, "Stuttering is a pregenital conversion neurosis in that the early problems of dealing with retention and expulsion of feces have been displaced upwards into the sphincters of the mouth" (as cited in Van Riper, 1982, p. 264).

One of the most often cited definitions is that of Wingate (1964). This definition is commonly used to describe subjects in clinical studies since it describes a comprehensive multitude of behaviors and attitudes that the clinician can expect to see across a wide variety of clients.

> The term "stuttering" means: 1. (a) Disruption in the fluency of verbal
> expression, which is (b) characterized by involuntary, audible, or silent,
> repetitions or prolongations in the utterance of short speech elements,
> namely: sounds, syllables, and words of one syllable. These disruptions
> (c) usually occur frequently or are marked in character and (d) are not
> readily controllable. 2. Sometimes the disruptions are (e) accompanied
> by accessory activities involving the speech apparatus, related or unre-
> lated body structures, or stereotyped speech utterances. These activi-
> ties give the appearance of being speech-related struggle. 3. Also, there

not infrequently are (f) indications or reports of the presence of an emotional state, ranging from a general condition of "excitement" or "tension" to more specific emotions of a negative nature such as fear,
embarrassment, irritation, or the like. (g) The immediate source of stuttering is some incoordination expressed in the peripheral speech mechanism; the ultimate cause is presently unknown and may be complex or
compound. (1964, p. 488)

Following years of study concerning the psycholinguistic features of stuttering and his conclusion that the language skills (word fluency, word association, storytelling) of people who stutter are atypical, Wingate (1988) proposed
that "stuttering is a deficit in the language production system, a defect that
extends beyond the level of motor execution . . . [and that] the defect is not
simply one of motor control or coordination, but . . . involves more central
functions of the language production system" (p. 239).

Many definitions of stuttering include the perceptual effect of the stuttering on a *listener* but fail to consider the reaction of the *speaker* that occurs
before, during, and following the stuttering moment. This is an important
shortcoming in some definitions because, as much and possibly more than
anything else, it is the *speaker's* response to the break in fluency that helps to
differentiate the fluency breaks of people who stutter from those who do not.

Perkins (1983) discusses this idea when he points out the problems associated with definitions of stuttering that depend on listener perception. Although
the listener is able to identify the acoustic features of the fluency break, he
or she is unlikely to distinguish the cognitive and affective experience of the
event. Thus, definitions that deal only with the surface (audible and visual)
features of the problem do not completely describe the stuttering experience. A comprehensive definition of stuttering must also take into account the
effect of the experience on the speaker. Van Riper acknowledged this when,
in 1982, he stated that "stuttering occurs when the forward flow of speech is
interrupted by a motorically disrupted sound, syllable, or word, or *by the
speaker's reactions thereto* [italics added] (p. 15).

How the speaker reacts—what he tells himself about his stuttering experience (or the possibility of stuttering)—helps to define himself and his speech.
In a related issue, Silverman (1996) takes a pragmatic approach when he discusses the *handicapping* effect of stuttering. He maintains that the number
of choices and activities that stuttering prevents the person from doing defines the degree of handicap. Citing several personal accounts (Attanasio, 1987;
Carlisle, 1985; Johnson, 1930; Murray & Edwards, 1980; Shields, 1989; Sugarman, 1980; Van Riper, 1984), he points out that the actual handicap that
can result from being a person who stutters can be considerably different
(often greater) than the surface features of the stuttering would indicate. It
is not uncommon for the handicapping effects associated with stuttering to
result from the speaker's reaction to his situation and his attempts to alter or
adapt to the problem, often in less than effectual ways.

Finally, the involuntary nature of the problem, with the associated loss of control and helplessness, is a crucial feature that defines the experience of being a person who stutters. Several authors agree that a fundamental and distinguishing characteristic of the stuttering moment is the *loss of control* by the speaker (Cooper, 1968; Manning, 1977; Manning & Shrum, 1973; Perkins, 1983). Note that the involuntary aspect of the syndrome is included in the previously discussed World Health Organization (1977) definition. While the concept of "involuntary" can be somewhat difficult to identify and measure, Manning and Shrum state that such a loss of control:

> can be extremely identifiable and specific to the stuttering client. The client is able to "know" whether he is completely "in charge" of his speech or whether "the block has assumed command." Certainly the stutterer could indicate to the clinician when such control has been achieved. In many instances, though, the experienced clinician is able to identify such control or the lack of it. (1973, p. 33)

Perkins (1983) argues that the involuntary nature of stuttering should form the core of the definition. In 1990 he suggested that although listeners can demonstrate reasonably good reliability in identifying the surface features of stuttering (but see also Ingham, 1990) a more valid and authentic indicator of stuttering is provided by the person who is producing (or attempting to produce) the speech. Because it is possible for the speaker to distinguish precisely whether he is in control of his speech, Perkins (1990) describes stuttering as being categorically different from nonstuttered speech.

> The essence of stuttering, in my view, is not what is perceived by listeners as stuttering in the acoustical signal, but rather what occurs in the production of stuttered speech. . . . Stuttering is the involuntary disruption of a continuing attempt to produce a spoken utterance. . . . From the stutterer's vantage point, however, the judgement is categorical: Either involuntary blockage has or has not occurred to some degree. If it has not occurred, then what sounds like stuttering to the observer would not feel like stuttering to the speaker. The reason that this distinction is categorical is because the proposed definition posits that loss of control of the ability to voluntarily continue a disrupted utterance is the essence of stuttering. If the disruption is not involuntary to some degree, then it is not a stuttered disfluency. Moreover, the stutterer would not react to it with apprehension, struggle, or avoidance if it were stuttered. (1990, p. 376)

Thus, Perkins sees stuttering as being qualitatively unique because the speaker, during a moment of stuttering, is not in control and feeling helpless (see Chapters 4 and 8 for examples). While this view may seem intuitively appealing, it has proven to be difficult to test (Martin & Haroldson, 1986; Moore & Perkins, 1990).

In summary, although the surface features of stuttering are sometimes clear and distinguishable, it would appear that some of the most telling features lie under the surface and reside in the more subtle cognitive and affective layers of the syndrome. As Conture (1990, pp. 17–20) suggests, there are many nonverbal features such as body movement, tension, and psychosocial discomfort that help to more precisely distinguish and define stuttering.

A comprehensive definition of stuttering by Peters and Guitar (1991) incorporates both the physiological capacities of the speaker as well as the adaptive learning that takes place. These authors define stuttering as "a disorder of the neuromotor control of speech, influenced by the interactive process of language production, and intensified by complex learning processes" (p. 18).

STUTTERING FROM A HISTORICAL PERSPECTIVE

Students may not always appreciate the value of learning about past models of stuttering etiology. Justification for studying such models is proposed by Silverman when he says:

> Our present views on both the etiology and management of stuttering are built upon the experience of the past. Clinicians who are unaware of how stuttering has been treated in the past are more likely to use intervention strategies that have been shown again and again to be of little or no long-term value than are those who have this knowledge. These strategies may produce a rapid reduction in stuttering severity, but the vast majority of clients on whom they are used are likely to relapse within five years following termination of therapy. (Silverman, 1996, p. 10)

There is some measure of support as well as conflicting evidence for nearly all theories of stuttering onset. In addition, there are exceptions to all attempts to explain stuttering behavior even in small subgroups of individuals (Daly, 1981; Schwartz & Conture, 1988), let alone across the variety of different stutterers. Since the conclusions about theories are tentative and subject to change with the availability of fresh data, Silverman (1996) suggests that the clinician must continuously evaluate each theory in the light of new evidence.

Wingate (1968) pointed out that the questions that are asked in a field are influenced by the *zeitgeist* (the spirit of the times). What is published is driven, to some degree, by what is fashionable as much as it is by the decisions of reviewers and editors. Those issues that are considered important enough to be supported by available funds are influenced by the zeitgeist. Questions are researched and the results of investigations generate further considerations along a line of inquiry. The zeitgeist gradually changes and the pendulum swings back and forth, often returning again to views that, at one time, were thought to have outlived their usefulness. Sometimes the published articles, particularly review articles, summarize research that has pursued a particular direction for a time. These review articles, in turn, have their own influence on the zeitgeist. Sometimes, review articles simply reflect and document a change in the zeitgeist that has already occurred.

There have been many attempts to formulate models that explain the onset of stuttering. One thing remains clear. In nearly all cases, stuttering is a multidimensional problem. Determining onset is complicated by the fact that there are no absolute definitions or criteria that enable the clinician to absolutely differentiate stuttered speech from nonstuttered speech and to identify those who are and are not stuttering (Ingham, 1984; Onslow, 1992). Using an interesting analogy, Conture (1990) compares stuttering to the common cold. That is, despite years of trying, no one has come up with a cause or a solution to the problem. There are a variety of explanations and a variety of remedies. Sometimes, for some people, a remedy will work. In other instances, possibly because of the interaction of the remedy and the person or the timing of this interaction, the remedy is less effective. Each treatment comes with its own cadre of supporters. Nevertheless, there appears to be no clear-cut cause and no consistent cure. There may be one difference, however, between the common cold and stuttering. The chances of successfully treating a cold may be somewhat better than altering the network of behaviors and attitudes that come together in the syndrome of stuttering.

Excellent descriptions of the long and fascinating history of proposed stuttering causation are provided by Van Riper (1982) and Silverman (1996). Perhaps the oldest view is that stuttering is a form of punishment for wrongdoing on the part of the child or the parent. Undoubtedly this view continues to be held today in some cultures and social-economic groups throughout the world. Stuttering has been around for a long time through human history.

The earliest recorded indication of stuttering is provided by the Egyptians, who used the term *nitnit* and represented the problem with a sequence of hieroglyphics (Faulkner, 1962). The verb *to stutter* appeared in a papyrus copy of a narrative dating from the Middle Kingdom of Egypt titled, "The Tale of the Shipwrecked Sailor" (DeBuck, 1970). Reading Figure 2–1 from right to left, the initial symbols represent the concept of *impediment* or *impede*, and the final portion, the *determinative*, indicates human speech.

Interestingly, the references to stuttering in this narrative tale of a high official returning to the royal court after a failed expedition include the sentences: "You must speak to the king with presence of mind. You must answer without stuttering! A man's mouth can save him. His speech makes one forgive him." In addition, as a sailor in the story makes his way about the island on which he is shipwrecked, he encounters a large snake who repeats sentences: "Who brought you, who brought you, fellow, who brought you? Don't be afraid, don't be afraid" (Lichtheim, 1973).

At the most basic level, models of stuttering etiology can be separated into physiological or psychological models or some combination of these two. We will first discuss stuttering as a physical problem, an idea that is again becoming favored.

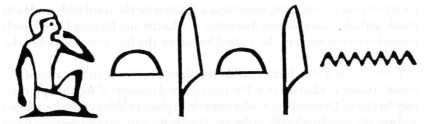

Figure 2–1. Reading from right to left are the Egyptian symbols indicating impediment followed by the determinative indicating human speech. (From Faulkner, R.O. (1991) A Concise Dictionary of Middle Egyptian. Reprinted by permission of The Griffith Institute, Ashmolean Museum, Oxford, England.)

STUTTERING AS A PHYSICAL PROBLEM

There is a long tradition in the literature of attributing stuttering to physiological processes not directly related to speech and language production. Nearly every structure of the body, whether associated with speech production or not, has been implicated in the search for a cause of stuttering. Examples include, but are not limited to, dryness of the tongue or problems in the hyoid bone, the hard palate, the uvula, the root of the tongue, the larynx, various aspects of the hearing mechanism including the higher auditory pathway, assorted bones of the head, the endocrine and autonomic nervous systems, and the central nervous system. Since the tongue is often involved during moments of stuttering, that structure has often been implicated as the culprit. According to Silverman (1996) the belief that an abnormality in the structure and/or function of the tongue causes stuttering appears to have been the most widely held one between the time of Aristotle and the Renaissance, approximately 1500 A.D.

Since one or more anatomical structures were thought to be implicated, it was not uncommon to recommend various forms of surgery for those who stuttered. Believing a spasm of the glottis to be responsible for stuttering, Johann Dieffenbach, a German surgeon, performed more than 250 operations on the tongues of people who stuttered in France and Germany in 1841. Performed without anesthesia, the operation involved a horizontal incision at the base of the tongue and the excising of a triangular wedge. Dieffenbach claimed that his operations were successful, except, of course, for those who died as a result of infection. However, his claims were not confirmed by others and the technique was rapidly abandoned by the end of the same year (Hunt, 1861). (Interestingly, the common houseplant Dieffenbachia, known for its bitter-tasting leaves, is named after this somewhat infamous surgeon.)

Other "cures" for offending parts of the anatomy included severing the hypoglossal nerve, piercing the tongue with hot needles or blistering it with embrocations, encouraging smoking as a sedative for the vocal folds, and both tonsil- and adenoidectomies. According to Blanton and Blanton (1936), such procedures continued in the United States for the first few decades of the twentieth century.

There is also a long history of placing objects in the mouth or against the throat in order to elicit fluency. The first reported example of such an approach may be that of Demosthenes, who was told to place pebbles under his tongue and practice speaking loudly to the sea. During the past several centuries there have been a multitude of devices (see Silverman, 1996; Van Riper, 1982) that likely facilitated fluency by both distracting the speaker from his habitual method of speech production and producing altered forms of phonation and articulatory timing. With few exceptions, these devices provided only temporary fluency.

One of the earliest and most influential examples of the constitutional view of stuttering was that proposed by Lee Edward Travis and his colleagues at the University of Iowa. Based on the earlier work of Orton, this theory held that people who stuttered lacked the unilateral dominance for speech production, which is usually located in the left hemisphere. It was proposed either that people who stutter made greater use of their right hemisphere for speech than nonstutterers (Moore, 1984; Moore & Haynes, 1980) or that the control of speech production and/or perception was shared by both hemispheres (Cerf & Prins, 1974; Curry & Gregory, 1969; Haefner, 1929; Oates, 1929; Ojemann, 1931).

More recent efforts to explore possible differences or deficits in the physical makeup of individuals who stutter have focused on more subtle tasks of speech and nonspeech activities such as auditory and visual tracking, finger tapping, and reaction time. Although there are exceptions, several authors have used a variety of tasks on which subjects who stutter perform less accurately or slower than those who do not. For example, stuttering subjects have been found to be somewhat slower in starting and stopping a sound when they hear a buzzer (Adams & Hayden, 1976; Starkweather, Hirschman, & Tannenbaum, 1976). Stuttering subjects have been found to be somewhat slower when reacting to respiration (exhalation) and articulation (lip-closing) movements. The results of number of studies (see Silverman, 1996, pp. 60–61) indicate that stutterers have slower phonatory reaction times (the time it takes to initiate or terminate phonation in response to a signal). Furthermore, in a related study, Cross and Luper (1983) found that stutterers are slower than control subjects at nonspeech movement, such as finger tapping.

Temporal-Processing Abilities

Another area where the results of several investigations have shown general consistency relates to the ability of people who stutter to process fine temporal features. The theme of these investigations is that stutterers experience a subtle breakdown in speech or speech-related functioning. This breakdown, particularly when the speaker is experiencing internal or externally generated stress, may result in a reduced ability to achieve fluency.

Kent's (1983) view of stuttering as a reduced ability to generate temporal patterns is a good example of this more recent view and indicates the return, during the later decades of this century, to seeing stuttering as a physiological problem. Kent proposed that stuttering is a result of a central nervous system disturbance that results in a "reduced ability to generate temporal patterns, whether for sensory or motor purposes, but especially the latter" (p. 252). For whatever reasons, stutterers seem to lack the ability to smoothly sequence the movement or gestures of speech. There is some indication that people who stutter perform less well than nonstuttering controls on tasks requiring the discrimination of subtle temporal differences in signals (Hall & Jerger, 1978; Kramer, Green, & Guitar, 1987; Toscher & Rupp, 1978). The suggestion is that those who stutter may be demonstrating a lack of central nervous function that allows for the control of both incoming and outgoing signals.

Related to this general line of thinking is the fact that many more males than females are found to stutter, with ratios of from three-to-one to five-to-one often cited (American Psychiatric Association, 1994; Andrews & Harris, 1964; Beech & Fransella, 1968; Bloodstein, 1987; Van Riper, 1982) The findings of Geschwind and Galaburda (1985) indicate the possibility that because of the secretion of testosterone during fetal development, males have more disorders involving less-than-ideal development in the left hemisphere. The result is less obvious hemispheric dominance for speech activities, and thus, a central nervous system that is more vulnerable to fluency disruptions.

Although researchers continue to find intriguing differences in speech related performances of subjects who stutter, the perplexing result continues to be that many of these subjects *do not* show any difference in performance. As Peters and Guitar (1991) point out, the differences, even when they can be noted, are not in and of themselves a direct cause of fluency breaks. Rather, these authors view such findings as conditions that provide fertile ground in which stuttering may grow. That is, such deficits may be neither necessary nor sufficient to *cause* stuttering (Bloodstein, 1995). It may also be, of course, that some of these differences may be a *result* of stuttering, particularly for adults who have been stuttering for decades.

Genetic Influences

It has often been noted that stuttering tends to run in families, a fact that suggests a genetic link for the disorder. This supposition for stuttering onset has gained support during recent decades and seems to tie in nicely with the above-mentioned proposal of an inability to precisely process temporal patterns. Investigations of family genetics and the characteristics of twin pairs suggest that, as for many other human characteristics, there may be genetic influences that at least predispose a person to develop stuttering. Andrews and Harris (1964) traced the family history of eighty stuttering children. They found that more males than females were likely to stutter, that females were more likely to have relatives who stuttered than males, and that stutterers were more likely than nonstutterers to have stuttering relatives. Investigators who have considered the occurrence of stuttering in identical twins (monozygotic pairs, with identical genetic makeup) and fraternal twins (dizygotic pairs, sharing only a portion of their genes) have found stuttering to occur more often for both children in monozygotic pairs than in dizygotic twins (Andrews, Yates-Morris, Howie, & Martin, 1991; Howie, 1981). The genetic term *concordance* indicates the presence of a particular characteristic for both twin pairs, and thus stuttering is said to have a higher concordance in monozygotic than dizygotic twin pairs. It is also the case, however, that some identical twins are also discordant. Howie (1981) found, for example, that six out of sixteen identical twin pairs did not result in stuttering in both subjects.

Kidd and his associates (Kidd, 1977; Kidd, Kidd, & Records, 1978; Kidd, Reich & Kessler, 1973) also found convincing evidence that the occurrence of stuttering follows familial patterns. These authors indicated that the occurrence of stuttering can be explained by a combination of genetic and environmental factors.

The ratio of stuttering in males and females may also interact with genetic loading for factors of fluency. The sex difference suggests that either males are more susceptible to stuttering and/or females are more resistant to it. It may be that females will stutter only with a higher degree of genetic loading and also be more likely to pass it on to their offspring. Similar findings have been noted in the familial history of cluttering, and there seems to be some interaction of these two disorders throughout the generations of families (Weiss, 1964). People who stutter are far from a homogeneous population, and it appears that some, particularly those with a strong familial history of stuttering, may possess a strong neurophysiological loading for the disruption of speech fluency. As we will discuss in subsequent chapters, these findings have strong implications for both treatment as well as long-term success and the possibility of relapse.

In summary, whatever predisposing factors may be inherited, they do not appear to be, in most cases at least, sufficient to result in stuttering. Such predisposing characteristics must combine with environmental factors for stuttering to not only begin but also develop. As Conture (1990) suggests, in this way, stuttering may be similar to asthma or migraine headaches.

Auditory Feedback

The nature of auditory feedback in those who stutter is another feature that has been the subject of research. Cybernetic theory holds that in a closed loop system, various forms of feedback are used to regulate the output of a system, as with a thermostat that controls the temperature of a building. The goal of a such a system, termed a *servosystem*, is to match what is intended as system output to the actual output and reduce any differences between the two (the error signal) to zero. If for some reason there is a distortion of the information arriving via the feedback loop, the error signal will be incorrect. When this occurs, the system tends to go into oscillation. Fairbanks (1954) and Mysak (1960) described the nature of such systems and interpreted many aspects of speech production in this manner. The basic idea was that, for speakers who stutter, the distorted feedback creates the misconception that an error has occurred in the flow of speech. Stuttering occurs when the speaker attempts to correct an error that has, in fact, not occurred.

Subsequent studies (Black, 1951; Lee, 1951; Neeley, 1961; Yates, 1963) provided some indication that what was occurring for speakers who stuttered was a distorted auditory feedback signal. They noted that for normal speakers, altering the auditory feedback by delaying the signal tended to produce stuttering-like behavior. For example, it was generally agreed that nonstutterers speak under delayed auditory feedback (DAF) in much the same way people do when they stutter. That is, the effect of DAF on normal speakers is to produce repetitions and prolongations of sounds, slowing of speech, pitch increases, and greater vocal intensity. In order to "beat" the effect of the delayed feedback, the speaker must disregard that signal, slow his speech, and focus attention to the undistorted tactile and proprioceptive feedback from his articulators that is available to him. When speakers who stutter respond (with or without DAF) in this manner, there tends to be a reduction in the severity of stuttering. Depending on how these fluency breaks are considered, there may also be a reduction in the frequency in stuttering (Hayden, Scott & Addicott, 1977). Because of these effects of DAF, some treatment programs have employed it as a way to establish fluency in some speakers (Ryan & VanKirk, 1974; Shames & Florance, 1980). Once the speaker has gradually learned to maintain improved fluency under the distorted feedback, the delay intervals are varied in the direction of instantaneous or normal feedback and the client learns to speak without using the device as he continues to use the slow speech along with an emphasis on proprioceptive feedback.

More recent reconsiderations of this view have failed to support the idea of an error in the feedback loop of subjects who stutterer. Postma and Kolk (1992) investigated the effects of error monitoring in eighteen adults who stuttered and a group of control subjects. The speakers were asked to detect self-produced phonemic errors under normal and masked auditory feedback conditions. The results failed to indicate that the experimental (stuttering) subjects performed less well than nonstuttering speakers in either the accuracy or speed of their error detection. They concluded that speakers who stutter possess a deficit in their ability to self-monitor the accuracy of their speech production. They further speculated that rather than a deficit in any speech-monitoring ability, speakers, and particularly those who stutter, may be experiencing prearticulatory errors, which they are attempting to covertly repair.

The Covert Repair Hypothesis

A recent extension of the above-mentioned view is the development and elaboration of what is called the covert repair hypothesis (Postma & Kolk, 1993). This hypothesis also makes use of a monitoring device that checks on the accuracy of speech and speech flow. A key difference, however, is that this monitoring performs a central or internal function rather than the auditory or proprioceptive sensory feedback loops characteristic of the models previously presented. In this model, monitoring is taking place during the formulation of the phonetic plan (see Figure 2–2) and *prior* to the actual (motor) implementation of articulatory commands. As a result of monitoring, a kind of prearticulatory evaluation takes place, which entails not only the *detection* of errors but also allows for their *correction*. Thus, the phonetic program is covertly repaired during the assembly of the phonetic plan but before the error is executed. Disfluencies are seen as side effects of this covert repair process. Postma and Kolk suggest that this covert process may be thought of in much the same way as overt self-repairing. That is, the process involves an interruption of speech production, a revising of the necessary movements, followed by a new attempt with a revised plan. This hypothesis nicely explains many of the disfluencies of normal speakers and had been extended to explain the fluency breaks in stuttering speakers, for both loci and type of intrasyllabic disfluencies. It also coincides well with a number of reports of phonological-processing abilities of subjects who stutter (Bosshardt, 1990; Bosshardt & Nandyal, 1988; Postma, Kolk, & Povel, 1990; Wingate, 1988). An analysis by LaSalle and Conture (1995) of the disfluencies produced by preschool children who stuttered provided preliminary support for the notion that both overt and covert self-repairs may interact with a child's ability to perform phonological encoding in a timely manner. This hypothesis appears to offer a number of testable ideas and is likely to generate a good deal of research during the next several years.

STUTTERING AS AN EMOTIONAL OR PSYCHOLOGICAL PROBLEM

Van Riper, after many decades of treating thousands of children and adults who stuttered, wrote a fascinating article in what was then called the *Western Michigan University Journal of Speech Therapy*. Written in 1974, the article was titled "A Handful of Nuts." From the many hundreds of clients he had seen up to that point in his career, Van Riper found only a very few who had severe emotional problems. These people, while they most certainly stuttered, also had emotional problems that were considerably more handicapping. His description of these clients makes for some exciting reading. As we shall see,

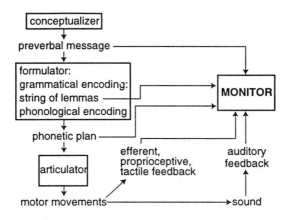

Figure 2–2.   Speech production with monitoring routes. Covert repair takes place during the formulation of the phonetic plan and prior to the translation of articulatory commands into speech movements by the motor system. (From Postma and Kolk [1993], p. 474. Copyright © American Speech-Language-Hearing Association. Reprinted by permission.)

however, there are relatively few people who have such deep-seated emotional problems that are directly related to their stuttering (see also Van Riper, 1979).

Through the 1920s many people who treated stuttering in this country were physicians, and many of these individuals held a psychoanalytic view of the disorder. Stuttering was viewed as a psychopathology, a symptom of a more deep-seated, psychological disorder. However, with the development of university speech and hearing centers and the creation of the National Association of Teachers of Speech in 1925 (the precursor of the American Speech-Language-Hearing Association) (Paden, 1970), fewer physicians provided treatment. The new clinicians, who were trained in the behavioral sciences, were less likely to hold a psychoanalytic view of stuttering (Silverman, 1996).

The neurotic or psychoanalytic explanation of stuttering also has been termed the *repressed-need hypothesis* (Silverman, 1996). Stuttering is seen as a neurosis. Individuals who stutter do so as a result of a repressed, neurotic, unconscious conflict. Stuttering behavior is seen as a symptom, which is symbolic of this conflict. The origin of the conflict is a central question, and there was no shortage of suggestions about the possible source. Some theorized that the source was psychosexual, a fixation of psychological development at an oral or anal stage of infant sexual development (Glauber, 1982). It was proposed, for example, that one who stuttered had not experienced oral erotic gratification as an infant, possibly due to a disturbance in the mother-child relationship. Others proposed a neo-Freudian view that the source of conflict was the result of inadequate interpersonal relationships (Barbara, 1965, 1982; Wyatt, 1969).

Many of these opinions sound strange and even preposterous to most speech-language pathologists. The chapter by Travis, "The Unspeakable Feelings of People with Special Reference to Stuttering," in the two editions of his *Handbook of Speech Pathology* (1957, 1971) are lucid examples of this viewpoint. This chapter likely stands as the high-water mark of this analytical perspective. It is unlikely that a client or parent will have access to the opinions about stuttering etiology expressed these chapters. However, the well-versed clinician should be aware of these views and have an opinion about this approach to fluency disorders.

Silverman (1996) indicates that an American physician named Edward Scripture (1931) was one of the first to combine psychotherapy and speech treatment that focused on changing specific speech habits. This combined approach is similar to that of more modern clinicians who are psychoanalytically based (Barbara, 1982; Freund, 1966; Glauber, 1982). According to Silverman (1996) there has been relatively little success reported by those using a psychoanalytic approach for treating stuttering. Brill (1923) indicated that after eleven years of treating a total of sixty-nine stutterers through psychoanalysis he was able to claim only five persons cured, one of whom was reported to have subsequently relapsed. There is the indication that Freud himself (Freund, 1966) did not believe that psychoanalytic techniques were particularly helpful in treating stuttering.

Related to the psychological status of children who begin to stutter, there has been considerable discussion in the literature concerning the characteristics of their parents. In order to determine the possibility that the parents of children who stutter are emotionally or psychologically different from parents of nonstuttering children, Adams (1993) reviewed thirty-five articles that contrasted the attitudes, traits, emotions, psychological adjustment, and child-rearing practices and behaviors of parents of children who stutter. Adams found some limited evidence that the parents of young stutterers may possess some attributes that could have a negative effect on young children who stutter. For example, Zenner, Ritterman, Bowden, and Gronhovd (1978) found that parents of young stuttering children may possess higher levels of both trait and state anxiety. Gildston (1967) noted that parents were perceived by some of the children who stuttered as being slightly less accepting. Quarrington, Seligman, and Kosower (1969) found that parents of young stutterers set lower goals for their children than those of normally speaking children. However, Adams found that the vast majority of investigations indicated no differences between the experimental and control parents. In fact, some investigations identified characteristics in the parents of young stutterers that are generally viewed as psychologically healthy—for example, parents of stuttering children were found to be less possessive and less likely to exert hostile control (Yairi & Williams, 1971).

Adams summarized his findings by addressing three questions concerning the home environment of children who stutter:

1. Do stutterers as a group grow up in a home environment that can validly be described as blatantly pathologic or unhealthy emotionally? Adam's answer was a certain no.

2. Do stutterers as a group grow up in a home environment that can validly be described as "emotionally unsatisfactory or conducive to maladjustment?" Adams's answer to this question was that he found little support for this idea.

3. Do children who become stutterers grow up in a home environment that, although not obviously pathologic, is nonetheless unique or different from the home environment of youngsters who develop normal speech? Adams's answer to this final question was also a certain no.

STUTTERING AS LEARNED BEHAVIOR

This view of stuttering onset has also been termed the *anticipatory-struggle model* (Silverman, 1992). The essence of this model is that stuttering is a learned behavior. This view, at least in an informal sense, also has a long history. Amman (1700/1965) was one of the first to state that stuttering was, in fact, a bad habit. In a precursor to the learning theories of the twentieth century, in the 1800s, Erasmus Darwin (grandfather of Charles Darwin) attributed stuttering to emotionally conditioned interruptions of motoric speech. Arnott (1928) believed that stuttering resulted from a learned "spasm of the glottis." According to Van Riper (1982), this was the most popular view of stuttering onset and development in both the United States and Great Britain from the middle to the end of the nineteenth century. For example, during this time Alexander Melville Bell (grandfather of Alexander Graham Bell) wrote a number of books suggesting that stuttering was learned. One important implication of this view was to place this problem within the arena of the educator rather than a medical professional (Bell, 1853). Dunlap (1932) also considered much of stuttering to be learned and recommended weakening the behavior by having the speaker stutter on purpose, or voluntarily stutter. However, these views of stuttering as a learned behavior were the exception during the early part of the twentieth century.

After several decades in which the zeitgeist favored physical and psychoanalytical views of stuttering etiology, there was a gradual change in viewing stuttering as learned behavior during the middle third of the twentieth century, from approximately 1930 through 1950. Many people were entering the field at this time with backgrounds in psychology, and the majority had received their training at the University of Iowa. Many of these scholars had a profound influence on the general field of communication disorders. This concentration of researchers, clinicians, and authors led to what has been termed the "Iowa Development" (Bloodstein, 1995). A second generation of clinicians included such individuals as Hugo Gregory, Joseph Sheehan, and Dean Williams.

Perhaps the most profound result of the early stages of the Iowa development was the diagnosogenic interpretation of stuttering onset as developed by Johnson. Having been influenced by the writings of Alfred Koszybski in his book *Science and Sanity* (1941) and his work in what was termed general semantics, Johnson developed a "semantic theory" of stuttering. General semantics is the study of the ways in which people use words to explain their lives and solve problems. Johnson's theory also became known as the semantogenic or interactional theory (Perkins, 1990), and it had both a profound and long-term impact in the area of fluency disorders. This theory held that stuttering evolves from normal fluency breaks that are overreacted to by the parents. Two sentences contained in *An Open Letter to the Mother of a "Stuttering" Child* states the essence of this view.

> The diagnosis of stuttering—that is, the decision made by someone that a child is beginning to stutter—is one of the causes of the stuttering problem, and apparently one of the most potent causes. Having labeled the child's hesitations and repetitions as "stuttering," the listener—somewhat more often the mother than the father—reacts to them as if they were all that the label implies. (Johnson, 1962, p. 2)

As the child attempts to stop producing these natural breaks in fluency, the result is both greater anticipation and increased struggle behavior. Johnson and his associates proposed that fluency breaks that started out as normal gradually became abnormal as a result of the penalties associated with this behavior. Eventually, the speaker "learned" to stutter in his unique manner and the problem became self-reinforcing, affecting many aspects of his life.

Certainly much of the stuttering that we see on the surface, and possibly some of what resides underneath, is learned. That is, we can learn ways of escaping from experiences of fear and penalty. Eventually, we can learn ways of interpreting events and of thinking about ourselves. We can learn to play the role of a person who stutters (Sheehan, 1970). Perhaps most apparent are the assortment of escape and avoidance behaviors that become accessaries to the experience of fluency breakdown. Escape behaviors are attempts to get away from the stuttering moment and include a multitude of activities including eye blinks, head nods, interjections, and a wide variety of tension and struggle activities. As the speaker is able to move away from the moment of helplessness or through the sentence, the behavior that appeared to facilitate this escape is rewarded. A powerful link is formed between these behaviors and the escape from the stuttering, one that is extremely difficult to weaken. Avoidance behaviors are related to the anticipation of stuttering. In anticipation of a difficult speaking situation, speaking partner, word, or sound, the speaker chooses to avoid or completely postpone the feared stimulus by using starter sounds or words ("ah, let me see") or timing and distraction devices (finger or head movement, audible or inaudible movements of the articulators). The point is that these behaviors gather around the initial fluency break, making it ever more complex, distracting, and handicapping.

As with other models, there are several studies that provide support and several others that do not. That is, normally speaking preschool children do tend to repeat and hesitate (Johnson & Associates, 1959; Yairi, 1981, 1982). A central question, however, is whether these early fluency breaks are normal: whether they are a function of formulative processing or whether they are indicative of a motoric break in the system. There are data to support both arguments, with Johnson and Associates (1959) arguing that the initial fluency breaks are essentially normal. Other researchers (Bloodstein, 1958; McDearmon, 1968; Van Riper, 1982; Wingate, 1988; Yairi & Lewis, 1984) suggest that the original fluency breaks are far from normal, both in terms of quantity and quality.

One of the more compelling studies indicating that stuttering can be created by misdiagnosing normal breaks in fluency is described by Silverman (1988b) in his accounting of an unpublished study conducted by Tudor in 1939 titled, "An Experimental Study of the Effects of Evaluative Labeling on Speech Fluency." It is clear why Silverman (1988b, 1996) refers to this investigation as the "monster study" and why the research was never published. Although the investigation was conducted prior to the development of the diagnosogenic theory, it provided a direct test of this hypothesis. The goal of the study was to see if labeling someone as a stutterer would influence the speaker's fluency.

Children living in an orphanage in Davenport, Iowa, were subjects. From a total of 256 children, 12 children were randomly selected. Ten children identified as stuttering during speech were also included. These children were divided into four groups. The first group of 5 children who apparently did stutter were designated by the experimenters as *not* being stutterers and the attempt was made to remove the label of *stutterer* from these children. The second group of 5 children who did stutter were designated by the experimenters as true stutterers, a label they endorsed. The third group consisted of 6 normally speaking children with what was determined to be normal fluency. The ages of these children were five, nine, eleven, twelve (2 children), and fifteen years. As described below, the label of *stuttering* was endorsed for these children. The final group of 6 normally speaking children were not given the label of *stutterers* and were complimented on their speaking ability (e.g., "You speak very well. Your speech is of very good quality").

The study lasted for three months. During this time, both the normally speaking children in the third group as well as their teachers and staff of the facility were told that these children were demonstrating classic signs of stuttering. For example, the children were told that they were found to be having:

> a great deal of trouble with your speech. The types of interruptions which you have are very undesirable. These interruptions indicate stuttering. You have many of the symptoms of a child who is beginning to stutter. You must try to stop yourself immediately. . . . Do anything to keep from stuttering. . . . Don't ever speak unless you can do it right. . . . Whatever

you do, speak fluently and avoid any interruptions whatsoever in your speech. (Tudor, 1939, pp. 10–11).

In addition, the childrens' teachers and staff were informed that:

these children show definite symptoms of stuttering. The types of interruptions they are having very frequently turn into stuttering. . . . Watch their speech all the time very carefully and stop them when they have interruptions; stop them and have them say it over. Don't allow them to speak unless they can say it right. (Tudor, 1939, pp. 12–13).

The children, the teachers, and the staff were consulted a minimum of once each month in order to reinforce the label of *stutterer*. Dictaphone recordings were made of all children for both reading and monologue speech at both the outset and conclusion of the study. Five judges rated the childrens' speech using a five-point, perceptual-fluency rating scale, and disfluencies were tabulated and placed into categories of syllable repetition, word repetition, phrase repetition, interjection, and pauses. Apparently no count was made of silent or audible prolongations.

Tudor provided a subjective analysis of the subjects from the third group by stating that by the end of the investigation, all six children showed varying degrees of speech disruptions and concern about their speech. According to Tudor:

They were reluctant to speak and spoke only when they were urged to. . . . [T]heir rate of speaking was decreased. They spoke more slowly and with greater exactness. They had a tendency to weigh each word before they said it. . . . [T]he length of response was shortened. . . . [T]hey became more self-conscious. They appeared shy and embarrassed in many situations. . . . They accepted the fact that there was something definitely wrong with their speech. Some hung their heads, others gasped and covered their mouths with their hands. (pp. 147–148).

As Silverman (1996) points out, these results were especially striking since five of the six children were beyond the age during which stuttering usually begins. The investigation appears to provide reasonably strong support for the essence of the diagnosogenic theory of stuttering onset and development.

However, a recent reexamination of the original study by Patton, Montague, and Buffalo (1996) suggests that, despite Tudor's interpretation, the results were not necessarily supportive of the diagnosogenic theory. In the first place, Patton et al. point out that there were several flaws in the Tudor investigation, including the lack of intra- and interjudge reliability measures for both the transcription of the recordings and the judges' classification of disfluency type. Second, reanalysis of the original data obtained by Tudor indicated that no significant differences across the four groups of children were found for either the perceptual fluency rating or any of the disfluency categories. Interestingly, this was true, not only for the scores obtained at the end of the experimental period, but also for those scores obtained at the outset. That is, statistical analysis of the data by Patton et al. revealed no statistically significant difference between subject groups at the beginning of the study before the experimental conditions were applied.

In the 1960s, stuttering as a learned behavior was formalized, in the form of both classically (instrumental) conditioning and operant (respondent) conditioning. Both approaches hold that the speaker gradually learns to stutter, but for slightly different reasons. With classical conditioning, the speaker learns to associate speaking with an emotional response. Just how this occurs is unclear, although some children may indeed have much more difficulty than others in achieving fluency. Alternately, it may be that some children experience highly penalizing responses to natural fluency breaks that may become tied to the experience of speaking. In any case, the child learns that speaking is, or can be, difficult and begins to both anticipate and struggle during breaks in his fluency. Again, whether the initial fluency breaks are indeed normal is a major issue of debate. If the initial breaks are normal, then the argument that stuttering can be learned is strengthened. If the initial or core breaks in fluency are not normal, however, learning would assume somewhat less importance. That is, it would suggest that, at least at the outset, something is not functioning normally in the speaker's speech production system.

Models of operant or respondent conditioning do not explain the onset of stuttering as well as they do the evolution of the behavior. Operant models propose that the fluency breaks of young children are shaped by the response they elicit. These theories propose that listeners respond to the child's fluency breaks by reinforcing their occurrence. The breaks are then gradually shaped into greater abnormality, with associated struggle and secondary characteristics. Operant models do well in explaining the great variety of secondary behaviors that develop with each individual. The avoidance and escape behaviors, while somewhat similar across all people who stutter, tend to be uniquely shaped by listener responses so that individuals tend to develop distinctive behaviors. The fact that these secondary behaviors are not regularly reinforced makes them particularly resistant to change since an intermittent schedule of reinforcement tends to strengthen behaviors, making them more difficult to extinguish.

Over time, the learned or secondary behaviors such as eye blinks, head movements, or gasping for air become part of an integrated and tightly bound pattern of behavior. In addition, it is suggested that negative reinforcement, or escape from punishment, is occuring. This may also be one explanation why the frequency of stuttering does not always decrease with what is perceived as punishment. That is, the "punishment" may help the speaker to escape from the stuttering moment by providing a highlighting affect (Cooper, Cady, & Robbins, 1970; Daly & Kimbarow, 1978).

Brutten and Shoemaker (1967) attempted to combine the best of the classical-conditioning and operant-conditioning models in the two-factor approach. They suggested that the initial fluency breaks occurred as a result of classically conditioned negative emotion being associated with the act of speaking. Via classical conditioning, learned, negative emotion disrupts the cognitive and motoric production of speech. The autonomic nervous system responds to this negative emotion. The development of secondary behaviors was the result of respondent or operant conditioning.

The high-water mark for traditional learning theories was likely a review article by Gerald Siegel published in 1970. Siegel, one of the foremost researchers in the field of behavioral science, pointed out that operant-conditioning models fail to adequately explain stuttering behavior in the laboratory, let alone in the real world. Although research has shown that it was clearly possible to manipulate the secondary behaviors of stuttering, clinicians had much less success in explaining the development and modifying the core behavior of the disorder, that is, the cause of the fluency breaks in the first place.

A final account of stuttering as learned behavior is Bloodstein's (1961, 1993, 1995) *continuity hypothesis*. Like the diagnosogenic theory, this view also proposes that stuttering develops from the normal fluency breaks produced by young children. However, misdiagnosis and negative reactions by one or more significant listeners are *not* part of the problem. Bloodstein suggests that both the tension and the fragmentation of fluency breaks increase as a result of communicative pressure. The development of stuttering is not a consequence of the child trying to avoid normal fluency breaks that have been mislabeled. As tension and fragmentation increase, especially for part-word repetitions, the pattern becomes chronic and the child is more likely to be identified as a stutterer.

THE CAPACITIES AND DEMANDS MODEL

One of the more recent paradigms used to explain the onset of stuttering is called the capacities and demands (or demands and capacities) model. This is a comprehensive model in that it considers both the capacities of the individual and the effects of his environment in the development of the disorder. Proponents of such a model propose that children who stutter possess a genetic or constitutional basis (or, at least, a predisposition) for fluency breakdown. This predisposition, along with environmental factors, combine to both originate and maintain the problem. Variants of this model were first proposed by Andrews and colleagues (Andrews et al., 1983; Andrews & Neilson, 1981; Neilson & Neilson, 1987). More recently, Starkweather (1987), Adams (1990), and Starkweather and Gottwald (1990) have provided theoretical elaboration.

In this model, the deterioration of fluency is viewed as reflecting an imbalance between the child's current capacities or abilities for fluency and the demands placed on the child in his environment. There is no disorder, and certainly nothing that could be termed a deficit. However, if the demands of the environment continue to exceed the capacities of that particular child, stuttering is more likely to occur. As Starkweather (1987) describes:

In this model, the capacities for fluent speech—the m
guistic and emotional skills that make easy speech p(
dren—interact with demands for fluency placed on the
communicative environment and by the child himsel
fluency grows, the expectations of parents and of the
Very young children are expected to be hesitant and :
Older children are expected to produce more wor(
more easily. In this way, capacities and demands for
neously increasing. If the environment demands more fluency than the
child can produce, stuttering will begin. Whether the stuttering will continue or remediate depends on whether a growing capacity to produce
fluent speech can catch up with the world's accelerating demands.°

The various capacities that have been suggested as necessary for achieving
fluency include oral and speech motor coordination, linguistic ability, cognitive ability, and social-emotional maturity. The demands from the environment
take the form of rapid thought processing, complex language formulation, rapid
speech, turn-taking behavior, and independent social behavior (Gottwald &
Starkweather, 1995; Starkweather, Gottwald, & Halfond, 1990).

Ratner (1995) indicates that there is some clinical support for this model
in the form of the *trading relationship* between fluency and associated speech
and language capacities. She notes that a proportion of children's nonfluen-
cies evolve from linguistic pressures that exceed their productive capacities.
That is, a fluent child sometimes begins to "stutter" following intervention to
enhance expressive language or phonological skills (Hall, 1977; Meyers,
Ghatak, & Woodford, 1990).

A SUMMARY OF MODELS

Perhaps a good way to complete this section on the theoretical views of stuttering
etiology is to paraphrase the comment of Conture (1990), who states that neither
the child's capacity alone nor his environment alone appear to be sufficient to cause
stuttering. In most cases, both components seem to be necessary for the problem
to develop. For example, Andrews, Yates-Morris, Howie & Martin (1991) found
that 71 percent of the variance contributing to the likelihood that one would stutter was accounted for by environmental factors, while 29 percent is accounted for
by the individual's unique environment (factors affecting the fetus and following
birth). Peters and Guitar (1991) agree that predisposing physiological factors interact with developmental and environmental influences to enhance the problem.

Many researchers have found that people who stutter possess one or more
predisposing characteristics that may, at the very least, set the stage for the
onset of stuttering. None of these features, in and of itself, is likely to directly
cause the problem. As mentioned at the outset of this chapter, if the etiology

° From Starkweather, *Fluency and Stuttering*. Copyright © 1987. All rights reserved. Reprinted
by permission of Allyn & Bacon.

yndrome was uncomplicated, the mystery of etiology would have been
ed long ago. In more extreme cases such as individuals undergoing injury
the central nervous system due to trauma, medication or disease, traumatic emotional damage including conversion neurosis (Roth, Aronson, &
Davis, 1989), or extreme environmental or communicative pressure, as in
the "monster" study described by Silverman (1988b), one or relatively few factors may bring about a chronic disruption of fluency. Rather, in the vast majority of cases it takes a critical mass of factors that combine to tax the system
over a critical time during the development of speech and language.

THE DEVELOPMENT OF STUTTERING

The nature of stuttering at onset has often been discussed in the literature and
forms the basis for many diagnostic decisions when assessing young children
who are suspected of stuttering (see Chapter 3). Rarely do the characteristics
of stuttering begin after the early childhood years, although some instances
of late onset will be discussed in Chapter 4. For this reason, stuttering has
often been called a disorder of childhood (Bloodstein, 1995; Conture, 1990,
Van Riper, 1982).

The hallmark of stuttering onset in children is the gradual development of
the distinguishing characteristics. Because these features usually develop
slowly and are highly variable, determining their presence in young children
can be a difficult clinical decision. Authors have noted that even during stuttering moments, young children who stutter produce relatively normal movement sequences (Caruso, Conture, & Colton, 1988). Furthermore, during
perceptually fluent speech, children who stutter are nearly identical to normally speaking children in terms of temporal onsets, offsets, and durations of
speech movements (Conture, Colton, & Gleason, 1988). The great overlap
in the behaviors of young, normally speaking children and those who eventually emerge as young people who stutter can make it difficult for the clinician to make precise diagnostic choices, let alone predict future performance.
There is no absolute standard for how often or how tense a fluency break must
be before it will be called stuttering. As much as anything, the designation of
stuttering may coincide with whether the child's manner of speaking takes
away from the effective communication of the message. If the quality of the
speaker's fluency begins to detract from the effective communication of the
message, it may be nearing the threshold of a problem.

The most common approach for differentiating the fluency breaks of young
children was developed by Wendell Johnson and his associates (Johnson, 1961;
Johnson & Associates, 1959) and modified by Williams, Silverman, and Kools
(1968). This scheme identified certain surface behaviors of stuttering into
the following categories:

- part-word repetition
- single-syllable word repetition

- multisyllabic word repetition
- phrase repetition
- interjections
- revision-incomplete phrase
- dysrhythmic phonation (sound prolongations within words, unusual stress or broken words)
- tense pause (barely audible heavy breathing and other tense sounds between words)

Although younger stutterers tend to have a higher occurrence of nearly all form types (Yairi & Lewis, 1984) the categories of part-word repetitions, word repetitions, dysrhythmic phonations, and tense pauses tend to occur most often (Silverman, 1974). Still, there is no fluency break that stuttering children produce and normal speakers do not. Yairi and his colleagues make use of what they call *stuttering-like disfluencies* (SLD) (e.g., Yairi, Ambrose, & Niermann, 1993), which include part-word repetition, single-syllable word repetition, and disrhythmic phonation, and contrast these with what they call *other disfluencies*, which include polysyllable word repetition, phrase repetition, interjection, and revision-incomplete phrases. These authors have suggested that some combinations of fluency breaks, such as SLD, may be more sensitive measures of early stuttering.

Researchers have also noted the tendency for children who stutter to produce fluency breaks in clusters (Colburn, 1985; Hubbard & Yairi, 1988; LaSalle & Conture, 1995; Silverman, 1973). That is, children in the early stages of stuttering often produce a sequence of between- or within-word breaks in close proximity to one another. For example, when contrasting the conversational speech of thirty young (average age of four years, three months) children who stuttered (CWS) with a control group of children, LaSalle and Conture (1995) found that 32 percent of the clusters produced by the children who stuttered were stuttering-stuttering (within-word disfluencies) sequences, while the children who did not stutter *never* produced such clusters in any of their 300-word speech samples. They also noted that the occurrence of clusters containing within-word disfluencies was positively correlated with greater severity of stuttering and, perhaps, chronic stuttering.

Van Riper (1982) also provides criteria for differentiating normal from abnormal fluency breaks (see Table 2–1). These often-cited guidelines distinguish stuttering and normal disfluency on the basis of speech characteristics and reaction of the speaker to forms of stress and awareness of the problem. It is apparent that more than speech attributes must be considered when differentiating between a normal speaker and someone who is stuttering. Because of the considerable overlap in the type of fluency breaks, it has been suggested that nonverbal behaviors also should be considered when describing the onset of stuttering. Conture (1990) suggests two types of nonspeech behavior that the clinician can look for: (a) body movement and tension and

(b) psychosocial discomfort and concern. Conture and Kelly (1988) found that young stutterers were more likely to move their eyeballs to the left or right or to partially or totally obscure their view of the listener by blinking. In addition, young children may indicate their frustration and anxiety about speaking. Although the young child may not be extremely concerned, he may be in the initial stages of thinking of himself as someone who has trouble talking (DeVore, Nandur, & Manning, 1984).

Conture (1990) suggests a sequence of development that corresponds closely with Van Riper's (1982) tracks of stuttering development (see Van Riper, pp. 94-108).

Alpha Behaviors

These are brief, subtle inefficiencies in speech production characterized by short within-word pauses, laryngeal catches, and articulatory arrests at the beginning of an utterance or at the transition between sounds and syllables. These subtle breaks appear to occur as a result of an interplay between the child's capacity for producing fluency and environmental stimuli or demands.

Beta Behaviors

These are oscillatory movements of the speech mechanism that are characterized by brief to lengthy repetitive productions. These are compensatory or coping reactions to the original Alpha factors and take the form of syllable repetitions, laryngeal adduction, and nostril flaring.

Gamma Behaviors

These are relatively tense and/or fixed speech movements that are viewed as coping reactions to the Beta activities. These behaviors take the form of fixed laryngeal adductory postures, labial contacts, and lingual posturing. These result in inaudible sound prolongations or a cessation of airflow or voicing. This stage is a significant step in the development of stuttering, marks a reduced likelihood for it that spontaneous recovery will take place.

Delta Behaviors

These are both nonverbal and verbal reactions to Beta, Gamma, and possibly Alpha behaviors and are seen as reactive speech and nonspeech behaviors. These coping reactions are in the form of such responses as pharyngeal muscle constriction, vocal fold lengthening (pitch rises), vocal fold shortening, blinking of eyelids, and eyeball movements.

Table 2–1 Guidelines for Differentiating Normal from Abnormal Disfluency. (From Van Riper, C. *The Nature of Stuttering* (2nd ed.). Copyright © 1982. All rights reserved. Adapted by permission of Allyn & Bacon.)

BEHAVIOR	STUTTERING	NORMAL DISFLUENCY
Syllable Repetitions:		
a. Frequency per word	More than two	Less than two
b. Frequency for 100 words	More than two	Less than two
c. Tempo	Faster than normal	Normal Tempo
d. Regularity	Irregular	Regular
e. Schwa vowel	Often present	Absent or rare
f. Airflow	Often interrupted	Rarely interrupted
g. Vocal tension	Often apparent	Absent
Prolongations:		
h. Duration	Longer than one second	Less than one second
i. Frequency	More than 1 per 100 words	Less than 1 per 100 words
j. Regularity	Uneven or interrupted	Smooth
k. Tension	Important when present	Absent
l. When voiced	May show rise in pitch	No pitch rise
m. When unvoiced	Interrupted airflow	Airflow present
n. Termination	Sudden	Gradual
Gaps (silent pauses):		
o. Within the word boundary	May be present	Absent
p. Prior to speech attempt	Unusually long	Not marked
q. After the disfluency	May be present	Absent
Phonation:		
r. Inflections	Restricted; monotone	Normal
s. Phonatory arrest	May be present	Absent
t. Vocal fry	May be present	Usually absent
Articulatory Postures:		
u. Appropriateness	May be inappropriate	Appropriate
Reaction to Stress:		
v. Type	More broken words	Normal disfluencies
Evidence of awareness:		
w. Phonemic consistency	May be present	Absent
x. Frustration	May be present	Absent
y. Postponements	May be present	Absent
z. Eye contact	May waver	Normal

In addition, Conture (1990) describes three possible patterns of development for young children who possess Alpha features. One possibility is the spontaneous resolution of the Alpha behavior. This is thought to occur for about 40 to 50 percent of children who begin demonstrating Alpha behaviors. Their fluency breaks are characterized as brief, often imperceptible. That is, they may have somewhat longer articulatory contacts and slightly slower trajectories to articulatory targets than controls. These children may exhibit cycles of Beta behavior, which eventually fade away. For whatever reasons, these children do not move to, and stay at, the next stage of stuttering development. They do not respond to the subtle motoric breaks with tense or fixed gestures. It may be important to note that for the most part, these children also have essentially normal articulation, language, and neuromotor development.

Another possible sequence has children reacting to the various Alpha features and progressing gradually through the Beta level. The difference for these children is that they will recover only with treatment. They also comprise about 40 to 50 percent of the total population of children who begin with Alpha behaviors. These children may demonstrate increased numbers of sound prolongations and associated nonspeech behaviors. It is likely consequential that they tend to also have some difficulty with articulation, deviant or delayed sound production, and phonological difficulties, as well as other language or voice problems (St. Louis & Hinzman, 1986). In an attempt to cope with the Alpha and Beta features, these children go on to develop Delta behaviors that make the problem even more apparent. Conture suggests that treatment intended to alter the Gamma behaviors will not solve the problem of the more central Alpha and Beta features.

A final progression is the rare instance in which a child begins stuttering in a nondevelopmental manner. That is, the onset is characterized by Gamma and Delta behaviors. This unique scenario is analogous to adults who begin to stutter as a result of psychological trauma.

Although this pattern of development assists in understanding how stuttering may evolve, there is a growing body of data that suggests that such development is not always the case. A microview of very early stuttering, children approximately two through five years of age, indicates a less predictable pattern of development. The longitudinal data accumulated by Yairi and his associates concerning onset and development (Yairi & Ambrose, 1992a, 1992b; Yairi, Ambrose, & Niermann; Yairi & Hall, 1993; Yairi & Lewis, 1984) suggest that stuttering in young children can reach an advanced form soon after onset. This early stuttering can take complex forms that include head and facial movements and long, tense, blocking behavior. Yairi, Ambrose, and Niermann (1993) conclude that, for many children, the peak of stuttering is reached during the first two to three months postonset. However, perhaps the most interesting finding is the observation that a substantial number of children show a dramatic decline in both the frequency and severity of stuttering within the first six months after onset (Yairi & Ambrose, 1992a; Yairi, Ambrose, & Niermann, 1993). Such recovery takes place without formal clinical intervention. Furthermore, a two-year follow-up of young recovered children studied by Yairi and Ambrose (1992a) indicated no instances of relapse. Their data make a strong case for continued recovery from stuttering during the early childhood years, a trend that is counter to a good deal of thinking about the developmental nature of the problem. Not only do such results seriously confound studies of treatment efficacy with this population of young stuttering children, it indicates caution concerning intervention decisions. Uncertainty concerning the developmental sequence of stuttering suggests the value of at-risk registers (to be discussed in Chapter 3).

CONDITIONS CONTRIBUTING TO ONSET

This section will consider two sets of conditions that have been related to the onset of stuttering. The first set of conditions are those that, while they have been considered in the literature, seem to have relatively little influence on stuttering causation. These conditions, although they may be prominent events in the child's life, simply coincide with the initial observation that the child is beginning to stutter. We will then discuss conditions that may have a greater effect on onset. These are factors that relate more directly to the child's capacities for producing fluent speech. It is important to understand that many investigations of young stuttering children are descriptive studies that do not allow an assumption of cause-and-effect relationships between the speaker or environmental characteristics and the onset of stuttering behavior. While there may indeed be a relationship between these events, the fact that they covary may instead only signify that another unknown factor or factors is causing this relationship.

Less Influential Factors

These factors have not been shown, at least to date, to have a strong influence on precipitating the problem of stuttering. In many instances, these factors are similar to the myths that tend to be associated with stuttering (see Chapter 7).

General Physical Development. Children who stutter have the same general physical makeup as children who speak normally. There is no evidence that children who stutter are distinctive in terms of general developmental milestones such as ages of teething and weaning, as well as developing the ability to dress and feed themselves, acquire bowel and bladder control, sit, creep, stand, and walk (Andrews & Harris, 1964; Cox, Seider, & Kidd, 1984).

Illness. On occasion, parents will report that stuttering began following an illness. As Silverman (1996) points out, if the illness affects the central nervous system, a cause-and-effect relationship between the illness and the onset of stuttering may be possible. However, children who stutter do not appear to have more illnesses than those that do not (Andrews & Harris, 1964; Johnson & Associates, 1959). Illness could influence the nature of stuttering in those who already stutter, for it may be difficult to maintain the energy to monitor speech production and use fluency-enhancing techniques when the child is sick and resistance and energy are low (Luchsinger & Arnold, 1965; Van Riper, 1978).

Imitation. This consideration of stuttering onset may be influenced by the culture of the speaker. For example, Otsuki (1958, as cited by Silverman, 1992) reported that in Japan, imitation was a major causal factor in 70 percent of his cases. In his review of clinical cases, Van Riper (1982) indicated that although there were several instances where imitation appeared to be involved in the onset of stuttering, only one case appeared to be attributed to this cause. The strongest argument against imitation is that the early forms of stuttering are highly dissimilar from the more advanced forms.

Shock or Fright. Parents may report the onset of stuttering following a traumatic emotional event (Van Riper, 1982). However, as both Van Riper (1982) and Silverman (1996) point out, in many cases, the initial signs of stuttering often preceded the suspected event. Rather than a cause of the stuttering, an event that happens to occur at approximately the same time as the stuttering was first observed serves as a marker of that time period. Parents may report the onset of stuttering associated with an event without knowing that their child had been stuttering for some time in school and other locations outside the home. Moreover, as Silverman indicates, in almost all cases, the "traumatic" events are not really very traumatic.

Emotional and Communicative Conflicts. Similar to shock or fright, some parents suspect that a variety of interpersonal and family stresses can bring about stuttering. There are, of course, many forms of emotional and communicative stress for children. The majority of authorities believe that, although such forms of stress may well aggravate the fluency breaks of children who have already begun to stutter, there is little empirical support for this form of causation. Children who stutter do not have a greater number of emotional conflicts than their normally speaking counterparts (Adams, 1993; Andrews & Harris, 1964; Bloch & Goodstein, 1971; Bloodstein, 1987; Johnson & Associates, 1959; Van Riper, 1982). Again, as with illness, shock, or fright, emotional or communicative stress undoubtedly contributes to breakdowns in the motor sequencing of speech (Van Riper, 1982).

Socioeconomic Status of the Family. The very few data that are available indicate that stuttering is present in all socioeconomic groups. Van Riper (1982) reviews many studies that report varying amounts of stuttering across both cultures and races. Gillespie and Cooper (1973) and Dykes and Pindzola (1995) report data showing a higher occurrence of stuttering in African-American populations. Undoubtedly, factors of social-economic and race interact with, and cloud, this issue. Bloodstein (1987) suggests that the occurrence of stuttering may be related to the imposition of high standards for the achievement of status and prestige, along with the intolerance of deviancy, values that may vary depending on the socioeconomic status of families.

Nationality. The occurrence of stuttering in technologically developed countries is typically reported at approximately .07 percent to 1 percent of the population. The occurrence is somewhat higher in several cultures throughout the world, due possibly to a combination of limited genetic pools and cultural responses to disfluency (Bullen, 1945; Lemert, 1953, 1962; Morgenstern, 1956; Snidecor, 1947).

More Influential Factors

Other factors do appear to have a somewhat greater influence on the likelihood of stuttering, although their precise impact remains unclear. Again, it is important to keep in mind that stuttering onset is most likely the result of a combination of intrinsic and extrinsic factors, and no one aspect is likely to decrease a child's capacity or increase the environmental demands to the point where stuttering will occur. Rather, these conditions may be best thought of as predisposing factors that can place a child at greater risk for both *precipitating* and *maintaining* stuttering (Silverman, 1992).

Sex. The higher occurrence of stuttering in males is one of the few consistencies about stuttering (Kent, 1983). The reasons why males consistently show a higher occurrence of stuttering may relate to boys being less adept at language and speech activities or less able to adapt to communicative stress. The previously mentioned findings of Geschwind and Galaburda (1985) suggest that young male speakers may have greater difficulty in achieving or maintaining fluency. In addition, as discussed earlier, there may also be a sex-related genetic influence that, at the very least, precipitates stuttering (Kidd, Kidd, & Records, 1978).

Age. Children who are approximately two through seven years of age are much more likely to begin stuttering than older children, adolescents, or adults. There is a much greater chance of stuttering onset before age five than after age seven. Andrews (1984) suggests that the risk of developing stuttering drops by 50 percent after age four, 75 percent after age six, and is virtually nil by age twelve. The onset of stuttering during the middle or late adult years is extremely rare and is likely to occur only in cases of neurological or psychological origin.

Genetic Factors. There is a long history of documentation that stuttering occurs with much greater than usual frequency in some families. Bloodstein's (1995) review indicates that the percentage of persons who have relatives on the maternal or paternal side who stuttered ranges from 30 to 69 percent.

Research during the past few decades has indicated a genetic component in selected groups of people who stutter (Cox, Seider, & Kidd, 1984; Johnson & Associates, 1959; Kidd, 1977; Pauls, 1990; Poulos & Webster, 1991; Sheehan & Costley, 1977; Yairi, 1983).

Twinning. A child is more likely to stutter if he is a member of a twin pair in which the other twin also stutters (Howie, 1981). This is especially true if the twins are identical. It is less likely that both members of a fraternal twin pair will stutter (Howie, 1981). These findings seem to be explained by a predisposition to stuttering that is genetically linked (Howie, 1981; West & Ansberry, 1968) and to family and environmental factors.

Brain Injury. Van Riper (1982) summarizes findings that report considerably greater than a 1 percent occurrence of stuttering with brain injury, especially for speakers with cerebral palsy and epilepsy. However, it can sometimes be difficult to distinguish motor speech and language problems (particularly word finding) from fluency breaks. In addition, speakers who are developmentally delayed often have a higher than usual occurrence of stuttering, especially those with Down's syndrome. Van Riper (1982) summarized the results of seven independent studies indicating prevalence figures ranging from a low of 7 percent (Schaeffer & Shearer, 1968) to a high of 60 percent for clients with Down's syndrome (Preus, 1973). Averaging across all seven studies and the two reported categories of "general retardates" and "mongoloids" results in a prevalence figure of 24 percent (standard deviation [SD] = 18.1). Of course, with this population, there is also a much higher occurrence of many speech and language problems, including cluttering. In addition, developmental delays and neuropathological influences can mask the identification of fluency disorders. Studies indicate that both verbal and nonverbal intelligence is slightly lower in stutterers in contrast to control subjects. For whatever reasons, individuals who possess less than normal cognitive abilities tend to have more fluency problems.

Speech and Language Development. There is an obvious interplay of factors such as intelligence, school performance, and language skills. Summarizing a series of studies by Andrews and Harris (1964), Berry, (1938), Kline and Starkweather (1979), Murray and Reed (1977), and Wall (1980), Peters and Guitar (1991) conclude that children who stutter typically achieve lower scores than their peers on measures of receptive vocabulary, the age of speech and language onset, mean length of utterance, and expressive and receptive syntax. In addition, children who stutter frequently also exhibit other communicative problems. Especially for these children, speech and language production *is* likely to be more difficult, and there is a higher probability that they will find themselves exerting increased effort when they are speaking.

Motor Coordination. There is some evidence that people who stutter have somewhat greater difficulty in fine motor coordination (Riley & Riley, 1984; Starkweather, 1987; Van Riper, 1982). At least part of the act of speaking is a motor skill, and any delay or deficit in this aspect could certainly adversely affect the development of normal fluency. There is, for example, some indication of a lack of appropriate interaction between laryngeal and supralaryngeal behaviors during fluent speech in young stutterers (Zebrowski, Conture, & Cudahy, 1985), which was confirmed by Borden, Kim, and Spiegler (1987). Such oral-motor difficulties could be especially problematic for children who have above-average linguistic skill as well as a strong desire to communicate.

CONCLUSION

The uncertainties about the possible causes of fluency disorders will continue for many years. Despite this, the clinician should be familiar with the possibilities that have been proposed and have a reasonable response to a question such as, "What causes stuttering?" Having considered the many possibilities for stuttering onset, it should be obvious that people who stutter are far from a homogeneous group. This may be one reason why there are so many divergent theories of stuttering onset throughout history. This also may help to explain why some speakers are more apt to recover than others, why treatment techniques that work well with one person do not work with another, and why relapse is an especially important issue with some clients. As a result of advanced technology as well as greater understanding of the human speech production system, there is increasing evidence of neurophysiological factors contributing to both the onset and maintenance of fluency problems. This is not to say that such factors indicate a deficit; they rather indicate reduced capacities for producing fluent speech and language. Such decreased capacities, in combination with environmental demands (particularly during a critical developmental period of speech and language acquisition), may result in chronic stuttering—but sometimes they do not. Following onset, fluency disorders usually follow a reasonably well-understood evolution. Current authors agree that the early diagnosis of stuttering dramatically increases the chance of therapeutic success.

RECOMMENDED READINGS

Shields, D. (1989). *Dead languages*. New York: Knopf.
Van Riper, C. (1974). A handful of nuts. *Western Michigan Journal of Speech Therapy*.

Van Riper, C. (1982). *The nature of stuttering* (2nd Ed.). Englewood Cliffs, NJ: Prentice-Hall. See ch. 5, "The Development of Stuttering," pp. 88–110; ch. 17, "The Nature of Stuttering: An Attempted Synthesis," pp. 415–453.

Van Riper, C. (1990). Final thoughts about stuttering. *Journal of Fluency Disorders, 15,* 317–318.

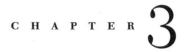

CHAPTER 3

Assessing Fluency Disorders in Children

PRELIMINARIES TO ASSESSMENT

Before discussing the assessment of children (in this chapter) and of adolescents and adults (in Chapter 4), we will present several concepts that have a primary influence on our decisions as we attempt to characterize nonfluent speech and handicapped speakers, regardless of age. The many differences between the assessment of younger speakers, who may or may not be starting on the road to stuttering, and those older speakers who have traveled the road for many years will become obvious. However, there also are many important similarities. It is the similarities, the primary concepts that unite the assessment process for younger as well as older speakers, that we will discuss first.

THE VARIABILITY OF FLUENCY

Our level of fluency varies widely across time and location. At times, we speak nearly automatically, with words flowing smoothly and effortlessly. On other occasions, particularly when we experience communicative or emotional stress, the smoothness begins to disappear and breaks in our speech take place, or at least they become more obvious. Although fluency varies for all speakers, its variability is even more pronounced for the person who stutters. In most instances, the stutterer is more likely than the nonstutterer to react sooner and to a greater degree to fluency-disrupting stimuli. At the other extreme, people who stutter are sometimes able to "turn on fluency." By avoiding feared sounds or words and "rising to the occasion," they are able to become uncharacteristically fluent. The great variability of stuttering behaviors is one of the facts about stuttering and something that contributes to the mystery of the disorder. The variability of stuttering behavior makes it difficult for listeners to become accustomed to the speaker, for it is not always possible to predict whether a person will stutter, and it is even less possible to anticipate the severity of the stuttering. It is also important to mention that the variability presents an especially difficult predicament for the person doing the stuttering. That is, the person who stutters cannot always be certain of the amount and degree of difficulty he will have in any given speaking situation. It is difficult for the stutterer to compensate for a handicap that is so inconsistent. Of the many communication handicaps that people may suffer, perhaps none is more variable than stuttering.

The high degree of intraspeaker variability makes the assessment of fluency more formidable than it may first appear. As Bloodstein (1987) states, "The great variability of stuttering from time to time under different conditions is liable to result in assessments that are unrepresentative" (1987, p. 386). Almost any assessment protocol will provide only a glimpse of the complexity. Many aspects of the fluency disorder will go undetected unless the assessment is conducted in a variety of speaking situations. The more these situations are similar to the daily activities of this person, the more likely we are to obtain a valid indication of the problem. Perhaps more than in any other communication disorder, the assessment of stuttering is an ongoing process that, by necessity, takes place over several assessment treatment sessions.

Characteristics of Normal Fluency

Another difficulty we face when assessing fluency is the lack of data describing the nature of fluency in normal speakers. For instance, we know relatively little about the fluency characteristics of normal children and their responses to fluency-disrupting stimuli. We know almost nothing about changes in fluency throughout the life cycle, particularly for older speakers (Manning, Dailey, & Wallace, 1984; Manning & Shirkey, 1981). Furthermore, few data have been accumulated about the fluency characteristics as a function of variables such as gender, race, culture, and social-economic level. Given the changing demographics of the United States, there are many important questions that should be asked concerning these variables if we are to be in a position to help clients who stutter (Cole, 1986, 1989; Cooper & Cooper, 1991b; Satcher, 1986; Waldrop & Exter, 1990).

In order to appreciate the nature of nonfluent speech production, it is necessary to understand the dimensions of fluent speech. Even the best of speakers speaking under ideal conditions are apt to produce breaks in the flow of words. Language and speech production is a complex task, and it takes years, possibly decades, of experience to do it well, especially under conditions of stress. As Van Riper (1982) and Starkweather (1987) have pointed out, it is fortunate that humans have the opportunity to practice speaking as much as they do.

Starkweather (1987) provides an elegant assessment of the research on the dimensions of fluent speech in both children and adults. The term *fluency*, derived from the Latin for *flowing*, describes what the listener perceives when listening to someone who is truly adept at producing speech. The speech flows easily and smoothly, in terms of both sound *and* information. There are no disruptions of the stream, and the listener can attend to the message—the overall effect of the performance—rather than considering how it was produced. The effect is similar to observing any accomplished athletic performance that requires complicated sequential movements, such as gymnastics, ice skating, diving, or swimming. The impression when observing such athletes is one of smoothness and ease. The individual segments of the performance are blended together, with no obvious transition from one movement to the next. There is a consistency to the behavior, and little or no tension is evident. As a matter of fact, it may look as though the performer is unencumbered by the force of gravity, almost floating, with relatively little effort being expended.

Most young adult speakers are able to achieve a level of speech production that results in a high level of fluency. Such fluency requires facility at a minimum of two levels of production: language and speech. Filmore (1979) described three types of language fluency, which are interpreted by Starkweather (1987) as syntactic, semantic, and pragmatic fluency. Starkweather adds a fourth component, which he describes as phonologic fluency. Speakers who are *syntactically* fluent are able to construct highly complex sentences. Speakers who are *semantically* fluent possess and are able to access large vocabularies. Speakers who are *pragmatically* fluent are adept at verbal response in a large variety of speaking situations. Starkweather's term *phonologically* fluent describes those speakers who are able to pronounce long and complicated sequences of sounds and syllables, including nonsense and foreign words.

Although *language* fluency is a prerequisite for the production of fluent speech, it is not the case that individuals who stutter are deficient in these aspects of language competence or ability. People who stutter do, however, exhibit difficulties in *speech* fluency.

There are several dimensions of speech fluency. Starkweather (1987) defines speech fluency in terms of continuity, rate, duration, coarticulation, and effort. *Continuity* relates to the degree to which syllables and words are logically sequenced as well as the presence or absence of pauses. If the semantic units follow one another in a continual flow of information, the speech is interpreted as fluent. If, however, the units of speech fail to flow in a logical sequence, information does not flow. Despite a continual flow of sound and the absence of pauses, the speech is not thought of as fluent, as in the following paragraph offered by Starkweather:

> What I mean, what I mean is, that, uh, when you, you, go to the, uh, store because, uh, you, you want some, need some, uh food or supplies or something, and, and, uh, the storekee—the man, clerk, who, who waits, well not waits, but serves, you know, gets some—something for you is, well, if he, if he, well if he is sort of, well, stern, or you know angry or something, then, well, then, I find it, well, I find it difficult to talk. (1987, p. 19)

Another aspect of continuity has to do with a disruption in the flow of sound in the form of pauses. The pauses in the sequence of speech can be viewed from several perspectives. Clark (1971) differentiates pauses as conventional and idiosyncratic. *Conventional pauses* are used by speakers to signal a linguistically important event. *Idiosyncratic pauses*, on the other hand, reflect hesitation or uncertainty on the part of the speaker. These pauses indicate a decision-making process concerning upcoming word choice, style, or syntax.

Pauses also have been considered as unfilled or filled. Unfilled pauses are characterized by a silence lasting *longer* than approximately 250 milliseconds (msec.) (Goldman-Eisler, 1958). This duration is suggested as a convenient threshold for normal silent intervals during fluent speech since normal word junctures rarely exceed this duration (e.g., the juncture necessary to distinguish *night rate* from *nitrate*). Filled pauses are characterized by essentially meaningless sounds such as "ah," "er," "uh," and "um." With filled pauses, the flow of sound continues, but again, the flow of information does not. Whether the speech is considered fluent depends on many other features, including the frequency of these pauses along with the occurrence of other aspects of fluency.

Rate of speech also signals the perception of fluency. Most people talk about as fast as they can, as indicated by Tiffany (1980), who noted that the maximum and ordinary rates of speech tend to be similar. Young adult speakers of English average approximately five syllables per second (Picket, 1980; Stetson, 1951; Walker & Black, 1950). Obviously, according to the speaking task, there is considerable variability in terms of such factors as formality of the speaking situation, time pressure, and interference from background noise or competing messages. There appears to be a reasonably wide range of acceptable rates in the judgment of fluency. It is well known that if communication failure is likely, such as when speaking in a noisy environment, speakers are likely to slow down (Longhurst & Siegel, 1973). Likewise, if a speaker is producing a lengthy utterance, the rate of speech is likely to be more rapid (Malecot, Johnston, & Kizziar, 1972). It is not surprising, then, that listeners provide speakers with a great deal of latitude in their judgments of nonfluency based on rate alone. That is, simply because the speaker is producing speech at a slow rate, everything else being equal, he is not likely to be evaluated as being nonfluent. Conversely, simply because a speaker is producing speech at a very rapid rate, he or she is not likely to be evaluated as being fluent. Although the rate of speech production is obviously one aspect of fluency, it does not appear to be a primary dimension. The flow of speech and information is based, not only on rate, but on a combination of many factors, and particularly the ease of production (as we shall see).

Duration of speech segments relates closely to the *coarticulation* of the segments, so we will discuss them concurrently. The duration of the consonants and vowels of a language varies considerably with speech rate and phonetic and linguistic context. For example, stressed syllables are longer than unstressed ones (Umeda, 1975). Sound segments are longer at the initiation and termination of syllables, words, and phrases (Fowler, 1978). Segment durations are dramatically influenced by position in the syllable (initial consonants are longer than syllable-final consonants), length of the word (segments are shorter with longer words), and sentence length (segments and words are shorter during longer sentences) (Huggins, 1978). Much of what occurs in terms of the duration of individual sound segments and words appears to be related to the speaker's anticipated flow of information during an utterance (Starkweather, 1987). That is, the speaker may not need to plan all aspects of the upcoming utterance in terms of the necessary respiratory, phonatory, and articulatory events. Rather, the speaker would only need to have some idea about the amount of information the utterance would contain. Once the intended information was anticipated, the relative length of the utterance and the corresponding duration of the units of the sentence would be consolidated into the planned production.

Closely related to the durational aspects of individual sound segments and words is the fact that, during speech there is a considerable overlap of the movements associated with speech sounds. Each sequence of speech sounds is the result of several coordinated gestures, each with its own associated movements. The movements will result in differing productions for individual sounds in terms of velocity of movement as well as the location and degree of contact. Because adjoining sounds and their associated gestures overlap temporally to the degree that the movements are not conflicting the sounds are coarticulated.

This overlap, or *coarticulation*, extends across many sound segments, both forward and backward in time (Kozhevnikov & Chistovich, 1965; Ohman, 1965). The effect extends forward in time because the speaker anticipates upcoming sounds and, to the degree possible, and assuming there are no competing movements taking place, begins to move the articulators into position to produce upcoming sounds. That is, the anticipation of upcoming sounds will influence the production of sounds currently being produced. The example is easily appreciated by contrasting the production of the words *see* and *sue*. The acoustic characteristics of the /s/ is clearly affected (note the typically high-frequency resonance) during the production of the /s/ in *see* as a result of lip flaring in anticipation of the /e/. In contrast, the quality of the

/s/ in *sue* has a much lower resonance as a result of lip rounding in anticipation of the upcoming /u/. This type of coarticulation may thus be thought of as anticipatory or forward (in time) coarticulation.

Coarticulatory effects also extend backward in time when the inertial effects of sounds that have already been produced influence the location and degree of contact of sounds currently being produced. An example of this effect would be a slightly more posterior lingual-alveolar contact for the production of the /t/ in the word *cat* than for the word *sat*. That is, the lingual-velar production of the already produced /k/ results in the tongue having to move a greater distance to the front of the oral cavity to produce the /t/. The place of contact for the /t/ in this case would be apt to be produced in a somewhat posterior position relative to the place of the /t/ in the word *sat*. This type of coarticulation may thus be thought of as backward (in time) coarticulation. These coarticulatory effects are greater when the speech rate is increased (Gay, 1978; Gay & Hirose, 1973; Gay, Ushijima, Hirose, & Cooper, 1974). The main point of all this for our discussion of fluency is that these coarticulatory, or overlapping, effects contribute to the timing and smoothness of the speech. In fluent speech, articulatory movements between the sounds, syllables, and words are done with ease. The transitions are smooth, and there is a continuous flow of overlapping sounds.

The final, and perhaps the most telling dimension of fluency, particularly as it relates to stuttering, is *effort*. Starkweather (1987) distinguishes two types of effort: effort associated with linguistic planning and that associated with muscle movement. Clinically, it may be that the listener's perception of effort, in combination with the other dimensions of fluent speech production already discussed, is the most sensitive indicator of fluent speech. As Starkweather suggests, "Fluent speech is effortless in two distinct ways: it requires little thought, and it requires little muscular exertion" (1987, p. 37). Fluent speech is characterized by little attention being paid to the process of production; speaking is "automatic." The focus is on what is being said, on the information that is being communicated from one person to another. The thought process in fluent speech takes relatively little time, while the execution of the speech takes somewhat longer. To the degree that the focus of the speaker is on *how* speech is being produced, there is a good chance that attention will be taken away from *what* is being said.

Finally, in terms of effort, Starkweather (1987) makes the insightful comment that the perception of effort and, thus, fluency is closely related to the force of contact between opposing articulators. Fluent speech and fluent speakers are characterized by little sensation of opposition or constriction of airflow. The air, the movements, and the sounds are produced with evident ease and smoothness. On the other hand, people who stutter are at the opposite end of the continuum of effort. Greater effort is associated with all the following: greater contact between articulators, greater impedance between the flow of air and the structures of the vocal tract beginning with the vocal folds, and greater subglottic air pressure. With the speaker producing speech in this fashion, it is likely that speech will be judged as nonfluent. The focus for these speakers, particularly during overt stuttering, is nearly completely centered on *how* the speech is produced.

Formulative versus Motoric Fluency Breaks

If fluency can be described as the easy, automatic, and continuous flow of sound and information, then the essence of a fluency disorder is the difficult, deliberate, broken sequence of sounds and/or information. Indeed, at the most basic level that is what happens in one form or another for both children and adults who stutter. There are many individual features of stuttering occurring on the surface that tend to obscure this central facet of the problem. These surface features are behaviors that speakers use to escape from, disguise, or minimize the handicapping effects of stuttering. These also, of course, are an important part of the stuttering behavior for each speaker. It is necessary to identify and map these features for each person. However, throughout the assessment and treatment of both children and adults who stutter, we find ourselves returning repeatedly to the fact that the essence of what the speaker is doing is preventing the easy, open flow of smooth and continuous speech.

The fact that normal speakers also exhibit many breaks in their fluency forces us to distinguish between normal and abnormal types of breaks, a task that has been a historical point of contention in the field for decades. Even the semantics of what to call the fluency breaks of normal and stuttering speakers has created difficulties. At the center of the controversy is whether the fluency breaks of nonstuttering speakers are qualitatively different than those of stuttering speakers. This fundamental question has received as much research attention as any issue in the field.

This issue is important for understanding the development of fluency breaks in the young child, particularly one who may be in the process of developing a pattern of stuttering. Because this is such an important issue, there has been considerable controversy over the differences, or lack thereof, in the fluency breaks of young stuttering and nonstuttering children. Much of the controversy stems from the fact that the very early stages of stuttering are difficult to investigate. As Yairi and Lewis (1984) point out, investigations of the fluency of young children have been beset by such problems as a reliance on parent accounts and the difficulty of obtaining speech samples in a natural environment. An even bigger problem, however, is the lag between the initial behaviors of stuttering and the referral for professional assistance. These problems have contributed to the conflict about whether the fluency breaks of young stutterers are indistinguishable from those of normal speakers (Glasner & Rosenthal, 1957; Johnson & Associates, 1959; Johnson & Luetenegger, 1955) or are different in many clinical aspects from normal speakers (Bloodstein, 1974; McDearmon, 1968; Van Riper, 1982).

We will take a moment to address the issue of whether the speech behavior of people who stutter and that of those who do not is essentially the same. That is, is it reasonable to consider the fluency breaks of stutterers and non-stutterers on the same continuum? While there are some who argue that the fluency breaks of stutterers and normal speakers are so distinctively different as to be mutually exclusive (Hamre, 1992), most investigators believe that the fluency breaks of all speakers fall on the same continuum (Bloodstein, 1992; Starkweather, 1992). Still others suggest that this discussion has gone on long enough and that it is time to move on to other explanations (Conture & Zebrowski, 1992; Ham, 1992; Van Riper, 1992a). People who stutter are, after all, making use of essentially the same speech production system as normal speakers. One would expect, even given some difficulties at one or more levels of this system, that there would be considerable overlap in the nature of the speech produced. Some people who stutter are clearly more distinguishable by both the amount and type of their fluency breaks. Some people who stutter do not do so in any observable way, at least they do not do so by producing the repetitions, prolongations, or blocking behavior of traditional stuttering. The discussions concerning the continuity or discontinuity between the surface behavior of people who stutter and those who do not are interesting, if somewhat esoteric. If the focus of our decisions during assessment and intervention is on the *person* rather than dogma of treatment or ideological positions it is clear that we must go beneath the surface and consider the affective and cognitive features of the speaker's fluency breaks.

The terms that will be used in this text will be *formulative* and *motoric fluency* breaks. We have chosen this nomenclature rather than terms such as *(normal) disfluencies, (abnormal) dysfluencies, stuttering moments,* and the like primarily because they present a clearer picture of what appears to be happening for stuttering as well as nonstuttering speakers.

Drawing from the writings of Starkweather (1987); Van Riper (1982), Bloodstein (1974), Yairi and Clifton (1972), and Gordon, Hutchinson, and Allen (1976), Manning and Shirkey (1981) suggested the use of these terms for describing the continuum of fluency breaks among speakers. Formulative fluency breaks are characterized by (1) breaks in fluency between words, phrases, and larger syntactic units (including whole-unit repetitions thereof), (2) lack of obvious tension during the breaks, and (3) interjections between whole-word or larger syntactic units. These breaks are typical of normal speakers. However, they are also present in the speech of stutterers. Motoric fluency breaks are characterized by (1) breaks between sounds or syllables (part-word breaks), (2) obvious tension in the vocal tract, (3) pauses with a possible cessation of airflow and voicing and (4) an excessive prolongation of sounds or syllables. These breaks are more typical of speakers who stutter but may also be present to a small degree in normal speakers.

With these terms in mind, we may begin to distinguish some differences in the fluency breaks of children and adults and in the patterns of breaks for stutterers as well as nonstutterers. The normally speaking young adult typically displays few motoric fluency breaks and only slightly more formulative fluency breaks (Manning & Shirkey, 1981). The relatively few studies conducted with older normal speakers provide preliminary evidence suggesting that formulative fluency breaks tend to increase somewhat during late adulthood and that motoric fluency breaks continue to be infrequent (Gordon, Hutchinson, & Allen, 1976; Manning and Monte, 1981; Yairi & Clifton, 1972).

The fluency breaks of young adult stutterers are made up almost entirely of motoric fluency breaks. In fact, there appears to be a notable absence of formulative (or normal) fluency breaks, a fact that may also be used to distinguish stutterers from normal speakers (Manning & Shirkey, 1981). It may be that progress in treatment is sometimes signaled by an *increase* in the frequency of formulative fluency breaks to levels typical of normal speakers. That is, as the person who stutters begins to consider the variety of ways of expressing a thought rather than dealing with the short-term problems inherent in avoiding or struggling through a motoric fluency break, formulative breaks may increase in frequency to normal or near-normal levels.

The fluency breaks of normally speaking children often contain a large number of formulative fluency breaks. Bloodstein (1974) suggested that such breaks may be a function of language learning. While motoric fluency breaks may occur, they are relatively infrequent. For the normally speaking child, the frequency of both formulative and motoric breaks decreases as the neurologic system approaches maturity and psycholinguistic abilities are developed. By early adolescence, the speaker will achieve the optimum level of fluency typical of the young adult (Manning & Shirkey, 1982).

In an attempt to decrease the effect of the usual delay between the onset and diagnosis of stuttering, Yairi and Lewis (1984) analyzed the fluency breaks of two- and three-year-old children within two months after the initial identification of stuttering behavior. Ten children identified as stuttering (five boys and five girls), were matched with a group of normally speaking children. A perceptual analysis was performed on audiotaped samples of spontaneous speech of all subjects, with intrajudge and interjudge agreements ranging from +.93 to +1.0. The results indicated much overlap in the type of fluency breaks of the two groups, especially for interjections and revision-incomplete phrases. The fluency breaks of the ten normally speaking children were characterized by a relatively even distribution across eight categories of fluency breaks. The most frequent fluency breaks for these normal speakers were, in order, interjection, part-word repetition, and revision-incomplete phrase.

Yairi and Lewis also found that the most frequent fluency breaks for the stuttering children were, in order, part-word repetitions, dysrhythmic phonation, and single-syllable repetitions. The stuttering children had more than three times the number of fluency breaks of the normal speaking children (21.5 breaks and 6.2 breaks per 100 syllables, respectively). The stuttering children had significantly more fluency breaks for all categories of breaks, although significant differences ($p < .05$) were found only during part-word repetitions and dysrhythmic phonation. It has been suggested that whole-word repetitions may be a precursor to part-word repetitions (Bloodstein & Grossman, 1981).

Finally, Yairi and Lewis found that the stuttering children distinguished themselves from the control subjects in the number of repetitions that occurred during the part-word repetitions. That is, while the normally speaking children rarely repeated a part-word repetition more than once (range of 1–2), the stuttering children typically repeated a portion of the word two or more times (range of 1–11). In a subsequent study, Ambrose and Yairi (1995) analyzed 1,000 syllables of 29 experimental subjects recently diagnosed (mean of 2.14 months postonset) as children who stuttered (average age, 34.76 months) and 29 control subjects (average age, 35.57 months). The young stuttering children demonstrated a significantly greater number of units per repetition ($p < .002$). The frequency per 100 syllables of disfluencies containing two or more repetition units for the experimental subjects was 3.70 ($SD = 3.77$), while for the control subjects it was 0.21 ($SD = .20$).

Surface versus Intrinsic Features

As we mentioned earlier in this chapter, the assessment of fluency disorders is made difficult by the natural variability of stuttering. Along with this great variability, the features of stuttering are often intricate and subtle, particularly with children; these are all reasons for the many debates over what is and is not stuttering (Hamre, 1992; Perkins, 1990).

Another problem in assessing stuttering is that what we see on the surface is only part of the problem. The surface behaviors of stuttering are reasonably obvious. These are behaviors that we can see and hear, such as the frequency, duration, and tension of stuttered moments, as well as the accessory features used by the speaker to postpone or escape from the moment of stuttering. Although not necessarily an uncomplicated perceptual task, these surface features of stuttering can be observed and recorded with some degree of accuracy and reliability. The variability of these features both within and across speakers complicates the task, and their variability may be further expanded with the introduction of treatment. Despite these dilemmas, it is worthwhile to identify and follow the quantity and quality of the surface features. At the very least we want to determine features such as the frequency and duration of both formulative and motoric fluency breaks, as well as the degree of tension and fragmentation. These surface behaviors provide one view of the problem as well as one measure of progress during treatment. However, even with children, and certainly with adolescents and adults, in order to obtain a valid indication of the speaker's handicap, we need to look below the surface. It is below the surface that we find the intrinsic features: the deep structure of the stuttering syndrome. They are the intrinsic aspects of the *person* who is doing the stuttering.

My experience as a school-age stutterer illustrates the importance of appreciating the intrinsic aspects of stuttering. All the clinicians who worked with me over the years knew about stuttering. They could identify stuttering moments and categorize the overt aspects of my surface behaviors. They helped me to understand, monitor, and, to some degree, modify these behaviors. On the other hand, most of the clinicians did not indicate to me that they understood much about the person who was stuttering. The fear and helplessness that were influencing the choices I made related to my speech were not obvious to them. Because the clinicians knew most about the surface features of stuttering, that was what we focused on. However, the best clinicians I encountered were those who not only knew about the surface features of the problem but also showed an understanding—an insight—about the deep structure and the intrinsic nature of the problem. They knew that at the center of my decision making was the fact that I felt helpless. I had no sense of being able to control my speech. Whether or not my stuttering reached the surface, it was taking place frequently as I constantly altered my choices and constricted my options because of the *possibility* of stuttering. Stuttering, in many instances, never reached the surface, but the choices I was making were examples of profound moments of stuttering even though they were not tabulated as a repetition or prolongation.

To understand the intrinsic nature of stuttering is to appreciate the loss of control that occurs with stuttered speech. Regardless of the surface behavior that occurs during a moment of stuttering, the person experiences a profound loss of control (Cooper, 1968, 1987, 1990; Manning, 1977; Manning & Shrum, 1973; Perkins, 1990). Although nonstutterers have breaks in their fluency, they rarely experience a distinct loss of control while speaking. However, everyone has experienced a loss of control during an athletic or physical activity. There is an instant when you perceive that you are not in control of your body, a fleeting moment when realize you have lost your balance. It is at this moment that you recognize that you are not in charge and cannot determine the consequences of your helplessness. There is, at this moment, a level of anxiety and even fear, and we know we are not in charge.

Such an experience is more likely to occur if you are taking part in activities that require some degree of precision, timing, and balance. Activities such as skiing, skating, paddling a kayak, and wind surfing are good examples. However, it is also possible to encounter similar situations during more common activities such as riding a bike, climbing stairs, walking or running, or even driving a car.

A common example for adults is the feeling you have when sliding out of control in your car through an icy intersection. During these moments one experiences a level of fear and helplessness such as occurs for the stutterer during a moment of stuttering. This loss of control can be both profound and discrete. It has been suggested that it is measurable (Moore and Perkins, 1990), at least by the person doing the stuttering. Whether a clinician can identify such a loss of control in another speaker has yet to be demonstrated empirically. Nevertheless, over the years several authors have suggested that it is possible for experienced clinicians to accurately identify such moments (Bloodstein & Shogan, 1972; Cooper, 1968; Manning & Shrum, 1973). In discussing the difficulty of identifying successful avoidance behavior by stutterers, Starkweather (1987) makes an important point that is perhaps even more pertinent to this discussion. He argues that although we may not have the means to apply rigorously scientific study to what we consider to be the essential features of an event it should not preclude our study of those features. " Our first duty as scientists is to be true to the validity of the phenomenon being observed. If we lack the means to examine it objectively, we cannot assume or pretend that it doesn't exist" (Starkweather, 1987, p. 122).

It sounds rather mysterious—being able to detect moments of helplessness, of loss of control, in another person's speech. How might this be accomplished? One way to become calibrated to the speaker is to note his or her body language. How do speakers stand or sit as they are producing fluent speech? Is the relaxed nature of their fluent speech reflected in their body position, in the location of their hands or their head? In contrast, what are they doing with their body when they are producing overtly stuttered speech? Moreover, what do they do when they are producing not stuttered, but also not quite fluent, speech? The body cues may be subtle and are likely to be unique to the speaker. Some clients may reveal their status by subtle nostril flaring, and others, by a slight alteration in the rate or tempo of speech. Fluent speech sounds smooth and feels smooth to the clinician as it is being imitated. However, if it sounds flat or has the "sticky" quality of a constricted vocal tract, the speaker is apt to be experiencing something less than complete control. The client's speech may be "fluent" in a traditional sense, but it is really just "not stuttered." This occurrence should sound and feel to the clinician as though the client is doing such talking on thin ice. He is not stuttering in the usual sense, but as a clinician who is becoming calibrated to the speaker, you will have the feeling that he is not completely in control of his speech. Moreover, when you ask the speaker, he will usually agree that he is not.

As we spend several sessions with such people, we will begin to understand how they are apt to express themselves during periods of fluent speech. Not only will we begin to anticipate the rate and tempo of their speech, but we will also begin to know what sentence structure and vocabulary they are apt to use. Moreover, when these patterns are not part of their speech, we may guess, often correctly, that they have avoided or substituted a word, or at the very least, that they have scanned ahead and are anticipating difficulty.

TWO BASIC PRINCIPLES OF ASSESSMENT

Although the assessment of fluency can be complex, it is useful to realize that much of what is done during both the assessment and treatment of stuttering can be reduced to two basic principles. Often, during both assessment and treatment, we find ourselves returning to these principles, particularly when we are not completely certain of our next clinical decision. First, and perhaps most important, it is helpful to remember that the more an individual who stutters alters the choices and narrows the options that are available in life, the greater the handicap of stuttering is apt to be. Clinicians, as well as people who stutter, need to appreciate this. Assessment must focus on determining the degree of such altered decision making in all its forms. In turn, treatment must increase the person's ability to make choices based on information other than the fact that sometimes he is apt to stutter. As the members of the National Stuttering Project proclaim in the title of their newsletter, the stutterer must learn to "let go" and live life as it can best be lived rather than basing decisions on the fact that, among other characteristics, he happens to be someone who stutters.

The second basic principle of assessment has to do with struggle behavior. That is, the more a speaker struggles, the greater the handicap. The clinician must determine how and to what degree a person is closing down or obstructing the speech production system in general and the vocal tract in particular. What is it about the source of energy and the vocal tract resonator/filter that is not being used efficiently (see Baken, 1987; Pickett, 1980; Zemlin, 1988)? How is the speaker preventing normal breathing, airflow, voicing, and articulation from occurring? What is he doing to prevent the transition from one sound or syllable to another? What is the speaker doing to keep himself from speaking (or stuttering) easily, openly, and smoothly? Much of what influences the clinician's assessment and treatment decisions can be based on these two principles: open decision making and open vocal tract on the part of the client.

THE ASSESSMENT OF YOUNG CHILDREN

As we discussed in the previous chapter, the developmental nature of stuttering suggests that stuttering emerges gradually, beginning with slight hesitations or Alpha behaviors (Conture, 1990) and slowly becoming more noticeable and complex. For reasons that are not completely clear, for some preschool and early school-age children, struggle, tension, anxiety, and even fear become part of the syndrome. The assessment of fluency in young children involves several important decisions. Using the suggested criteria discussed in the previous chapter, the clinician must first make a judgment about the nature of the child's fluency and whether it is within reasonably normal limits. Since, as we have discussed, there is no absolute standard for differentiating normal from pathological levels or types of fluency breaks, this judgment can be somewhat nebulous. Add to this uncertainty the great natural variability of fluency in a young child and the issue becomes even more complicated. Because children are in the process of maturing neurologically, physiologically, and linguistically, they tend to have greater variability of performance for all behaviors, including speech and language. This is un-questionably the case for speech fluency. The cyclical nature of stuttering in young speakers has been frequently discussed (Bloodstein, 1995; Conture, 1990; Starkweather, 1987; Van Riper, 1982). Such variability suggests at least two things. The good news is that it is generally easier to change behavior that is variable because treatment is much more likely to be successful when the behavior is relatively new (Starkweather, 1992; Starkweather, Gottwald, & Halfond, 1990). The bad news is that this same variability often makes ob-taining a valid sample of fluency difficult.

Assuming that the child's fluency breaks are considered to be abnormal, the next decision is whether the syndrome is likely to continue developing so that greater effort and struggle will become part of the pattern; will this manner of speaking become chronic? Given all this information, the clinician will make a decision about whether to initiate treatment. Finally, the clinician will make a choice about the degree of intervention. As we will discuss in subsequent chapters, intervention can be implemented at many levels. In-tervention can take the form of prevention that seeks to keep the beginning stages of primary stuttering from developing into secondary stuttering, by which time the behaviors are obviously under way. The goal, of course, is to keep stuttering from reaching its tertiary or full-blown state, and to avoid the impact of the associated handicapping effects. Because treatment has been shown to be extremely successful with young children who are still in the ini-tial or primary stages, a wise decision at this point is critical. The longer one waits, the longer it will take to treat the child and the possibility of a success-ful long-term treatment outcome swiftly decreases.

If a preschool child presents with part-word repetitions (especially if they are rapid), prolongations with tension, obvious restriction or even complete blockage of airflow or voicing, the diagnosis and the decision to intervene are manifest. Nonverbal signs of struggle in the form of eye, head, or gen-eral body movement may also indicate the need for intervention. However, if these signs are less evident, the best clinical choice is questionable. A fam-ily history of stuttering and the parents' concerned response to the child's dis-rupted fluency will likely point to intervention as the clear choice. Parental judgment of a child's speech difficulty should be considered a fundamental part of a diagnosis of stuttering (Conture & Caruso, 1987; Onslow, 1992; Riley & Riley, 1983). On the other hand, if there is no family history of stuttering and the parents and other caregivers are unconcerned about the child's speech, it *may* be advisable to monitor the child for approximately three months, as investigations by Yairi, Ambrose, and Niermann (1993) suggest that there is a tendency for children to recover within three months follow-ing onset. Still, the ideal window for intervention will contract, and it may be that intervention, even in the absence of great parental concern, is the best choice.

Conture (1990) proposes that intervention is called for if there is a pattern of within-word fluency breaks on predictable parts of speech. The pattern of disfluency, even though cyclical, should persist over a period of several months and be associated with certain sounds, syllables, words, or speaking situations. The clinician also will want to assess and consider the possible effect of other aspects of the child's speech, language, and oral-motor proficiency, using such measures as the Oral Motor Assessment Scale (OMAS) developed by Riley and Riley (1986). This measure determines the accuracy, smoothness, and rate of a child's articulatory movements and motor sequences. The child's overall capacities may influence the ability to maintain fluency, particularly under forms of communicate or emotional stress.

Information is obtained from many sources during the evaluation of young children. Case history information about the child's general development, family history, speech and language history, academic performance (if the child is of school age), and social and emotional status are all important for assessing the trade-off between the child's capacities and demands for fluent speech. Speech samples will hopefully be obtained during the formal evaluation, assuming the child will cooperate. Additional speech samples from representative situations outside the clinic setting can also be obtained either prior to or following the evaluation in the form of audio- or videotapes. A reasonable goal is to obtain a 300- to 500-word sample produced in a natural setting. Frequency counts of fluency breaks can be in either percent syllables stuttered (%SS) or percent words stuttered (%WS) can be obtained and the type of fluency breaks analyzed. Andrews and Ingham (1971) suggest that %WS can be converted to %SS by multiplying %WS by 1.5.

ELICITING FLUENCY BREAKS

There will be occasions when the very behaviors the clinician wants to observe and evaluate are not present. Although this also may occur during the assessment of adults who stutter, it is more often the case with children. On the day and time of the evaluation, the child may fail to exhibit the behaviors that concern the parents or the teacher. On such occasions the clinician must at least attempt to elicit these behaviors. The clinician assessing the young child must be prepared to introduce various forms of communicative stress during the assessment. She must be uninhibited enough and unafraid of stuttering in order to elicit these fluency breaks. Moreover, she must understand that by eliciting such breaks, she is not going to hurt the child. Furthermore, minimal examples are all that are required. Of course, if it becomes necessary to elicit fluency breaks from children in this fashion, parents or others who may be observing the evaluation should be informed of what is intended so that they will have an understanding of what is taking place.

There are many benign techniques the clinician may use to elicit fluency breaks in children. Essentially, what we are doing is creating a speaking situation where, temporarily at least, the demands we are placing on the child exceed his capacity to use his speech production system (Starkweather & Gottwald, 1990). The clinician may, for example, turn away from the child as he is describing an event or activity to the clinician. Loss of the listener's attention is often a powerful technique for eliciting fluency breaks in children (Johnson, 1962; Van Riper, 1982). The clinician may ask the child to respond quickly to a series of questions or ask him to answer somewhat abstract or difficult-to-answer queries (Guitar & Peters, 1980), such as, "How far is it from here to your home and how do you get there?" "What does your father or mother do at work?" Depending on the age of the child, he could be asked to read from books that are somewhat above his grade level (Blood & Hood, 1978) or asked to describe a series of pictures which are presented at a rapid rate so that he is unable to formulate a complete response. The clinician can also, of course, interrupt the child's response prior to completion, although this is not often necessary. Other listeners may be brought into the room or additional listeners can take the role of distracting or interrupting the child. Typically, only one of these activities is necessary to elicit examples of fluency breaks.

These techniques must be performed with appropriate understanding and sensitivity by the clinician as well as others who may be involved. However, these and other forms of communicative stress will sometimes be necessary to impose if fluency breaks are not otherwise present during the assessment. Of course, it is not necessary to elicit many of these breaks. Once a few examples have been obtained, the clinician can consult with the parents to determine if these breaks are indeed the behavior they have observed and are concerned about. (We cannot assume that the fluency breaks we elicit are of the same form and degree that the parents have seen before.)

In some instances, despite our best attempts, we are unable to obtain samples of the fluency breaks that the child is apparently producing at home. It is usually possible to reschedule another assessment during a time when the child is experiencing more difficulty or we may observe the child in a more natural setting at home or in school. Another possibility is to ask the parents to make an audio- or videotape of the child as he is experiencing fluency breaks. This step may be recommended even before the formal assessment so that some preliminary analysis of the child's speech can be started prior to the initial meeting.

In any case, consultation with the parents, grandparents, teachers, or other concerned persons who were involved in making the referral is a basic part of the initial assessment procedure. We often need to explain the process of speech and language acquisition as well as to differentiate between normal and abnormal fluency breaks. There are several booklets that may be helpful in this regard to parents, teachers, or interested others. These are listed in Appendix C.

INDICATORS OF AWARENESS

Another difference between the assessment of fluency in children and in adults is the child's lack of ability to describe the frustration and anxiety related to fluency failure. Some children are not aware of their fluency breaks. Others are keenly aware of their speech difficulty, but do not know how to express their helplessness, frustration, and anxiety. We cannot assume a lack of these intrinsic features simply because a child is not able to express them. Based on their experience with many young children, Rustin and Cook (1995) point out that some preschool children are very clear about the difficulties they experience. There are ample research findings indicating that young children who stutter develop a negative attitudes toward communicating (deNil & Brutten, 1991), as well as fears and avoidance behaviors (Conture, 1990; Peters & Guitar, 1991; Williams, 1985). Bloodstein (1960) observed that parents reported consistent difficulty on specific sounds or words as early as 2.5 years. For many years clinicians chose not to intervene directly on the speech of the child if he or she did not express a complaint (Cooper, 1979). However, although young children may not verbalize their speech difficulties, their feelings will be reflected in such behaviors as pitch rise, tension, prolongations, schwa substitutions, and cessation of airflow and voicing (Adams, 1977a; Van Riper, 1982; Walle, 1975). When a child demonstrates such behaviors, it can be assumed, to some degree at least, that he is aware of, and searching for ways to deal with, the problem. The child is attempting to overcome the loss of control inherent in stuttering. He may be ready to try nearly anything to avoid that experience. In such a case, regardless of the child's age or ability to verbalize his feelings, the decision to intervene is clearly appropriate.

FLUENCY BREAKS THAT SIGNAL CHRONICITY

Yet another important difference between assessing children and adults is the issue of chronicity. Without treatment, an adult stutterer is not likely to significantly change his level of fluency. For the young stutterer, however, there is a real possibility that the stuttering behaviors will cease. Although the estimated number of these young speakers who obtain fluency without intervention varies widely from approximately 40 percent to 80 percent (Cooper, 1972; Starkweather, 1987; Van Riper, 1982; Young, 1975), it appears that a significant number of children do "recover." It is important to point out that these relatively high rates of spontaneous recovery have come under question in recent years (Martin & Lindamood, 1986; Ramig, 1993a).

Determining which young stutterers will someday spontaneously recover is even more difficult than determining whether a young speaker is, in fact, a stutterer, for in attempting to determine whether a young child's stuttering will become chronic, we are attempting to predict the future. In making the decision about chronicity, we have even less data on which to draw than we have to distinguish between normal and abnormal fluency breaks.

One important consideration is the gender of the child. Andrews et al. (1983) report that from five to ten times more males than females stutter. Certainly this would seem to be the case based on the ratio of males to females who come to treatment centers. Recent data suggests, however, that gender may be more of an indicator of recovery from, rather than occurrence of, stuttering. That is, recent studies of young male and female children (ages 2 to $2\frac{11}{42}$ years old) indicate that the gender ratio is fifty-fifty; young boys and girls are equally as likely to demonstrate abnormal fluency breaks. However, as Starkweather (1987) points out, by the ages of 7 or 8, a clear difference begins to emerge; more boys than girls continue to manifest difficulties with fluency. Recovery, even without formal intervention, appears to be likely during the preschool years.

Some information about the timing of possible spontaneous recovery from stuttering is suggested by the classic longitudinal study of English children living at Newcastle-on-Tyne reported by Andrews and Harris (1964). One thousand children were followed for fifteen years and examined for a variety of health problems including stuttering. Most of the children studied began to stutter by the age of 5. No child began stuttering after the age of 11. Approximately one-third of the children demonstrated nonfluency from ages 2 to 4. Another third began to stutter at an average age of 7.5 years but continued to do so for only two years. The final third of the children began stuttering during the age range of 3 to 6 and children continued to stutter. Following a review of these data, Starkweather observes:

> The children who became chronic stutterers, however, were all stuttering between the ages of five and one-half and six and one-half. In other words, a child who begins stuttering during the preschool period has a reasonable chance, about 50 percent, of recovering soon. The same is true of a child who begins stuttering later, after age seven. But if a child begins stuttering at a young age, and the problem persists into the five and one-half to six and one-half year range, there is a good chance that it will become a chronic disorder. It looks as though there is a critical period, somewhere between age five and age seven, during which the patterns of speech become automated or habituated so firmly that it is difficult later to change. And if stuttering is present during this period of time, it too will be difficult to change later on.°

Cooper (1973) developed a checklist that may be of some help in determining those factors related to chronicity. This checklist is scored on the basis of the number of "yes" responses to questions concerning the historical, attitudinal, and behavioral aspects of stuttering in children. Based on the findings of McLelland and Cooper (1978), two to six "yes" responses are indicative of possible recovery, seven to fifteen "yes" responses indicate the need for continued monitoring of the child, and sixteen to twenty-seven "yes" responses

---

° From C. W. Starkweather, *Fluency and Stuttering.* Copyright © 1987. All rights reserved. Reprinted by permission of Allyn & Bacon.

are predictive of chronicity. Essentially, it appears that the more abnormal the speech in terms of tension and fragmentation (Bloodstein, 1960, 1987; Schwartz, Zebrowski, & Conture, 1990), the less likely the chance that the child will recover from stuttering. In addition the Stuttering Prediction Inventory (SPI) (Riley, 1981) was developed in order to determine the likelihood of chronicity. These may be valuable adjuncts to the diagnostic procedure with young children, but to date, there have been no longitudinal investigations that allow for the accurate prediction of future fluency.

A final comment concerns the issue of spontaneous recovery of young stutterers. Although authors agree that many speakers recover from stuttering, few have questioned whether these same speakers are more likely to begin stuttering again later in their adult years. It is relatively rare to find speakers who begin to stutter as adults. Most often, stuttering is a gradually developing problem beginning in the early years of speech and language development. It may be, however, that some people who begin stuttering later in life are those people who also stuttered as children, spontaneously recovered, and later, apparently in response to one or more stressful events, began to experience breaks in their speech. We have seen a few such adults where a reoccurrence of stuttering seems to be the most likely explanation for a relatively late "onset" of stuttering.

PARENT PARTICIPATION IN ASSESSMENT

In the sections of this book where we discuss the treatment of young children (Chapter 5) and suggestions for counseling (Chapter 7), much will be said about the importance of parent participation in the treatment of young children. Assessment procedures should include some measure of parent interest in actively participating in the treatment of their child. However, there will be occasions when parent involvement during assessment will be nonexistent. The motivation for initiating treatment may be minimal if the family physician or friends and family members suggest that the problem will likely go away by itself (Ramig, 1993c). In contrast to Rustin, who is reluctant to recommend treatment without parent involvement (1987; Rustin & Cook, 1995), Ramig contends that even in cases where parents cannot or will not become involved in treatment, the clinician should enroll the child.

Rustin and Cook (1995) suggest several questions the clinician can use to discover the nature of the family and of parent-child interaction. Though the questions themselves are important, the most important aspect of the interview process is the clinician's style and ability to be flexible and creative as she interacts with the parents. As Caruso (1988) describes, the intent is to follow the parent's lead, all the while probing for areas of interest and concern. As Rustin and Cook indicate:

In the interview, we learn about the rules and regulations in the child's life, the parents' attitudes toward child rearing, pertinent issues within the parental relationship, the problem-solving strategies employed, and the place the disfluency problem holds within the family. The interview is structured in such a way that the basic and noncontentious case details are gathered in the early stages of the process, with a gradual move toward more sensitive and emotional material as it progresses. (1995, p. 129)

Many inventories, scales, and procedures have been developed for evaluating the quality of both the surface as well as the deep structure of the syndrome (see Appendix A). Many of these measures are helpful for obtaining both data-based and criterion-referenced information for assessing fluency disorders. However, the variety of surface behaviors and intrinsic features that come together in stuttering do not always lend themselves to a realistic or valid analysis. Individual stutterers rarely fit the descriptions, situations, and categories present on any single measure. Many of these scales do provide helpful information that will prove useful as we make decisions concerning the initiation of treatment, the selection of a treatment strategy, and the phasing out or termination of formal treatment. However, assessment must go beyond all these procedures. No matter how many formal measures we administer or what we are able to discover during the initial meeting, we must recognize through what a small window we view the speaker and his problem. As much as with any other human communication disorder, the assessment of fluency disorders is an ongoing process. The process of assessment, while most intense during the initial stages of treatment, continues through treatment and into the posttreatment period, when the stutterer is likely to experience relapse (Silverman, 1981). In order to continue making good clinical decisions, the clinician must continue to obtain data concerning all aspects of the syndrome. The data obtained by using any number of assessment protocols are no substitute for the clinician's ongoing observation of the child's daily behavior in naturalistic settings.

MAKING USE OF AN AT-RISK REGISTER

Determining the probability of chronic stuttering is particularly difficult in young speakers. Given the results of the longitudinal research with very young stutterers by Yairi and his associates described in Chapter 2, the decision about whether to intervene can be especially dificult. A possible strategy for improving the decision-making process is the use of an "at-risk" register (Adams, 1977b; Onslow, 1992). These authors suggest that such a strategy will decrease the occurrence of the false positive and false negative errors in the identification of young stuttering children who may or may not be showing the early signs of chronic stuttering. A false positive decision occurs when a normally speaking child is incorrectly identified as a child who stutters. A false negative decision occurs when a child who stutterers is incorrectly identified as a normally speaking child. The goal of any such process, of course, is to make accurate choices—true positive identifications of the disorder. While decreasing the likelihood of either type of the two possible errors is desirable, a false negative identification is a more serious error. That is, a false positive identification could result in a child receiving some less-than-vital assistance in producing fluent speech, something that should be no great cause for concern (Onslow, 1992). On the other hand, a false negative decision is an error of greater consequence, given the evidence that treatment for more advanced stuttering is considerably more time-consuming and prone to failure and relapse (Bloodstein, 1987; Costello, 1983; Onslow, 1992). Thus, as Onslow (1992) recommends, the process leading to negative identification should be conservative, while the process resulting in positive identification should be relatively liberal. It has been suggested that the negative identification of communication disorders may result in the inefficient use of health care services (Andrews, 1984). However, Onslow comments that this view is not held for other communication disorders and questions both the logic and the ethics of withholding treatment from young children who stutter. In addition, he suggests that clients who are seen in the clinical setting may be more severely affected than nonclinical cases and less prone to recovery without intervention. Finally, he points out that because of the overall inefficiency of treating cases of advanced stuttering, accurate early identification may actually improve the overall efficiency of service delivery.

The development of an at-risk register is described by both Adams (1977b) and Onslow (1992) and is depicted in Figure 3–1. This strategy involves three

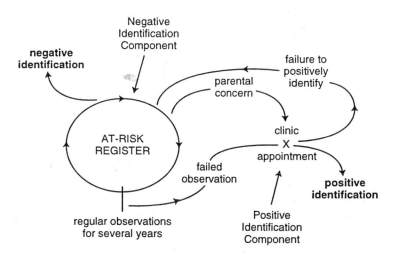

Figure 3-1. Diagram of strategies to identify early stuttering, in which positive identification and negative identification are separate processes. (From Onslow [1992], p. 25. Copyright © American Speech-Language-Hearing Association. Reprinted by permission.)

basic elements: the at-risk register and both negative and positive identification components. When stuttering is suspected, the parents bring the child to a clinic for a formal evaluation. The parents are requested to bring audio- or videotapes of their child's speech made in a natural environment, indicating the fluency characteristics of concern. The identification of a problem is based on the perception of stuttering by the clinician (or clinicians) and the parents. If a parent considers that a child is stuttering but the clinician fails to perceive stuttered speech in the clinic or in the recording, the child is listed in an at-risk register. In an instance where a clinician perceives stuttered speech but a parent does not, positive identification occurs if a second clinician perceives stuttered speech. . . . If the second clinician does not perceive stuttered speech, then the child is placed in an at-risk register (Onslow, 1992, p. 25).

Those children listed in the at-risk register are observed on a regular basis for a period of months or years. Onslow suggests that ongoing evaluations can take a variety of forms, including telephone conversations and face-to-face interviews with parents or questionnaires mailed to the home. Another tactic is to have the parents periodically call the clinic and respond to a series of questions that might indicate forms of speech fragmentation, tension, or struggle. Those children who pass the ongoing evaluations will continue being included on the register until a negative identification is made. How long this process should continue is a primary question, but based on Bloodstein's (1987) literature review, Onslow suggests a possible upper limit of twelve years. A child is moved to the positive identification component if, at any point, a parent becomes concerned and a formal evaluation is again scheduled. A child who is routed to the positive identification component but fails to be positively identified is moved back to the register.

Onslow makes the important point that the use of an at-risk strategy places no pressure on the clinician to make either a positive or a negative identification. If there is uncertainty concerning the diagnosis, the child is listed on the register and, if necessary, will remain there until a decision is made. However, as we suggest on several occasions in this text, if the clinician is in doubt, intervention is likely to be the safest decision in the long run.

CONCLUSIONS

Even for normally speaking young adults, fluency is often highly variable. This is particularly true for adults and, especially, children with fluency disorders. The great variability of a speaker's fluency across time and speaking situations combines with the often subtle differences between normal and abnormal fluency breaks to make the determination of stuttering difficult. Following the suggestions of several authors, it is recommended that normal fluency breaks may be best thought of as primarily a result of formulative or linguistic uncertainty. These breaks usually occur between words or larger linguistic units and are produced with little or no physical or emotional tension. Stuttering or motoric breaks are discussed as primarily a result of lags, mistiming, or a lack of required sequencing in the movements of the human speech-production system. These breaks tend to occur within words and syllables and are often produced with obvious physical tension and emotional anxiety. Diagnostic decisions must take into account, not only the surface behaviors that are observed and recorded but also the intrinsic attitudinal and cognitive features of the underlying problem. Assessment involves discovering what the speaker is doing with his or her speech production system that makes speaking so difficult, but the clinician also must determine how the speaker is making decisions and limiting life choices based on the possibility of stuttering.

The assessment of children is made more intricate due to developmental changes in the child's physical system and the cyclical nature of stuttering for young speakers. Furthermore, the formation of negative attitudes is somewhat more difficult to determine for young speakers. There appears to be a critical period from approximately age five to seven, during which children may recover from stuttering. Parents and significant other caretakers play an important role in the assessment process, providing both historical and developmental information as well as indicating patterns of interpersonal communication. At-risk registers may help the clinician increase the accuracy of identifying young chronically stuttering children and decrease the likelihood of making both false positive and false negative judgments.

RECOMMENDED READINGS

Peters, T., & Guitar, B. (1991). *Stuttering, an integrated approach to its nature and treatment.* Baltimore, MD: Williams and Wilkins. See Ch. 6, "Assessment and Diagnosis," pp. 155–174 (on the assessment of the preschool child).

Onslow, M. (1992). Identification of early stuttering: Issues and suggested strategies. *American Journal of Speech-Language Pathology, 1* (4), 21–27.

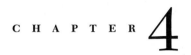

Assessing Fluency Disorders in Adolescents and Adults

PRELIMINARIES TO ASSESSMENT

We now turn to assessing stuttering in its more obvious form. Generally, although not always, both the surface- and deep-structure stuttering are more severe and more obvious in adolescent and adult speakers. On occasion, young children will display well-developed tension (sound prolongations and body movements) and fragmentation (within-word fluency breaks), which are typically associated with advanced or established stuttering (Schwartz & Conture, 1988). Usually, however, older speakers show greater complexity of behavior and demonstrate more obvious fear. Adolescents and adults have coped and adjusted to the problem for years. Thus, the features of their stuttering, especially those having to do with concealing of the problem, are more complex and sophisticated. Adolescent and adult speakers have had time to develop patterns of avoidance that mask the surface features, and therefore, the basic question to be answered during assessment is not whether formulative or motoric fluency breaks are occurring. Instead, the focus now is on the nature of stuttering and the handicapping effects of the problem with *this* particular person.

SEVERITY VERSUS HANDICAP

Sometimes, in an attempt to lessen the impact of stuttering on their lives, adult speakers will shape their speech into a pattern of symptoms that resemble other problems such as motor-speech disorders, voice disorders, language disorders, or even emotional disturbances. That is, he will refuse to speak or will speak in such a way that, although it is obvious that something is wrong, it is not clear that stuttering is the problem. Because of the tension in his voice or the fact that he is speaking in a slow and painstaking manner, it may appear as though he has a voice or word-finding problem. If a speaker is particularly adept at avoiding feared sounds and words, specific people, or speaking situations, he may rarely if ever be perceived as a person who stutters. He may, however, be thought of as someone who is introverted, shy, lazy, or somewhat peculiar. He may be seen as a person who is a bit strange because he uses sentence structures, rates, and intonation patterns that are idiosyncratic or inappropriate. He will not respond in expected ways to simple questions, pretending he did not hear the question or does not know the answer when it is obvious he does. He may avoid saying his own name or introducing friends or relatives when it is appropriate to do so. He will make excuses so that he will not have to participate in work, school, or social activities. He will do the same things normal speakers do when they want to avoid aversive stimuli. As speakers develop such ways of adjusting to stuttering, they are sometimes able to mask the stuttering entirely or at least obscure the severity and the true nature of the problem.

When determining the nature and severity of the stuttering syndrome with older speakers, the clinician is again faced with the natural variability of surface behaviors. Although this variability is not likely to be as great as with children, obvious fluctuations do occur in both the quantity and quality of stuttering in most adults who stutter. It is good to keep in mind that the formal evaluation may yield a relatively narrow view of these behaviors. The experienced clinician knows that she is unlikely to capture all the surface and intrinsic features of the problem in a single diagnostic interview. This variability is to be expected and, in fact, is an important diagnostic feature in distinguishing the normal (developmental) adult stutterer from individuals who present a sudden onset of stuttering following an emotional or physical trauma, as discussed in the final sections of this chapter.

Although it is not possible to obtain all the necessary information in a single attempt, we can obtain a good *sample* of the surface behaviors and can begin to understand the deep structure of the person's response to his fluency problem. The process of assessment will continue for many sessions. In the more difficult speaking situations, the person is likely to exhibit stuttering behaviors not seen previously or display behaviors that, although they may have been noted before, now occur with greater frequency and intensity. As the clinician begins to calibrate herself to the new client (a process that will take several sessions), additional features become apparent.

The severity of stuttering as suggested by the surface features does not necessarily correspond to the degree of handicap. The person's response to the problem—what he tells himself about it—is a critical indicator of handicap (Emerick, 1988). We have seen many people who, by any standard, would be judged as having a severe fluency problem based on the nature of the surface features of their speech production. They have frequent moments of stuttering with obvious tension and struggle behavior. However, it is as though they are not inclined to be handicapped. They make all or mostly all their decisions based on information other than the possibility of stuttering. It is probable that people who respond to their stuttering in this fashion never seek our help in the first place. At the other extreme, we have seen adults who stutter only infrequently, with relatively little tension or obvious struggle. Their stuttering moments are exceedingly brief, hardly noticed by their listeners. Nevertheless, they are devastated by these moments. The fact that they are a person who stutters, even though they do so rarely, is a serious problem. For them, stuttering is a handicap that cuts across all aspects of their life, vocationally, academically, and socially. These two examples are end points of a continuum and, of course, most speakers who stutter fall somewhere between these extremes of response. Simply stated, we need to map both the surface behaviors of stuttering for this speaker as well as the intrinsic nature of the problem.

THE NONREPRESENTATIVE SAMPLE OF CLIENTS

Many people who stutter do not seek formal treatment and instead make it through life by compensating and adjusting to the problem (Manning, Dailey, & Wallace, 1984). These people clearly stutter but, for one reason or another, they do not seek professional help. They may not be aware that treatment is available, or for some, the cost of treatment may be prohibitive. For others, it may be that the thought of treatment is so aversive that they would refuse treatment even if they can pay for it. For most of these people who stutter, however, it may be that they do not seek assistance because the handicap of stuttering is not sufficiently great.

Although there are no data to indicate how many never seek formal help, there is little doubt that a significant proportion of individuals who stutter never have contact with professional treatment centers. Consequently, these people never serve as subjects for the research on which we base our understanding of the problem and form our rationale for many of our clinical decisions. Perhaps it is good to keep in mind that our knowledge about stuttering and the people who stutter is based on a nonrepresentative sample of the total population of stutterers. Furthermore, it is likely that this sample is skewed in favor of people who come to recognize that they need help and are able to obtain assistance.

ASSESSING INTRINSIC FEATURES

In Chapter 3 we discussed the nature of the intrinsic features of stuttering. These features directly relate to the cognitive and affective aspect of the problem. Because of their very nature, these covert features of the person are more difficult to identify and quantify. It takes several sessions before the clinician will become calibrated to this person and recognize such features. Because surface behaviors are more easily observable, there is a tendency to spend the majority of the assessment procedure on these features. However, and this is especially true with adults, the intrinsic features must also be identified and eventually modified if long-term success is to be a reality (Emerick, 1988; Guitar & Bass, 1978).

Identifying Loss of Control

As we become attuned to the client, we can begin to identify the three levels of fluency discussed in Chapter 1: stuttered, unstable, and fluent. These levels of fluency tend to reflect the degree of control by the speaker. By pantomiming—by imitating his speech production with our mouths—we can begin to distinguish when the speaker is at each level of control. We can begin to sense when he is experiencing some lack of control over his fluency and identify those moments when stuttering does not quite reach the surface.

At times, during seemingly fluent portions of speech, the person is, at best, on the edge of control. As discussed earlier, in order to prevent overt stuttering, speakers may substitute and rearrange words. Although the speaker may be producing "nonstuttered" speech, he is not in control and is far from producing the effortless, smooth, and continuous speech that characterizes authentic fluency. An experienced clinician—especially one who is familiar with how the speaker is capable of expressing himself in terms of rate, tempo, and syntax—can detect this loss of control in the midst of unstable speech. The clinician may be able to key into the brief pauses or slightly sticky moments present in the unstable speech. Although there are no clear-cut signs of overt stuttering, there will be subtle signs that the individual is not in control. There is a slight hesitation prior to the onset of a word. The clinician notices a momentary prolongation or stickiness during the initial portion of a word or a word that is close to, but does not quite provide, the meaning the clinician has learned to anticipate. The client's body language may indicate a brief moment of fear during the production of a word that is not as smoothly articulated as the speaker is capable of producing it. Of course, one of the best ways to identify or confirm these unstable events is to ask the speaker to do so.

One of our adult clients indicated a loss of control in her speech by involuntary rapid eyelid fluttering, both during obvious moments of stuttering as well as during her moments of unstable speech. These eye movements assisted the clinician in identifying each instance when, although the client produced the word fluently in a technical sense, there were obvious surface features that suggested instability. She was slightly constricting her vocal tract, minimally slowing her movements, and using somewhat more effort to produce in sequence the sounds of the word. Furthermore, she consistently agreed with the clinician's assessment that a loss of control occurred during each of these events.

It may be that many of the differences that have been noted in the acoustics of stutterers' "nonstuttered" speech reflect this lack of control. Researchers have observed a number of differences in the fluent speech of stutterers of various ages, including brief pauses (Love & Jefress, 1971), centralized formant frequencies (Klich & May, 1982), fundamental frequency variations (Healey, 1982), vocal shimmer (Bamberg, Hanley, & Hillenbrand, 1990; Hall & Yairi, 1992; Newman, Harris, & Hilton, 1989), voice reaction times (Cross, Shadden, & Luper, 1979; Reich, Till, & Goldsmith, 1981), and voice onset, initiation, termination times (Adams & Hayden, 1976; Agnello, 1975; Hillman & Gilbert, 1977; Starkweather, Hirschmann, & Tannenbaum, 1976). These acoustic characteristics may reflect brief moments where control was lost and unstable speech occurred. If investigators, rather than considering only stuttered or nonstuttered speech, were to consider as a third category that of perceptually unstable speech, these acoustic measures may yield even more distinctive results.

In any case, it is important for the clinician to be able to identify these intrinsic aspects of stuttering. Many moments of stuttering do not coincide with the speaker's overt breaks in fluency. This is obviously the case when a word is avoided, and it is also the case during the production of unstable speech. This is important for the clinician to appreciate during treatment, for although she may think she is reinforcing fluent speech, she may, in reality, be rewarding something far less. If we base our decisions to reward the client based only on the surface behavior, we could easily be reinforcing avoidances, word substitutions, and most of all, a profound feeling of helplessness.

Testing the Link between Control and Fluency

There is another important aspect of the relationship between fluency and control. Just as a stuttering speaker may be wildly out of control as he circumvents possible stuttering moments and manages to sound fluent, it is also possible for him to speak in an overtly stuttered manner and be in complete control. In other words, the clinician can show him that it is possible to stutter on purpose in an open, easy fashion and be totally in charge of his speech mechanism. Being able to voluntarily stutter with complete control serves to break the remarkably strong link between the experience of stuttering and that of helplessness. The speaker begins to consider, usually for the first time, that it is possible to stutter and not feel helpless. It is possible to stutter and not to be afraid. It may even be possible to stutter in a different, easier, more fluent manner.

By attempting a bit of such voluntary stuttering during the assessment process, the clinician may determine the degree of fear associated with the moment of stuttering. If the client can follow the clinician into some experimental forms of easy, open stuttering, it suggests the possibility that the client is somewhat desensitized about stuttering and may be reasonably assertive once intervention begins. During the assessment, we need to begin identifying the occurrence of these moments of control loss—even the tiny ones—during nonstuttered speech. We need to identify the way that this speaker indicates a loss of control because we want to determine if these moments decrease as a result of treatment. As clinicians, we need to consider how the frequency of these subtle moments of stuttering during "fluent" speech correspond to the frequency of the more overt aspects of stuttering. Moreover, we need to factor in the presence of these subtle moments of stuttering in the form of unstable speech as we consider decisions to terminate formal treatment. The client should be able to identify the presence of these events after formal treatment is completed, since they may well be the first sign of an eventual relapse.

Assessing the Client's Decision Making

Perhaps the most important of the intrinsic features of stuttering is the nature of the decision making by the person who stutters. As we discussed in Chapter 1, these are the choices a person makes based on the *possibility* of stuttering. Most especially, we want to examine the narrowing of the options that can take place in the attempt to avoid stuttering. Herein lies the basis of the handicap for individuals who stutter; the life choices they make or fail to make, based on the fact that they are people who stutter.

As with the issue of control, it will take several treatment sessions to become calibrated to the client's lifestyle and manner of expressing himself before the clinician can begin to appreciate the client's decision-making paradigm (Hayhow & Levy, 1989). The person who stutters, even after becoming aware of these choices, is not likely to associate some of them with the syndrome of stuttering. It may be that these choices have become a way of thinking about himself: "It's just the way I am." He may explain that he is shy and does not like to talk to strangers: "I don't want to take part in class. I don't like to speak in front of groups. I don't like to use the phone. I'd rather mind my own business and would prefer not to introduce myself to strangers." (Indeed, to some degree that may be the case; not everyone who is free from stuttering is a highly verbal or interactive person.)

It takes time in treatment and a clinician who appreciates the possible extent of these choices before the client will begin to identify his subtle decisions. It takes a clinician who will provide security in the form of insight about the problem before the client will feel free to explore this aspect of the syndrome. Of course, it does little good to ask the client to stop making these choices at this point. The goal early in diagnosis and treatment is to help the client identify and acknowledge that specific choices to hide or avoid the stuttering are being made. As the person comes to appreciate this aspect of the problem, one reasonable response is to begin gradually making *different* choices in selected speaking situations.

Once the speaker begins to see the impact of choices made to avoid the possibility of stuttering, he may begin to make different decisions. It is important to note, however, that as this form of avoidance behavior decreases during treatment, there is also the real possibility that the frequency of fluency breaks will increase. Although the person is making progress as a result of treatment, the problem, as observed by those who do not understand what is occurring, may appear to be increasing in severity. Because the stutterer is now taking part speaking situations that he previously avoided, there are more opportunities for stuttering to reach the surface. The person is making better choices but, for the moment at least, he may be (overtly) stuttering more. In this instance at least an increase in the frequency of stuttering can be appropriately interpreted as a sign of progress in treatment (see Chapter 7).

MAPPING THE SURFACE FEATURES OF STUTTERING

The surface features of adults who stutter are relatively easy to evaluate. At the most basic level, there are three categories of behavior that may be used to determine the severity of overt stuttering—frequency, duration, and tension.

Frequency

The frequency of fluency breaks is often one of the most obvious aspects of the problem. Sometimes, a greater frequency of stuttering indicates a greater severity of the problem; sometimes it does not. Although the frequency of the fluency breaks is an aspect of the problem that is relatively easy to tabulate, it is also the feature that can be the most deceiving. For some speakers, the frequency of fluency breaks may be the least valid way of viewing the problem.

One of the most accurate and efficient ways to tabulate the frequency of stuttering is to determine the percentage of syllables (%SS) or words (%SW) stuttered. It is efficient because, with relatively little practice, it is possible to reliably count the frequency of breaks during both reading and conversational speech; that is done by shadowing the production of syllables by the speaker and indicating those syllables on which stuttering occurs. Stuttered syllables can be indicated with a keyboard or by hand by marking dots and dashes for fluent and stuttered syllables, respectively. It is a reasonably accurate procedure for indicating fluency because it is generally agreed that the timing of speech movements are closely related to syllable-sized (as opposed to word-based) units (Allen, 1975; Starkweather, 1987; Stetson, 1951).

Although it is advisable to tabulate %SS or %SW during both conversational speech and reading activities, it is good to remember that these values tend to be highly variable, depending on the speaking situation and the reading material. For example, speakers who are adept at avoiding or substituting words may have a greater frequency of stuttering when reading because they are unable to avoid or substitute sounds and words. For these speakers, on the other hand, conversational speech provides the opportunity to alter or substitute words, possibly yielding a smaller %SS value than would otherwise be the case.

Although the frequency of fluency breaks is usually positively correlated with other estimates of stuttering severity, it is important to appreciate that the frequency of these breaks also may be negatively related to the actual severity of the problem. That is, *speakers who substitute words, circumlocute portions of sentences, or avoid words and speaking situations may be stuttering severely but simply do not demonstrate their problem in an overt manner.* Thus, although the overt frequency of stuttering (what appears on the surface) may be low, the actual handicap may be quite severe. In fact, a speaker may not be producing any obvious fluency breaks. However, he may be continually making choices to alter the words and the manner by which he is communicating. Those choices, although they may not indicate that the person is stuttering, many times communicate (or miscommunicate) other aspects about the person. As one adult client said: "They never knew that I was stuttering. They just thought that I was weird."

Cooper (1985) has referred to the hazards of viewing stuttering primarily in terms of the number of fluency breaks as the "frequency fallacy." Persons who stutter and who choose not to raise their hand in the classroom in spite of knowing the answer, not to ask for directions or assistance, not to order a particular item in a restaurant, not to use their spouse's name during introductions, not to place or answer a telephone call (especially in a crowded room), or not to use a paging or intercom system at the office are still stuttering unnoticed. Unlike the tree falling in the forest, there is no sound. But such choices are examples of serious moments of stuttering. These stuttering moments are insidious because they have a subtle, but powerful, influence on the person's quality of life.

Duration and Tension

The duration and tension of observable stuttering contribute much to the sense of severity. The speaker may exhibit relatively few moments of stuttering. However, if these moments last for several seconds or are associated with considerable muscular tension as well as other nonverbal behavior (Conture, 1990), they severely detract from the person's ability to communicate. Often, the tension and duration associated with a fluency break are closely related in the sense that greater tension tends to result in longer moments of stuttering. As tension increases, and particularly if it is focused at a particular point in the vocal tract (lips, tongue, velum), a tremor is likely to occur. Tremors can be profound and unnatural occurrences involving the rapid oscillatory movement of an articulator. The rate of oscillation is often faster than one could produce voluntarily. The effect is dramatic, and these occurrences contribute much to the cosmetic abnormality of the problem.

Another possible result of greater tension is a stuttering "block." If the tension is great enough and the moment of stuttering lasts sufficiently long, the vocal tract may become occluded and airflow will cease. Although closure often takes place at the level of the vocal folds (the source of the periodic modulation of air in the vocal tract), obstruction at any supraglottal point will result in partial or complete cessation of airflow and, thus, voicing.

A good way to clearly think about what is taking place during a moment of stuttering is to consider what is physically occurring in the vocal tract in terms of the source-filter approach to speech production (Fant, 1960; Kent & Read, 1992; Pickett, 1980). That is, the clinician can ask herself: "What is the speaker doing to disrupt the source of energy, the air supply from the lungs? How is the speaker preventing the modulation of this source of energy at the level of the vocal folds? How is he constricting or occluding his vocal tract so as to adversely affect the resonant characteristics of this system?" An understanding of the anatomy and physiology, as well as the acoustics, of the speech production system will enable the clinician to apply her knowledge in the assessment of what the stuttering speaker is doing to make the process of sequencing from one speech segment to another so difficult.

As the treatment progresses, it will become important for the client as well to take this perspective about his speech production system. We cannot assume that the structure and function of the speech production system are even vaguely understood by the client. Thus, it will be useful for him to acquire some basic anatomical and physiological understanding. By doing so, speech production becomes less mysterious and the client begins to understand that he has the ability to make some of his own decisions as he uses this system. He is not as helpless as he may feel in the midst of a moment of stuttering. In addition, by understanding the nature of this system, he is able to develop a heightened sense of proprioceptive feedback concerning the respiratory, phonatory, and articulatory integration necessary for fluent speech production. As he begins to develop an understanding and, literally, a feel for what he is doing (or not doing) with his system, he can begin making decisions that will make the process of speaking (or stuttering) easier and smoother.

Measurement of tension has been accomplished using a variety of techniques including galvanic skin response (GSR), electroencephalography

(EEG), and, most typically, electromyography (EMG) (Van Riper, 1982). Most clinicians are not likely to have access to such equipment. Fortunately, however, it is not usually necessary to have a high level of precision when measuring tension in the clinical setting. The experienced clinician is able to identify the sites and rate the degree of tension with reasonably good consistency. Because tension and duration are often closely related, easily made measures of duration can yield an indication of the tension that is occurring. Formal measures of duration, such as spectrographic or waveform analysis, while helpful, are not usually necessary. The degree of tension and the duration of the fluency breaks may also be reflected in the rate of speech in words or syllables per minute, with lower rates indicating greater severity.

When determining the severity of stuttering, it is important to understand that no single measure will provide the broad-based assessment necessary to capture the nature of this complex syndrome. The tabulation of the most prominent behaviors, as well as frequency, tension, and duration, is a beginning. The degree of abnormality shown by the person as he struggles is indicated by both verbal and physical movements prior to, and during, a fluency break. These behaviors, and especially those at the extreme of the person's inventory of overt behaviors, may only be apparent during the most difficult speaking situations. The clinician may rarely see these behaviors in the clinical setting. Any behavior that, at one time or another, helped the person to escape from a stuttering moment, including extreme or even bizarre movements of arms, hands, legs, torso, may be incorporated into the struggle. Nothing can be ruled out, and virtually nothing should be a surprise to the experienced clinician. Certainly, for those speakers whose speech is characterized by such behaviors, the presence of these behaviors must be included in the overall determination of severity.

Fragmentation

One other way to think of the prominent features of stuttering behavior is the degree to which a word is fragmented. As discussed in Chapter 1, fragmentation of the word—a within-word fluency break—is a fundamental feature of nonfluent speech. There is no question that, on occasion, fluent speakers fragment words, especially when they are under communicative or emotional stress. People who stutter tend to do it more often and sooner in response to stress.

Bloodstein describes stuttering in its most basic form as "speech transformed by tension and fragmentation." He even goes so far as to suggest that "without tension there can be no stuttering" (1993, p. 137). Certainly, tension is an obvious feature of stuttering and contributes greatly to the perception of severity.

As Bloodstein (1993) points out, the fragmentation of movement tends to occur prior to, or early in the performance of, a difficult motor task. It is a natural aspect of what takes place when stutterers attempt the difficult (for them) task of saying a word. Nearly all stuttering occurs during the initiation of a word or a syntactic unit of a sentence or phrase. Speakers who stutter appear to be doing, to a more extreme degree, what nonstuttering speakers do. Why stutterers respond to the formidable task of language acquisition and production by fluency failure characterized by tension and fragmentation remains *the* most intriguing question of the discipline.

Subtle Surface Features

We have discussed the intrinsic features of stuttering in Chapter 3 and in the earlier sections of this chapter. What we will discuss now are those features of stuttering that, although on the surface, can be extremely subtle. They are subtle enough that it takes an experienced clinician some time to detect them. We might think of these as surface features that are closely connected to the intrinsic decision-making process.

Avoidance. To the degree that a person who stutters successfully performs avoidance behaviors, he can give the appearance of a mild, even nonexistent, fluency disorder. To the degree that he is unable to use avoidance behaviors successfully, the speaker will provide the portrait of a severe stutterer.

It takes energy to successfully avoid the feared stimuli of past fluency failure. There are people, words, sounds, and environments that elicit the anticipation of stuttering. It takes effort to scan ahead for these stimuli, and it takes even more effort to elude them as they come along. Some clients come to us feeling tired of the ordeal. These people often show relief when we suggest to them that they "give themselves permission to stutter."

Speakers who are especially adept at avoidance behavior have been called covert (Starkweather, 1987) or internalized stutterers (Douglass & Quarrington, 1952). It has been suggested that there are relatively few of such stutterers. However, we have seen many clients who are so adept at avoidance techniques that few people with whom they come in contact suspect they are speaking with a stutterer. They are able to hide the overt nature of their problem, so they do so. It can hardly be stated too strongly that avoidance is a poor strategy for stutterers who have a high frequency of motoric fluency breaks. Because changing to another word often results in stuttering on the new word, there is no advantage to the strategy. In some instances, stutterers will even find themselves stuttering on a postponement such as "ah" or "um."

Substitution. Substitutions are a most obvious form of avoidance. Another word is substituted for the feared sound or word, and the meaning of the sentence changes. Sometimes it changes only a little (dog/poodle, white/vanilla). Sometimes it changes a lot (tea/coffee, X-ray/radiology, no/yes). At the very least, substitution results in the utterance of a less precise or appropriate word for the context of the sentence or the situation (e.g., saying "hi" versus "hello" when answering an office telephone or not giving your full name or the complete name of the company when answering the phone at an office).

Based on our experience, it appears to be a good prognostic sign of whether substituting words in this manner is frustrating to the speaker—if he recognizes the lack of choice, the lack of precision the substituted word provides, and the degree of helplessness that is occurring. Again, on the surface, nothing abnormal has occurred—but of course, a moment of stuttering has taken place.

The following example illustrates the impact of this form of decision making on the part of the person who stutters. Several years ago we worked with a college student whom we will call Richard. Although he was a starting running back for a nationally ranked football team, he attended the university on an academic scholarship. During a group treatment meeting, he described a speaking event that took place when he was in junior high school. Rich had taken a quiz in class, which was then graded by a student in the adjoining aisle. His paper was returned, and he saw that his score was a 95. The teacher went up and down the rows of desks, asking each student in turn to report his or her grade. When it was his turn, Richard stood and tried to say, "ninety-five." After enduring a speech block for several moments, Richard decided he would be less likely to stutter if he said "eighty-five." And then he became stuck on that number. He quickly chose to say "Seventy-five!" The teacher recorded the grade, and Rich sat down. No one in the room suspected he had stuttered, but of course, a profound moment of stuttering had indeed occurred under the surface.

Postponement. As the person who stutters approaches a feared word or sound, there is often a moment of hesitation. It is much like hesitating prior to making a difficult leap over an obstacle. Sometimes the hesitation is subtle, taking the form of a slight pause. The speaker may be considering alternative words or thinking of different ways to structure the sentence in order to avoid using the feared word. Other times, particularly before uttering words that have resulted in severe stuttering in previous speaking situations, the speaker will use a series of sounds or words to postpone the attempts to initiate the word. Postponements are most likely to occur with words that cannot be easily avoided, such as names, addresses, school or place of employment. These events may take the form of formulative fluency breaks, for example, whole word or phrase repetitions or insertions of such words and phrases as, "ah," and "you know," into the flow of speech. While these sounds and words are, in fact, formulative breaks, their presence is a result of an upcoming or anticipated motoric break. Many times, these sounds or words are produced rapidly, providing an indication that they are a postponement rather than a formulative fluency break. In anticipation of possible stuttering, the speaker is pushing back the initiation of the feared word.

If the speaker makes frequent use of these postponements, especially if they include some tension, it makes listening to the speaker extremely difficult, even unpleasant. These extra sounds and words, while maintaining a continuous flow of sound, fragment the flow of information. They are justifiably called *junk words*, for they litter the speech of people who stutter to the point that listeners, if given the option, will flee. Often, as a result of treatment, clients are able to decrease the use of such postponements and starters. Even though the speaker may show no change at all in the frequency of stuttering, the perceptual effect is one of enormous improvement. There are fewer postponements, information flow is improved, and the speech is much easier to listen to.

The Client's Self-assessment

The perceptions of the speaker who stutters are likely to be the most important aspect of any assessment of severity or handicap, particularly for the adult. One of the simplest, yet most helpful, techniques for obtaining an initial perspective of the client is to have him respond to a series of questions designed to survey the range of the stuttering behaviors. These questions provide an opportunity to sample behavior and lead to a brief period of trial therapy, an important aspect of the assessment process.

In preparation for asking these questions we can draw a simple scale with equal-appearing intervals (like the one at the top in Figure 4-1), with 0 off the scale at left representing "no stuttering," 1 representing "Mild" and so on to 8 at the right representing "Severe stuttering." We place the scale in front of the person and ask him to indicate the point on the scale that best represents his overall, or average, stuttering (indicated by AVERAGE and its arrow, as an example of a mark a speaker might make on such a scale). Just this act of giving the client the pen and placing the scale in front of him is the first step in assigning him responsibility for his speech. It may well be the first time he has directly addressed his stuttering, particularly in an objective manner.

Once the client marks the point on the scale that indicates his average level of severity, we next ask him to indicate the point on the scale that best rep-

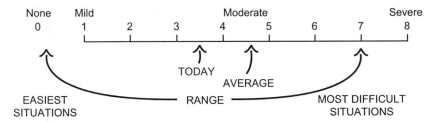

Figure 4-1.   Scale with equal intervals for determining the current, average, and range of stuttering behavior during the assessment of adolescents and adults.

resents the sample of speech that we are hearing at the moment. Although these points may, of course, be identical, often they are not. By asking these two questions, the clinician is able to demonstrate to the client that she understands the highly variable nature of stuttering.

We then ask the client to indicate the range of stuttering behavior. How far up and down the scale does his stuttering range? What point on the scale indicates the quality of his speech is in the best of speaking situations? For many speakers, this point represents no stuttering at all. We then ask him to indicate the point on the other end of the scale that represents his speech in the most difficult or feared speaking situations.

Once he has identified a range of behavior, we can make some observations about his speech and begin a short period of trial therapy. We can determine, for example, whether our view of the surface features of his stuttering coincides with his perception of severity. If it does not, and if the client perceives his stuttering to be very different than does the clinician, it may indicate that some time should be spent during treatment to explain the nature of stuttering and put the client's stuttering into a broader perspective. Most people who stutter, unless they have attended group therapy, have not had the opportunity to observe a wide range of stuttering behavior. Therefore, it is not surprising that their view of the problem is more constricted than that of the clinician.

Assuming that the client has indicated a range of severity on the scale, we are able to inform him that, in many ways at least, his stuttering is typical and reasonably normal behavior for someone who stutterers. That is, because of the variability and the nature of his stuttering, he is not likely to be stuttering because of some deep-seated psychological problem. Of course, before issuing such a statement, the person's case history should be reviewed and his overall response to the evaluators should be considered. By explaining this to the client, we provide an important service to someone who, in many instances, may have regarded himself as being far from normal. Moreover, depending on what he has read or been told about stuttering as a psychological problem, he may have had some doubts about his psychological well-being.

Next, using this information, we conduct some trial therapy. We ask the person to stutter along with us. This is very likely the first time he has been asked to do this fearful behavior on purpose. The very act of asking the client to willingly stutter demonstrates an unafraid, assertive, investigative attitude on the part of the clinician. Such a willingness to lead the way is highly motivating to many clients. In any case, it provides the first opportunity to explore and vary a behavior that for too long has seemed uncontrollable.

If the client has been stuttering during the evaluation, we already have an example of his stuttering at the moment. However, what is his speech like during a less stressful period? Is he able to demonstrate several examples of mild stuttering? Many clients will initially respond to the task, "Show me an example of mild stuttering," with a description of what happens to his speech.

Instead, we want an *example* of the stuttering. Can he willingly achieve this level of stuttering? Finally, can the person demonstrate, perhaps on his own or following our lead, the more moderate or, possibly, severe examples of his stuttering? Is he able to replicate his stuttering to the point that voluntary stuttering changes to real, "out-of-control" stuttering?

The degree to which the person can follow the clinician into stuttering speech tells us much about the client's levels of anxiety and motivation. These activities provide a preliminary indication of how much effort will be required for him to approach, experiment with, and manipulate his stuttering. We can assess the degree to which the speaker can step away from the moment of stuttering and describe some of his behaviors. The accuracy with which he is able to describe, or better yet, pantomime, moments of stuttering indicates his levels of anxiety and inhibition. Can he correctly identify occurrences and types of stuttering? Can he discriminate between the physical and emotional characteristics of real versus voluntary stuttering? Is he willing to venture with us across the threshold of control to see how he can survive during a *deliberate* moment of real stuttering? If the person is unable to follow us in our attempts to experiment and vary the stuttering in this fashion, the process of treatment is likely to be more arduous. These relatively simple activities provide valuable information about the nature of stuttering as well as the person who stutters.

Determining the Client's Desire for Change

Virtually all clinical authorities agree that the motivation of the person who stutters is a critical aspect of a successful treatment outcome (Van Riper, 1973). Motivation can also be regarded as a covert aspect of stuttering for, as with the loss of control, motivation can be difficult to identify and quantify. The person's commitment to change and growth should be assessed prior to, as well as throughout, the process of treatment. Depending on past successes and the client's response to new and difficult challenges, motivation will vary greatly between and within clients and in individual clients at various times.

One thing that does not accurately, or at least completely, reflect a person's level of motivation are the statements made during the assessment or treatment sessions. Many clients make sincere and honest statements of commitment. They say things that lead us to believe they are highly motivated. These are similar to the announcements we make when deciding to do things like diet or train for an event such as a marathon. While it is pleasant to hear these declarations of commitment during the assessment interview, if we place too much importance on such statements, we will be deceived. Our advice is to beware of the person who sounds overly committed. It is one thing to talk about making an arduous journey and quite another to take each difficult step along the way.

It is both natural and necessary to be motivated at the outset of treatment. The fact that the person has come to a treatment center for evaluation is an important step in acknowledging the problem. Moreover, there is some indication that even taking that first step results in desirable changes in both the surface and deep structure of the problem.

In determining a person's level of motivation, we first need to appreciate that entering into any new challenge can often be a frightening experience. This is true whether we are starting at a new school, beginning a new job, or challenging ourselves in nearly any other sense. There is a real element of risk as well as of partial or complete failure. In order to consider such challenges, we must reach some level of self-esteem and security. What we may be looking for in potential new clients is a person with a quality of "mental toughness" and a high degree of "psychic energy" (Cooper, 1977), who is willing to fail a bit during the process of change. Often, of course, this is not the case. It is typical for someone to have doubts and anxiety when initiating treatment for stuttering. As clinicians, we need to acknowledge this possibility to the client. This is not to suggest that we only enroll highly motivated people in treatment, but the client's true level of motivation does provide an indication of the progress we can expect once treatment is initiated.

It is easy to be motivated before the trek begins, but it often becomes more difficult once you begin climbing. As clinicians, we should take some time during the initial meeting with the client to provide a clear picture of the journey. The client may be overly enthusiastic, in part because he does not understand the nature of the treatment process. He does not understand that you are not going to cure him and that he is the one who must run the laps and do most of the sweating. Once he begins to appreciate how difficult it is to change his behavior and the way he views his problem, the initial high level of motivation may fade. We do not want to deplete the high level of motivation that is likely to be present at the outset of treatment, for the client will need to draw upon this reserve. We do, however, want to provide the potential client with a realistic view of the journey.

One practical suggestion for determining a person's level of motivation is to describe examples of the more difficult tasks he will be asked to complete during treatment. These can be explained in some detail or demonstrated during a short period of trial therapy. In addition, there are questions that may be asked to tap a potential client's level of motivation, which will force a realistic consideration of the current priorities in his life. For example, we can ask the person how much treatment is worth to him; how much would he be willing to pay for treatment? Is it worth $5, $25, or $50 per hour? Aside from the fees associated with this treatment center, how valuable, in real money, is this service for him at this time? How far would he be willing to drive to receive treatment: five, fifty, one hundred miles each way? There is a threshold that people will not exceed for treatment. That threshold, in dollars or miles, indicates the person's level of motivation. Such questions at first appear to be contrived, possibly even unethical. However, we have found that these thresholds of money or distance often provide an indication of the eventual level of motivation that clients demonstrate once in treatment.

One reason why persons who stutter often experience rapid change during an intensive, residential treatment program is the motivation necessary in order to attend. Not only may the cost of such programs represent a reasonably large financial commitment, the person also must often make significant social, educational, or vocational adjustments in order to attend such programs. If someone is serious enough to take his vacation time, spend a portion of his savings, and move some or all of his family to the location of an intensive treatment for several weeks, it is a good indication that he is highly motivated.

Another important consideration when assessing motivation is the time in the life cycle of the person who stutters. As with many aspects of life, the timing is crucial. As anyone knows who has attempted to convince a junior high school student who stutters to enroll in treatment, some people just do not want help—or at least they do not necessarily want it when we want to give it to them. The timing of when their lives cross ours can be decisive. Successful treatment is not simply a result of doing more or different things, but of doing the right things at the right time (DiClemente, 1993). The moments when people come to us for help can provide insight into their motivation and readiness for change. Where they are in the process of changing is critical for successful intervention. Recent research in the process of self- and assisted change suggests that a person's location on a continuum from self-reevaluation/contemplation of change to action/maintenance of change is a powerful factor in predicting a successful treatment outcome (DiClemente, 1993; Prochaska, DiClemente, & Norcross, 1992). It is a good idea to ask questions such as: "Why are you here today and not six months ago? Or why not a year from today? What is it that prompted you to ask for help at this time?"

The answers to such questions are important in the overall determination of motivation and especially readiness for change. Sometimes people refer themselves for treatment when they finally realize that their speech is preventing them from career advancement. Frequently they come for help when they are facing a major speaking event such as a presentation or a ceremony in which they must take part. In some instances adults come to us at times when they experience landmarks during their life cycle. That is, after people complete a period of their life, such as schooling, a job, a career, or a marriage, they tend to stand back and consider the current options (Sheehy, 1974). They now have an opportunity to do something about a problem that has been put into the background for much of their lives. Even without the occurrence of a landmark event, such reassessments are likely to occur in middle age. As Newgarten indicates, middle age is characterized by "self awareness," "heightened introspection," and "restructuring of experience" (cited in Kimmel, 1974, p. 58) Moreover, as Sheehy (1974) suggests, mid-life is often characterized by a reexamination whereby a person questions many views of the self and others. At this time, he or she is more likely to readjust old responses to lifelong problems (Sheehy, 1974; Vailant, 1977). Adopting new approaches to old problems is possible at any time during the life cycle, of course, but it seems to be most frequent during the decades of the forties and fifties. It could be that if individuals in that age range are interested in treatment, significant progress can result. It would seem that, even if there was no significant change in the vocational or social aspects of their lives, there is the potential for a significant improvement in the quality of life.

On the other hand, there is little information available about older individuals who stutter (Manning & Shirkey, 1981). Manning and Monte (1981) suggest that few stutterers beyond the age of fifty desire treatment. Manning, Daley, and Wallace (1984) found preliminary evidence indicating that, in most instances, these stutterers have learned to adjust to their problem and, although the problem does not appear to diminish in severity, it represents less of a handicap for older speakers. The authors obtained the attitude and personality characteristics of twenty-nine stutterers ranging in age from fifty-two to eighty-two. Although these speakers scored approximately the same as young adult stutterers on scales assessing approach and performance speaking behaviors, the large majority of the older stutterers perceived their stuttering as less handicapping now than when they were young adults. While a few subjects indicated the desire for treatment, most responded by indicating that stuttering had become less of a problem with increased age. In view of the volumes written on the topic of stuttering, the lack of knowledge concerning the nature of stuttering in older speakers is unfortunate. It would seem that, in order to completely understand the nature of this communication problem, it is necessary to appreciate the development of the disorder throughout the life cycle.

Assessing Atypical Fluency Problems

Each individual who comes to the assessment process presents a unique combination of surface features, attitudes, and motivation. The nature and needs of each client change as a function of the treatment process. However, while all clients are unique in themselves, it is useful to consider some broader categories of people with fluency problems.

The large majority of adolescents and adults seen for the assessment of fluency problems are people who have a history of developmental stuttering. They are perhaps best described by Van Riper (1971, 1982) as Track I stutterers, with essentially normal histories of speech and language development in all respects except for their fluency: for whatever reasons, they happen to stutter. Van Riper and others have described another related category of people with fluency problems defined as Track II. These individuals not only have something less than normal fluency, they also have difficulty in one or more areas of speech and language ability. Thus, they display a variety of other concomitant problems. Blood and Seider (1981) noted that 68 percent of 1,060 stutterers being treated in elementary schools had other speech, language, hearing, or learning problems. Articulation disorders were the most frequently reported concomitant problem. Just how these other communication problems relate to the onset or maintenance of fluency disorders is unclear.

Although the large majority of people who stutter show one of the above-mentioned developmental patterns, there are other speakers who comprise a relatively small but important group of people with somewhat atypical fluency disorders (St. Louis, 1986).

Neurogenic Stuttering. The fluency problems of this group of people have been referred to as *organic stuttering* (Van Riper, 1982), *cortical stuttering* (Rosenbek, Messers, Collins, & Wertz, 1978), and *neurogenic stuttering* (Helm, Butler, & Canter, 1980; Silverman, 1992). Other terms such as *neurogenic acquired stuttering, acquired stuttering, neurological stuttering,* and *stuttering of sudden onset* have also appeared in the literature. In such cases, the fluency breaks appear to result from damage to the central nervous system. The onset may be sudden, following head trauma, strokes, cryosurgery, drug usage, or anoxia, or the symptoms may develop slowly, as in degenerative disorders, vascular disease, dementia, viral meningitis, or dialysis dementia (Helm, Butler, & Canter, 1980; Helm-Estabrooks, 1986). One or both hemispheres may be involved, although the left hemisphere appears to be the more likely to be implicated (Rosenbek, Messert, Collins, & Wertz, 1978). Although there may be a variety of other language and speech disorders associated with these speakers (e.g., dysarthria, apraxia, and aphasia), Rosenbek et al. suggest that this form of stuttering need not accompany other speech or language problems.

The fluency breaks of these speakers are different in both number and type. Although these speakers stutter on an unusually high percentage of their syllables, they indicate relatively few secondary escape behaviors. Unlike developmental stutterers, fluency breaks occur, not only on initial sounds and syllables, but also in medial and final positions of words, for example "gre-e-en" and "sto-o-ore." In comparison to developmental stutterers who are more likely to have fluency breaks on content words, neurogenic stutterers are equally likely to stutter on function and content words. They do not show improved fluency with successive readings of a passage (often referred to as the *adaptation effect*). While these speakers may be annoyed about their speech fluency, they are not as likely to show anxiety or fear as the more typical stutterer. That is, in comparison to more typical stutterers, they share some of the same surface features, but few of the intrinsic features. Another unique characteristic of these speakers is the lack of fluency likely to result from fluency-enhancing conditions that tend to immediately eliminate stuttering, such as choral speaking, rhythmic speech, singing, prolonged speech, whispering, and silent speech (Andrews et al., 1983). For example, Perkins (1973) noted that of over one hundred stutterers, the only person who did not show a reduction in stuttering under such conditions was a woman who was later diagnosed as suffering from a neurological disorder.

Certainly this subcategory of individuals with fluency problems does not represent a homogeneous group, for there are wide varieties of speech characteristics, etiologies, and psychological and physiological influences, as well as speech-language disorders associated with the stuttering. Partly because these patients are likely to have so many problems and partly because they are not typically referred to the speech-language pathologist, it appears that these speakers are more common than would be apparent by most of the literature (Helm, Butler, & Canter, 1980; Rosenbek, Messert, Collins, & Wertz, 1978).

Psychogenic Stuttering. Another subcategory of stutterer who is also relatively uncommon is the psychogenic stutterer. There are, as Van Riper (1979) suggested, only a handful of emotionally ill people who come to us with the complaint of stuttering. To be sure, many of the people we will see are deeply troubled by what they correctly perceive as an extremely frustrating and threatening problem. Many of the behaviors displayed by individuals who stutter are neurotic and compulsive. The devices that enable avoidance and escape from the stuttering moment are far from normal. However, as Van Riper (1982) suggests, these behaviors are most appropriately interpreted as resulting from the fact that the person happens, for whatever reasons, to stutter. The behaviors are not likely to be the symptoms of some deep-seated conflict.

There is convincing evidence indicating the clinical value of attending to self-concept and self-esteem, interpersonal interaction, and role changes if we are to assist people in becoming less handicapped by stuttering, especially if long-term success is our goal (Guitar & Bass, 1978). Nevertheless, the large majority of people we assess for stuttering are fairly normal and do not differ psychologically from a matched group of nonstuttering speakers (Goodstein, 1958; Sheehan, 1958).

There are, however, some people with more severe emotional problems in any randomly selected group of people. An understanding of the characteristics of psychogenic stuttering allows a reasonably clear-cut identification. In many cases, the psychogenic stutterer has a history of emotional problems and may be currently receiving professional help for his problem.

As with the organic stutterer, the onset of stuttering behavior is typically sudden, with no previous history of fluency problems. In addition, the onset of fluency breaks may occur following an emotionally traumatic experience. When stuttering behaviors are first noticed, they tend to be well developed and do not show the typical gradual increase in complexity and severity seen in children who stutter into adulthood. In addition, one of the more striking aspects of the stuttering is its stereotypical nature. That is, the fluency breaks tend to remain reasonably consistent in frequency, tension, and type, regardless of the speaking situation. In contrast to the person whose stuttering is developmental in nature and whose overt stuttering behaviors tend to be highly variable, there tends to be little change for these speakers. There are few, if any, occasions where stuttering is absent, even during such fluency-producing situations as unison speech, singing, speaking alone, or speaking with a unique rhythm, intensity, or dialect. Fluency, or at least nonstuttered speech, is easy to elicit from even the most severe Track I or II stutterer. However, psychogenic stutterers tend to "hold onto" their stuttering in the sense that both the frequency and the form show little change, regardless of the speaking situation or speaking task. For example, like neurogenic stutterers, these clients typically show no adaptation effect with successive readings of the same material. It is almost as though they have chosen a particular "brand" of stuttering and for a time at least that is the way they are going to speak.

There is some agreement that the grouping termed psychogenic stuttering can be further subdivided into two categories. The first category, similar to Van Riper's (1982) Track III stutterer, is a person with a relatively mild emotional problem, which tends to be brought about by an emotionally traumatic experience. The stuttering behavior comes about suddenly, with no previous history of fluency problems. Stuttering, in this case, may be characterized as the symptom of a specific emotional event and often manifests itself as a conversion neurosis. The other category, similar to Van Riper's (1982) Track IV stutterer, represents the impact of a more profound emotional problem. There is no single, obvious emotional trauma but rather a history of emotional problems. Again, the stuttering behavior appears to be a symptom of a more deep-seated emotional disorder. An example of each type of psychogenic stutterer may help to clarify the nature of stuttering in these cases.

Several years ago we had the opportunity to interview a woman in her early thirties who complained of stuttering. Approximately three weeks prior to our assessment, she had been raped. One week following the attack, she lost her ability to speak, and when she began speaking again three days later, she was stuttering. She reported no personal or family history of stuttering. At the time of the assessment interview, she was stuttering on nearly every word. The frequency of her fluency breaks was uniform throughout the interview and consisted almost entirely of tense prolongations of whole words. We were unable to elicit any periods of fluent speech through using a variety of fluency-enhancing activities.

The experience of a sudden onset of stuttering following a traumatic incident is probably the most obvious aspect of this form of psychogenic stuttering. The person appears concerned about his speech, and he may show much tension and struggle behavior. His response to the traumatic experience takes the form of a conversion neurosis. There is a good possibility that over time, or possibly with the help of psychological counseling, normal speech will return.

We also had the opportunity to interview a forty-one-year-old man who complained of a sudden onset of stuttering. This man's fluency and behavioral history coincided with Van Riper's Track IV (psychogenic) stuttering. As was the case with the woman, this man also had no previous history of fluency disorders. However, there appeared to be no single traumatic event preceding the onset of his disrupted fluency. This man had, however, been receiving ongoing inpatient treatment at a local Veterans Administration hospital for a variety of emotional disorders.

As with the woman described here, we were unable to get this client to produce fluent speech using a variety of fluency-enhancing activities. Instead, the frequency of his stuttering was consistent throughout the assessment interview. His fluency breaks consisted of one- and two-unit repetitions produced at the same rate as the rest of his speech, rather than at a relatively more rapid pace. Although he explained that he was very concerned about his fluency problem, he showed no struggle or tension related to the fluency breaks, nor did he report any avoidances or fear associated with this problem. Perhaps the most interesting aspect of his stuttering was the way he watched listeners as he stuttered. He constantly maintained eye contact, and while we cannot say for sure that he "enjoyed" watching his listeners for their reactions, he certainly did not appear embarrassed or upset by his fluency breaks. He seemed to remain detached from his stuttering. As with the woman, it was apparent that stuttering was not his most important problem. However, while the woman's speech seemed to be reflecting a somewhat temporary emotional reaction to a specific trauma, this man's speech appeared to be one of many symptoms related to a more general and longer-term emotional problem.

As we have indicated, this type of person who stutters (Track III and IV) is rare within the population of people who stutter. If, however, we suspect that stuttering is not the most important or basic problem, but rather a reflection of an emotional disorder, we will refer the person to an appropriate professional.

Cluttering. A final type of fluency disorder that we will discuss is *cluttering*. The term itself distinguishes such speakers from the groups of stutterers we have discussed previously. The term also provides a practical description of the speech and language abilities of these individuals; their language and speech are cluttered and chaotic. Speech is difficult to understand, and sometimes unintelligible, not as a result of fluency breaks but because the speech is unorganized and produced at an extremely rapid rate, a condition known as tachylalia.

Cluttering has been discussed for many years in the European literature (Weiss, 1964), but following a thirty-year lapse of concern about this complex communication disorder throughout the world, there has been a renewal of interest (Daly, 1992, 1993; Silverman, 1992; St. Louis, 1986; St. Louis & Myers, 1995). Because we tend to find what we are looking for, and because few clinicians have been looking for cluttering symptoms, few clients have been identified by speech-language pathologists. As awareness is increasing, however, more people with this syndrome are being discovered. As Daly (1986) suggests, clinicians in this country are beginning to consider cluttering as a clinical entity, and the problem is beginning to receive more attention. Daly (1992) reported that approximately 5 percent of the clients he had seen over twenty years were pure clutterers, speakers who presented without features characteristic of stuttering. When he included those clients who showed a combination of both stuttering and cluttering features, the occurrence increased to 35 to 40 percent.

Several definitions of this disorder have been offered that emphasize slightly different views of etiological and behavioral aspects of the problem. All authors agree that the problem is complex and involves many aspects of perception, learning, and expression (both verbal and written). Weiss (1964, 1967) considered cluttering to be the consequence of a central language imbalance that affected all language modalities. Luchsinger and Arnold (1965) described cluttering as an inability to formulate language, with associated organic, familial, and aphasic-like symptoms. St. Louis and Rustin (1992) describe the problem as a speech-language disorder, characterized by abnormal fluency that is not stuttering and rapid and/or irregular speech rate. The definition found in the American Psychiatric Association's *Diagnostic and Statistical Manual of Mental Disorders, Third Edition-Revised* (DSM-III-R) (1987) states:

> The essential feature of Cluttering is a disturbance of fluency involving an abnormally rapid rate and erratic rhythm of speech that impedes intelligibility. Faulty phrasing patterns are usually present so that there are bursts of speech consisting of groups of words that are not related to the grammatical structure of the sentence. The affected person is usually unaware of any communication impairment. (pp. 85–86)

Finally, Daly (1992) provides a behavioral description that includes the most basic features of the problem:

> Cluttering is a disorder of speech and language processing resulting in rapid, dysrhythmic, sporadic, unorganized, and frequently unintelligible speech. Accelerated speech is not always present, but an impairment in formulating language almost always is. (Daly, 1992, p. 107)

Of the groups of stutterers we have discussed, clutterers appear to be most like the neurogenic stutterers in that a pattern of "organicity" runs through the constellation of symptoms. Weiss (1964) and Arnold (1960) suggest a genetic basis for the disorder. In addition, several authors have pointed out that the symptoms have much in common with learning disabilities (Daly, 1986; St. Louis & Hinzman, 1986; Tiger, Irvine, & Reiss, 1980).

Extensive lists of cluttering features have been provided by Weiss (1964) and St. Louis and Hinzman (1986). As a result of a review of the current literature by St. Louis and Hinzman (1986), they accumulated a list of sixty-five different characteristics. Many features listed overlap and tend to provide a confusing picture of receptive and expressive problems that characterize these clients. Daly (1992) suggests five basic features that describe the essence of the disorder: (1) excessive rate of speaking, (2) inattention to grammatical details, (3) delayed speech and language development, (4) poor reading comprehension, and (5) unorganized writing. Another key feature that seems to pervade all aspects of expressive language is a nearly complete unawareness of the problem.

The writing of clutterers is typically rapid and disorganized, characterized by a combination of rapid speech, misarticulations, fluency breaks, and use of words that are out of place, superfluous or meaningless—termed *maze behaviors* by Loban (1976). Daly (1986) recommends procedures for obtaining writing samples during the diagnostic interview, and suggests (1992) that seeing cluttering in written form exemplifies the problem.

Both during writing and in speaking, these clients lack the ability to attend to the details of a task; indeed, this is reflected in all aspects of their expressive communication. It appears that they are taking a gestalt view of communication; they have difficulty, for example, describing individual aspects of an activity or event. Only with concentrated effort are they able to attend to the individual words or punctuation on a page of text. Their oral reading sounds as though they were demonstrating speed reading aloud; it is as if they were attempting to produce the entire page of text in a single utterance. Their speech is explosive. They speak in rapid bursts with louder than normal intensity at the outset of the utterance and then decrease to a murmur. In addition, the already rapid rate of speaking often accelerates as they produce longer sentences (Daly, 1986).

Often, the most prominent feature of cluttering is a rapid rate of speech. The speakers seems to be in a hurry, even driven, often displaying a compulsive and tense demeanor even when not speaking. Furthermore, there are no pauses between words or sentences; the punctuation is disregarded. The speaker pauses only long enough to take a breath—and then only because he must breathe—and then moves swiftly onward. Sounds and syllables are omitted, seemingly as a function of the urgency to produce the utterance. Sounds are sometimes added and misarticulated, particularly /r/ and /l/ (Daly, 1993). Although the fluency breaks are a prominent feature, they appear to be the result of the speaker's rapid rate of speaking rather than an attempt to avoid moments of stuttering. The intrinsic features of the stutterer, which include loss of control, helplessness, and fear, do not appear to be operating here. In fact, a primary characteristic of the disorder is the speaker's unawareness that there is any problem at all (Bloodstein, 1987; Daly, 1992; Weiss, 1964). Unawareness does tend to be a characteristic of pure clutterers. It is important to point out, however, that for those clients who appear to present a combination of both cluttering and stuttering symptoms, fear of specific sounds and words as well as avoidance behavior may be present.

It is clear that individuals diagnosed as clutterers and those diagnosed as stutterers have several features in common. In fact, there are a number of speakers who display both stuttering and cluttering characteristics (Daly, 1986; St. Louis and Hinzman, 1986). This combination of speech behaviors occurs most often in children (Bloodstein, 1987). Indeed, Weiss (1964) suggested that stuttering often is the result of the child's attempts to stop cluttering.

Fluency breaks are characteristic of both cluttering and stuttering. However, while whole-word and phrase repetitions are present in the speech of clutterers, the majority of the breaks take the form of rapid repetitions of one-syllable words and the first sound or syllable of polysyllabic words. Moreover, in contrast to the fluency breaks of stutterers, there does not seem to be greater tension associated with the repetitions than is already occurring during the nonrepeated speech.

When the overall patterns of speech, affective behavior, and cognitive nature of the client are considered, the differences between these two groups of speakers become even more obvious. Perhaps the most striking difference is the clutterer's nearly complete unawareness of the problem. Furthermore, to the degree that he becomes aware of a problem, he may deny the abnormalities of his speech. This response, along with their personality characteristics, makes these clients difficult to work with. They tend to be intolerant of interruptions (Van Riper, 1992b) and suggestions to monitor their production, an essential ingredient of treatment strategies. In addition, they may have immature responses, a short temper, and a history of emotional problems. As Daly (1992, 1993) points out, they provide a challenge to our ability and our patience.

Another difference between these fluency problems will become apparent during a short period of trial therapy. People who stutter typically have more fluency breaks when asked to monitor their speech. The more attention stutterers pay to how they are speaking, the more difficulty they are likely to have. With clutterers, on the other hand, if they are able to monitor how they are speaking, there is immediate improvement. As long as they monitor their output, they are able to speak slowly, clearly, and without fluency breaks, even when under communicative pressure. The problem is, however, that their ability to closely monitor their production is short-lived and usually can be maintained for only a few minutes. Stutterers, on the other hand, nearly always have much more difficulty, at least early in treatment, when they closely monitor their speech production or when speaking under pressure. Much of the treatment for cluttering centers on getting the speaker to monitor his speech production. The person who stutters, on the other hand, must learn to not only monitor but also modify his behavior.

A final difference between clutterers and stutterers concerns the disrupted flow of information in the speech of clutterers. Sound may be flowing, albeit at an excessive rate. However, information flow is absent, or nearly so. The information is disorganized, and speech is characterized by hesitations, repetitions, use of poor grammar, and a profound lack of smooth and flowing muscular coordination. They demonstrate word-finding difficulties consistent with problems in formulating language. This may not be obvious in a diagnostic session or even early in treatment. Stutterers sometimes demonstrate what appear to be word-finding difficulties but are, instead, word avoidances, substitutions, circumlocutions, or recoil behavior, as they back away from feared words or pause as they pretend to think of the word.

It is likely that a greater awareness of the various forms of atypical stuttering would result in a greater proportion of people who stutter falling into these categories. While such speakers comprise a relatively small percentage of the total population of people who stutter, it is important to identify them in order that the most appropriate intervention strategy be initiated.

Finally, although not typically classified as a disorder of fluency, there have been a few authors who have suggested that spasmodic dysphonia shares many of the same characteristics as stuttering. Silverman (1996) in his text *Stutter-*

ing and Other Fluency Disorders includes comments concerning the etiology, diagnosis, and treatment for this unique and complex disorder. Spasmodic dysphonia is a poorly understood disorder of laryngeal motor control affecting speech production. (Comprehensive descriptions of this problem are found in Aronson, 1992, and Brodnitz, 1976). Because of the uncertainty about the etiology of this disorder, there is debate over whether it should be classified as a fluency disorder.

The core of the disorder is reflected in the spasmodic functioning of the vocal folds. The speaker's speech is characterized by abductor or adductor spasms that result in a breathy and/or effortful and strained vocal quality (sometimes associated with vocal tremor). The laryngospasms are associated perceptually with severe abnormalities of voice quality, prosody, and fluency (Aronson, Brown, Litin, & Pearson, 1968; Wolfe, Ratusnik, & Feldman, 1979). Because of these vocal stoppages and the tremor activity, spasmodic dysphonia has been likened to "laryngeal stuttering" or "stammering of the vocal cords" (Aronson, 1973; Luchsinger & Arnold, 1965; McCall, 1974; Salamy & Sessions, 1980). Based on perceptual judgments of naive listeners, Silverman and Hummer (1989) proposed that spasmodic dysphonia be reclassified as a fluency rather than a voice disorder. On the other hand, Cannito and Sherrard (1995) used traditional clinical measures to determine rate and fluency characteristics of twenty adult females diagnosed with spasmodic dysphonia. Although these subjects, on average, spoke significantly slower and produced more fluency breaks than a matched group of normal speakers, they exhibited a wide range of fluency phenomena. Cannito and Sherrard felt, on the basis of their data, that the observed differences in fluency were but one associated feature of a group of heterogeneous symptoms. In addition, the distribution of fluency breaks exhibited by their subjects was uncharacteristic of stuttering in that part-word repetitions were often in syllable-final position and prolongations occurred not only within syllables but also between syllables and words. These authors concluded that although spasmodic dysphonia speakers certainly display fluency breaks, this fluency disorder is easily differentiated from traditional stuttering. These findings coincide with those of Salamy and Sessions (1990), who concluded that spasmodic dysphonia and stuttering are different disorders.

CONCLUSION

Because of the developmental nature of stuttering, its occurrence in adolescents and adults may be more obvious than it is in young children. Generally, but not always, the problem becomes more severe with age, as the speaker enters into more competitive speaking situations. Still, there is much variability across situations and listeners. The severity of stuttering, as indicated by such surface features as frequency, duration, tension, and avoidance, does not necessarily indicate the handicap experienced by the speaker. Thus, the clinician's sensitivity for determining and appreciating the client's helplessness and loss of control associated with the stuttering experience is crucial. Determining the quality of the client's nonstuttered speech is also important, for it may be smooth and easy or, instead, characterized by many elements of instability. An assessment of the client's motivation and readiness for change is crucial for the success of what is likely to be, at the vary least, an arduous adventure.

Atypical fluency disorders present a somewhat rare and unique challenge to the clinician. The many differences between the more typical developmental stuttering and speakers who clutter or present with neurogenic or psychogenic stuttering may lead one to question whether these problems should even be considered as fluency disorders. In any case, assessment is an ongoing procedure that is likely to continue well into the initial stages of the treatment process.

RECOMMENDED READINGS

Daly, D. A. (1993). Cluttering: Another fluency syndrome. In R. Curlee (Ed.), *Stuttering and related disorders of fluency*. New York: Thieme Medical Publishers, pp. 179–204.

DiClemente, C. C. (1993). Changing addictive behaviors: A process perspective. *Current Directions in Psychological Science*, 2 (4), 101–106.

St. Louis, K. (Ed.). (1986a). *The atypical stutterer*. New York: Academic Press.

CHAPTER 5

Treatment of Young Children

INTRODUCTION

This chapter discusses strategies and techniques for helping the younger child who is beginning to stutter. The major focus is the child from approximately age two through age twelve. There are far more children who stutter than adolescents or adults. As discussed in Chapter 3, the literature strongly suggests that by the early teenage years, there is a notable decrease in the number of individuals who stutter. Thus, by far the largest number of potential clients with fluency disorders are to be found among children in their preschool and early school years (Conture, 1990). For years, writers in the field of fluency disorders have suggested that clinicians will have the greatest impact by providing service to this group of clients (Van Riper, 1982).

Although a child's chronological age is a factor influencing the behavioral features and severity of the stuttering syndrome, age is not as meaningful as the length of time stuttering has been taking place. As Conture (1982) puts it, the age of the stuttering is usually more meaningful than the age of the child. Children as young as two or three years old can present with strikingly complex stuttering behaviors and exhibit high levels of tension, struggle, and fear. Furthermore, the longer children have been stuttering, the more likely it is that the problem will become chronic. This may be especially true if the child continues to stutter throughout ages of five to seven, which constitute the *critical period* (see Chapter 3) during which stuttering may become habituated.

Both the amount as well as the directness of clinical intervention with preschool stutterers has clearly increased during the last decades of this century. According to Gottwald and Starkweather (1995), this is partially a result of the implementation of federal legislation in 1975 of Public Law 94–142, calling for the education of all handicapped children, and in 1986 of Public Law 99–457, requiring early intervention for children three to five years old. There may be at least one other factor contributing to increased interest in early intervention. The results of research findings with young children, particularly those of Yairi and his associates (Yairi, 1981, 1982, 1983, 1993; Yairi & Lewis, 1984) have documented many of the characteristics of very early childhood fluency breaks. Furthermore, Yairi and Ambrose (1992a, 1992b) have noted that 75 percent of the risk for stuttering onset occurs before the age of three years, five months. The increased understanding of early childhood stuttering, in combination with successful intervention for children who are seen as soon as possible after stuttering onset, has made it clear that such treatment offers the best chance for altering the development of the problem. As we shall see later in the following pages, such early intervention has been found to be both effective and long-lasting.

CONSIDERATIONS WHEN TREATING YOUNG CHILDREN

Many of the strategies and techniques used with older clients can be applied, in some cases with only minor alteration, to younger children. Of the two major strategies, fluency modification approaches are most often used. However, stuttering modification techniques may also be appropriate. Particularly with younger clients, the techniques used with these two general strategies become quite similar. That is, both strategies emphasize fluent responses, and both have the ultimate goal of spontaneous fluency. In addition, just as with older speakers, it is also important to consider and modify possible emotional and psychosocial features of the problem.

There are, of course, many salient distinctions between intervention with children and with older clients. In earlier chapters it was shown that fluency is highly variable with young children, a fact that makes both assessment and therapeutic progress somewhat more difficult to track for this age group. There is always the question of how much behavioral change is due to treatment and how much is due to the natural variability of the behavior. Other important differences when working with younger clients are:

1. Children are functioning with neurophysiological systems that are far from adult-like and still in the process of maturation.

2. Depending on the child's level of awareness and reaction to the stuttering experience, the clinician may select treatment techniques that are less direct than those used with adults.

3. Parents and a variety of other professionals, and particularly the child's classroom teacher, have a substantial role in the treatment process.

4. The clinician will more likely place greater emphasis on the evaluation and possible treatment of the child's other communication abilities including language, phonological, and voice problems.

5. The likelihood of achieving spontaneous or automatic fluency is much greater for young children than for adults.

6. There tends to be somewhat less effort needed for helping the child to transfer and maintain treatment gains into extratreatment environments.

7. Relapse following formal treatment is not usually a serious problem, as it is with adult clients.

All these features combine to produce a number of clinical choices that the clinician must consider. One of these is the directness of the intervention process.

INDIRECT VERSUS DIRECT STRATEGIES

During the first seven or eight decades of this century in the United States, the treatment used with young children who stuttered was indirect; the children themselves were not the recipients of the intervention activities. Rather, the significant adults in the child's environment—the parents, family members, grandparents, and teachers—were advised concerning procedures for altering the child's environment. The choice of this general approach was due to the many cautions from authorities who strongly recommended that the clinician not do anything to make the child aware of the problems he seemed to be having with his speech. Clinicians were extorted not to bring the child's attention to his disrupted speech or to respond in any way that might associate speech with negative emotion. This view was especially popular during the decades of the 1940s through the 1960s and coincided with the prominence of the diagnosogenic theory of stuttering onset and development (see Chapter 2). A series of quotes from a popular textbook of the time by Eisenson and Ogilvie (1963) reflect the then-current thinking about intervention for the early or primary stages of stuttering. Described by Bluemel in 1932, primary stuttering is seen as a transient phenomenon during which the child does not yet show awareness of his problem or demonstrate special effort during speaking.

> Emphasis in the treatment of the primary stutterer is to prevent him from becoming aware that his speech is in any way different from that of others around him and a cause for concern. (p. 318)

> Essentially, therefore, the primary stutterer is to be treated through his parents if he is not of school age. If he is of school age, teachers as well as parents become the recipients of direct treatment. (p. 318)

Parents were instructed to respond in the following ways:

> If the child is a primary stutterer or is showing any of the speech char-
> acteristics associated with stuttering, it is essential that signs of parental
> anxiety be kept from him. Do not permit the child to hear the word
> stuttering used about his speech. Do not . . . do anything that makes it
> necessary for him to think about speaking or to conclude that he is not
> speaking well. (p. 323)

Johnson's 1962 "Open Letter" contained this statement: "Do nothing at any
time, by word or deed or posture or facial expression, that would serve to call
Fred's attention to the interruptions in his speech. Above all, do nothing that
would make him regard them as abnormal or unacceptable" (p. 3).

Finally, Van Riper, in the first edition (1939) of his popular text, *Speech Correction: Principles and Methods*, wrote, "The way to treat a young stutterer
in the primary stage is to let him alone and treat his parents and teachers."
With such cautions, few clinicians and parents were likely to intervene directly
and assist a young child with his communication problems. The fear was
that direct intervention could make the stuttering more severe, a fear that
permeated the decision-making process for clinicians. Doubtless, there
continue to be many clinicians who continue to hold such views and are
overly cautious when deciding whether treatment is appropriate for young
children.

Even if a young child is producing frequent fluency breaks, a less direct
strategy is often used during the initial period of treatment. This is especially
the case for the child whose fluency is characterized by relatively easy breaks
with low levels of tension or struggle and who is generally unaware of any
speaking difficulty. With indirect intervention, the clinician takes no direct action to modify specific features of the child's speech. Parents and significant
others are counseled and provided with information concerning the developmental nature of language and fluency. The clinician will likely spend as
much or more time working with the parents as with the child. The major
focus of an indirect strategy is to make speech enjoyable for the child and to
adjust those environmental factors that tend to disrupt his fluency. By decreasing demands, desensitizing the child to fluency-disrupting stimuli, and
giving rewards for open, easy, and forward-moving speech, the child is guided,
step-by-step, toward increased fluency.

Treatment is likely to be more direct if the child is experiencing tension
and struggle behavior or fragmenting multisyllabic or, especially, monosyllabic
words. In addition, the child may be exhibiting the nonverbal characteristics
of more developed stuttering such as breaking eye contact with the listener
(Conture, 1990). For these children, the clinician will be more straightforward in demonstrating specific activities for enhancing fluency and modifying moments of stuttering. A number of authors (Gregory, 1995; Healey &
Scott, 1995; Peters & Guitar, 1991) have indicated that fluency modification

techniques are more likely to be used at the outset of treatment. Depending on the success of these techniques, stuttering modification techniques may also be employed. A more direct approach to modifying stuttering consists of identifying stuttering events, contrasting both fluent and stuttered speech and having the child intentionally produce both forms. The clinician will select the most appropriate activities along a continuum of directness according to the needs of the child and his response to treatment.

Regardless of how directly the clinician works to alter the child's speech, treatment for young children who stutter should be characterized by a high degree of reassurance and encouragement by the clinician. Conture (1990) holds that these clinician characteristics cannot be overemphasized. The treatment environment must be highly supportive as the child is guided into the exploration of his speech and himself.

The clinician's choice about the directness of treatment depends more on the characteristics of the child's problem than on his age. As discussed in Chapter 3, however, regardless of the directness of the treatment strategy, it is better to intervene rather than wait for the problem to go away. Although clinicians or parents need not be alarmed or seek immediate help, it is widely agreed that early intervention is an influential factor in the success of treatment (Adams, 1984; Gottwald & Starkweather, 1995; Peters & Guitar, 1991; Starkweather, 1987; Starkweather, Gottwald & Halfond, 1990). Nonetheless, as Conture (1990) points out:

> Unfortunately, some professionals, who do not have enough experience or interest in stuttering, will use up precious time in the early stages of the development of the child's stuttering problem and only refer to a more qualified professional when the child is showing signs of a worsening and, generally, more habituated speaking problem. (p. 126)

THE ROLE OF THE PARENTS

Clinicians have known for many years that parents play a central role in the successful management of stuttering with young children (Bluemel, 1957; Wyatt, 1969). Since stuttering is most often a developmental disorder beginning during childhood (Bloodstein, 1987; Conture, 1990; Van Riper, 1982) the problem unquestionably involves the parents. Conture (1990) wisely points out that parents need to be rewarded for their insight and courage when they ask for help. The last thing they need is for the clinician to lecture or reprimand them for their previous patterns of parent-child interactions. Parents should be informed at the outset that they have not caused this problem to occur and are not totally responsible for eliminating it. However, as a good deal of research has demonstrated, parents can be shown how to assist in altering the child's environment so that stuttering behavior is not maintained.

Parents are significant listeners in the child's environment and have a powerful influence on the child's attitudes and speech behaviors.

Ratner (1993) provides a helpful metaphor that may be used to explain the nature of stuttering to parents. She points out the similarities of stuttering to allergies or juvenile diabetes. "Parental behaviors are not presumed to play a role in the onset of either allergies or juvenile diabetes. However, it is clear that the response of parents to these disorders can either mitigate or aggravate their consequences" (p. 238).

To the degree that parents are able to adjust the child's environment in regard to such problems (e.g., exposure to allergens or adjustments in diet), the symptoms will become less severe. As with stuttering, the maintenance of the symptoms, if not the etiology, can be significantly affected by actions taken by the child's parents.

It is the consensus of many clinicians who have achieved success with young children who stutter that parental involvement in treatment is crucial (Conture, 1990; Conture & Schwartz, 1984; Ham, 1986; Peters & Guitar, 1991; Riley & Riley, 1983; Rustin, 1987; Starkweather, Gottwald, & Halfond, 1990). Rustin indicates that, if there is going to be any realistic chance for therapeutic success, the parents must play a major role. She states that "without the involvement of parents, clinicians become powerless to help the child beyond the confines of the clinic room" (Rustin, 1995, p. 125). Likewise, Ramig (1993c) and Bronfenbrenner (1976) state that without the parents' ability to eventually develop the capability to help their child, the effects of treatment will likely deteriorate. Parental involvement not only assists the child in making behavioral and cognitive changes but also permits a form of mental hygiene to occur for the parents. Through counseling and parent group contact, the parents can accumulate the necessary information to become stronger and more confident about helping their child (Rustin & Cook, 1995). Although it may not be necessary for the clinician to spend a great amount of time desensitizing the young child to his fluency breaks, other people in the child's environment including grandparents and teachers, often receive great benefit from these activities (Silverman, 1992). It is also worth considering that increasing numbers of children from nontraditional families are being seen in clinical facilities. In such cases, the major caregiver may not be the child's actual parent. Whoever takes on this role, however, will play a central role during the stages of assessment, change, and maintenance.

Lest it sound as though the author is sitting in an ivory tower as this is being written, it should be pointed out that although having active parental involvement is an exemplary goal, it is not always possible. Ramig (1993c) points out that parents have many priorities, including work schedules and financial survival, which may well be regarded as more important than the status of their child's fluency. Particularly in rural or poor urban areas, there may be no way to contact the parents by telephone, the parents may not be able to read or write, or English may be a second language. If there is only one parent in the home, transporting the child to treatment may be difficult, or the single parent may not be able to afford services.

In order to assist the parents in understanding the problem and making good decisions on their own, the clinician can provide behavioral models as well as information. The clinician needs to be cautioned to go slowly. As discussed in Chapter 7, when counseling parents, it is easy to provide too much information too quickly (Conture, 1990; Luterman, 1991). As a result, parents can quickly become overwhelmed and discouraged. Rather than lecturing the parents, it is more effective to follow their lead by listening to their questions and responding to, and expanding on, the issues they want to know about. Once they have an opportunity to read informative pamphlets, see instructional videotapes, and observe treatment being conducted with their child, they will be much more likely to provide many insightful ideas and suggestions.

Stages of Parent Involvement

Ramig (1993c) suggests three possible stages of parent involvement during fluency treatment for young children: facilitating communicative interaction, and educational counseling, involving parents as observers and participants.

Educational Counseling. During this stage the clinician explains the difference between normal disfluencies and not-so-normal fluency breaks by discussing the surface characteristics of the child's behavior (see Table 2–1). Parents can be informed that, although the etiology of stuttering is not completely understood, a great deal is known about the dynamics of the problem and much can be done to influence the increase or decrease of associated features. As parents begin to understand the problem, they will become less anxious. The clinician's early role during treatment is to demystify an undesirable situation and give the parents something concrete to do beyond simply feeling helpless. The booklets listed in Appendix C will provide answers to many of their questions. For some parents, the increasing access to information about fluency disorders on computer internet systems is likely to be appealing (see Appendix C).

Through informed and reasonable counseling, parents will come to understand that, with a minimum of care, they are not likely to "do any damage" to their child. The child's parents will eventually become less inhibited and more likely to do reasonable and helpful things. Moreover, they will learn it is generally much better to acknowledge the obvious rather than behave as though the child's stuttering was something too awful to discuss openly and frankly.

Ramig (1993c) also suggests that during this initial stage of parent counseling, the clinician consider discussing the many myths that are commonly associated with stuttering and take the responsibility to correct these distorted views. Possibly the most common myth is that parents, by omission or commission, are the likely cause of their child's stuttering. As many authors have pointed out (Conture, 1990; Peters & Guitar, 1991; Rustin, 1987; Van Riper,

1982), parents often accept guilt for the problem, assuming they had a major role in the etiology. At the very least, there is often a level of frustration with a situation that requires formal intervention for a handicapping condition (Luterman, 1991). As Ramig (1993c) suggests, the reduction of possible feelings of guilt by the parents should be viewed as a major contribution of clinicians. Group meetings of parents provide an invaluable forum for dealing with these frustrations, as in this way parents begin to realize that they are not alone. The more experienced parents can provide support and share concerns and therapeutic concepts that are especially helpful (Berkowitz, Cook, & Haughey, 1994; Ramig, 1993c). Detailed descriptions of child and parent group dynamics may be found in Conture (1990, pp. 113–118).

Examples of other myths include beliefs that children stutter in order to gain attention, that once a child begins to stutter he is destined to a life of stuttering, that stuttering is always caused by some underlying psychological or emotional problem, and that stuttering can be transmitted from one family member to another by imitation or simply by hearing others (Ramig, 1993c).

Although it is not necessarily considered a myth, many clinicians tend to believe that as a group, parents of stuttering children behave differently than those of normally speaking children. As Ratner (1993) points out, however, there is no evidence for this view or for the opinion that the parental interaction style is related to the severity of a fluency disorder. Furthermore, no correlations were noted between stuttering severity at initial assessment and parental conversational behaviors of speech rate, frequency of questions, and interruptions. In addition, Weiss and Zebrowski (Weiss, 1993; Weiss & Zebrowski, 1992) found that parents of stutterers do not produce significantly more requests than parents of nonstutterers.

Facilitating Communicative Interaction. Ramig (1993c) suggests that this second stage helps the parent to develop interpersonal styles that will be conducive to fluency enhancement. The overall communication and interpersonal characteristics of the child, as well as the child-parent interaction style, should be continuously evaluated. These characteristics include linguistic as well as paralinguistic variables, many of which have been studied in recent years in an attempt to determine their effect on childrens' fluency (see Kelly, 1994, for a recent summary). Such studies have investigated the rate of the speech (Conture & Caruso, 1987; Kelly, 1994; Meyers & Freeman, 1985); parent responses to the child's fluency breaks, both verbal and nonverbal (LaSalle & Conture, 1991); the amount and type of interruptions of the child's speech by the parents (Meyers & Freeman, 1985); turn-taking behaviors and response-time latency (Kelly, 1994); and the complexity of the questions posed to the child (Stocker & Usprich, 1976); as well as the tendency for the parent to provide verbal and nonverbal corrections to the child as he is speaking (Gregory & Hill, 1980). As these features are identified, the parent can be shown how to alter some interactions. For example, the mother can be shown how to slow her speech, provide more time for turn taking, interrupt the child's speech less, and positively reinforce the child for using his fluency-enhancing techniques.

Conture and Caruso (1987) and Ramig (1993c) advocate the use of "Mr. Rogers" speech (referring to the soft-spoken television figure) as a prototype for slower, smoother speech and longer turn-taking pause times. Silverman (1996) suggests having the parents view videotapes of themselves and their child while the clinician points out both the undesirable and desirable ways they are responding to their child's fluency breaks. For example, the parents may be speaking rapidly and frequently interrupting or indicating by their body language (e.g., breaking eye contact) that they are not interested in what their child is saying. During an obvious or severe stuttering moment they may unconsciously freeze or show anxiety or concern. They may have a pattern of asking their child difficult or abstract questions that require complex responses. On the other hand, of course, the parents may also be doing many appropriate things, including modeling slow, easy speech and responding with an unafraid attitude to stuttering behavior. Videotapes of clinician-child interactions also can be used to demonstrate desirable parent behavior.

Clearly, the clinician plays a primary role in modeling better speaking behaviors, both inside and outside the treatment sessions. Ramig (1993c) suggests that it may be important to alter sources of family stress that appear to contribute to fluency breakdowns. Events such as arguments or conflict, financial problems, sibling rivalry, and responses to various illnesses may have an influence on the child's fluency. Of course, in some instances referral to other professionals is appropriate.

Parents as Observers and Participants. Ramig's third stage of involvement gets the parents actively involved in the treatment process. The participation of both parents is assumed to be the ideal situation, although there is minimal research on the role of the father in this process. Ramig (1993c) indicates that even if only one parent is able to take part, the result is still likely to be beneficial for the child. Initially the parent's role is to observe the interaction of the child and clinician as the clinician models changes in the above-mentioned interpersonal communication variables. The clinician may also demonstrate strategies for expanding the child's fluency or modifying moments of stuttering. As treatment progresses, the parents gradually begin to take part in the sessions by joining in with the clinician and the child. Gradually, the parents are included in treatment activities and eventually instructed to interact with the child on their own.

TREATMENT TECHNIQUES

Although most current authors writing about treatment for young children recommend reasonably direct treatment, there is some question as to whether practicing clinicians feel the same way. Based on several recent surveys of professional clinicians (see Chapter 1), some practicing clinicians continue to be hesitant, or at least highly cautious, about working directly with young children who stutter. Whether the clinician chooses to work indirectly or directly with the younger child, however, the essence of treatment consists of both facilitating the child's capacities to produce easily fluent speech and reducing the demands placed on the child that result in fluency disruption. Certainly, the clinician will have many related goals, such as decreasing the child's response to fluency-disrupting stimuli and increasing his assertiveness and risk-taking ability.

USING THE CAPACITIES AND DEMANDS MODEL

Conceptualizing treatment from a capacities and demands framework, as described in Chapter 2, can provide the clinician as well as parents, teachers, and other professionals, with a comprehensive and clear direction of treatment. We will approach treatment for young children from this framework. That is, we will discuss things the clinician can do to increase the child's capacity to produce smooth language and speech. We can assist the child in achieving a measure of control over a speech production system that is in the process of maturation. In many instances, working on the capacities side of the equation is all that is necessary for young children who have only recently begun to struggle with their fluency. For some children, changes in the communication environment may need to be considered, while for others, a more direct modification of stuttering will occur. These children are more likely to have a family history of fluency disorders or one or more other problems that make communicating or learning more demanding. In such cases, treatment may take somewhat longer. Conture (1990) suggests that most children will take approximately twenty weeks (with a range of ten to thirty) of weekly therapy before they are ready for dismissal. He also advises, however, that the clinician should be careful not to force treatment into a parent's busy schedule. The clinician should be prepared to give both the parents and the child an intermission from weekly treatment sessions and be available for parents during such intervals.

In any case, a realistic goal of treatment with most young children is a high level of spontaneous or normal fluency (Conture, 1990; Healey & Scott, 1995; Peters & Guitar, 1991). The future for fluency is bright for such children who receive early intervention. Although this is often the outcome of treatment for young children who are in the early stages of stuttering, a quote from Healey and Scott (1995) provides a larger view of the syndrome with which we are dealing, as regards even the young child:

> We are reluctant to base treatment effectiveness exclusively on pre- and posttreatment fluency data. This seems to be a rather narrow definition of "success." Some children in our program have demonstrated

increased levels of fluency but were unable to achieve a positive attitude about themselves as fluent speakers. (1995, p. 153)

As with adults, focusing on the child's fluency may provide the clinician with a restricted view of the syndrome and a narrow definition of progress. To be sure, high levels of fluent speech may be achieved by focusing only on the surface features of the child's behavior. However, there is little question that, even for young children, both affective and cognitive changes as well take place during effective treatment. Of course, the young beginning stutterer is not as likely to have developed the self-concept of a handicapped speaker, and thus the clinician may not need to formally intervene to produce these intrinsic changes. Nonetheless, monitoring such changes will provide the clinician with a larger window of progress and promote long-term success.

Gottwald and Starkweather (1995) provide an outstanding clinical suggestion that coincides nicely with the title of this text. Their comment emphasizes the importance of clinical decision making with young children. They recommend that the clinician devote the first ten minutes of each treatment session to reassessing the child and his current needs. Certainly, the clinician will go into each session with a long-range plan and specific treatment techniques at the ready. However, by first observing the child in a natural environment and noting the type and quality of his fluency characteristics, including speech rate and secondary behaviors, the clinician is more apt to make better decisions that are focused on the immediate needs of the child rather than trying to fit the child into preselected activities.

As discussed earlier, the two major approaches to fluency treatment come together with young children. The similarities and differences of these two approaches are shown nicely in Figure 5–1, developed by Ramig and Bennett (1995).

Regardless of which overall treatment strategy is chosen, it is the clinician who will be the "catalyst" for change (Silverman, 1992), providing the child with better models for speaking and the child and others with valuable information that will give them more control over their situation. The clinician can provide the child with skills for changing his speech as well as enhancing their own self-esteem and feelings about who they are.

Peters and Guitar concisely describe the basics of treatment for the young stuttering child.

We believe that, if we can provide the beginning stutterer with a sufficient number of positive and fluent speaking experiences during treatment, this fluency will generalize to more speaking situations. . . . This increased fluency will also reduce the opportunities the child has to respond to any remaining disfluencies with tension, frustration, or possibly escape and starting behaviors. The combined effect will be to allow time for the child's physiological system to mature and for normal fluency patterns to become stabilized. (1991, p. 274)

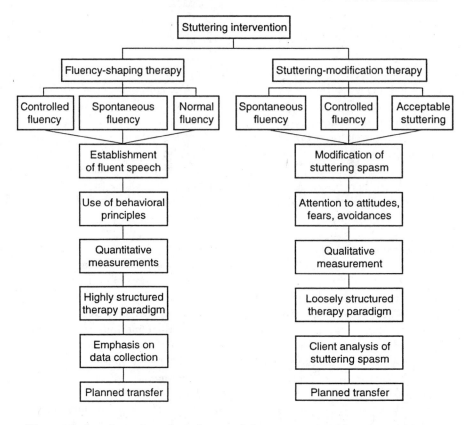

Figure 5–1.   Speech goals and general characteristics of fluency- and stuttering-modification procedures. (From Ramig and Bennett [1995], p. 140. Copyright © American Speech-Language-Hearing Association. Reprinted by permission.)

Increasing the Child's Capacities

Enhancing Fluency. Fluency-enhancing procedures provide the child with techniques for both initiating and enhancing his fluency. As described in Chapters 1 and 2, the clinician cannot always assume that because the child's speech is nonstuttered, it is necessarily fluent. Speech that is to be expanded and reinforced should have high-quality fluency, which is characterized by smooth and effortless production.

Techniques for creating and promoting fluency go by several names. These techniques have been called *fluency-initiating gestures* (FIG), *fluency-enhancing techniques, fluency-facilitating movements*, and *easy speech*. Regardless of the names for these techniques, they consist of procedures to help the child more efficiently manage the breath stream, produce gradual and relaxed use of the vocal folds, use a slower rate of articulatory movement, make gradual and smooth transitions from one sound to another, produce light articulatory contacts, and keep an open vocal tract in order to counteract constrictions resulting from tension. Many of these behaviors are already characteristic of parental or child-directed speech (slow rate, more leisurely turn taking, shorter utterances, more frequent use of paraphrase) (Ratner, 1993). Puppets or games and cartoon pictures can be used to facilitate these behaviors. Conture (1990) suggests the use of cursive writing as an analogy that a child will easily understand. The child is shown how to smoothly make the transitional writing movements between letters at the same time that he is saying the sounds of the word. Not only is the clinician able to demonstrate the value of easy and flowing (versus hard and erratic) movement during serial motor tasks, it also gives her an opportunity to show the child that his speech is something *he* is *producing* rather than something that is happening to him.

It is interesting to note that although young children usually respond with greater fluency to slower and less complex speech produced by the parent or the clinician, the reasons for this effect are not well understood. To say to a parent, "Slowing down may help your child to be somewhat more fluent," is correct, but we do not understand why this holds true (Ratner, 1993, p. 244). Ratner submits there may be some higher-order conversational or interactional factor in operation. It may be that the pragmatic aspects of communication come into play more than the actual complexity of language. For example, Weiss and Zebrowski (1992) found that responsive utterances were significantly more likely to be produced fluently than assertive utterances. In addition, slowing down speech and using less complex sentence structure is likely to facilitate turn taking.

Going beyond the specific techniques used, Ramig and Bennett (1995), provide a list of suggestions for the clinician, parents, and teachers when using a fluency-modification approach with younger school-age children. The clinician and everyone else (including parents and teachers) involved in the intervention process should:

1. Use basic and understandable terms when explaining and demonstrating what you want the child to do. These terms (e.g., "turtle speech," "rabbit speech") should be used consistently when identifying target behaviors and reinforcing the child's actions. Regardless of the methods used, children need to have terms and concepts that enable them to think about their speech and language (Cooper & Cooper, 1991a).

2. Model, rather than instruct, the child about how to perform specific target behaviors.

3. Model slow and easy speech when interacting with the child in a variety of treatment and extratreatment settings.

4. Model slow and easy body movements when interacting with the child, again in a variety of treatment and extratreatment settings. These movements can be coordinated with easy, slow, and smooth body movements. Such activities are especially good to use at the outset and completion of the treatment sessions.

5. Reinforce the child's accomplishments and feelings of self-worth in the context of as many experiences as possible.

Gottwald and Starkweather (1995) provide a succinct description of a combination of approaches, which includes the goals of both fluency enhancement, reduction of demands, and desensitization of the child to normal fluency breaks:

> Depending on the child's specific needs, the clinician may use a reduced speech rate, many silent periods and pause times, and the language stimulation techniques of self-talk and parallel talk, but at a slow rate. Also, the clinician may reduce the number of language demands made on the child, including limiting questions requiring complex answers and reducing implied expectations for ongoing oral communication. Finally, the clinician will use normal disfluencies, such as whole word and phrase repetitions. (p. 122)

Fluency modification approaches are especially useful if the clinician is using an indirect approach. The basic goals are described by a variety of sources (Conture, 1990; Luper & Mulder, 1964; Peters & Guitar, 1991; Van Riper, 1973).

Modifying Stuttering. For many children, it may be enough for the clinician to make use of some or most of the above-mentioned techniques for modifying fluency. In other instances, the clinician may decide to go to the next level and provide the child with techniques for helping him move through a stuttering event. With some young children, Van Riper (1973) does not recommend teaching the child to directly modify his stuttering moments. Rather, by using fluency-facilitating activities, the clinician assists the child in reaching a basal level of fluency in the treatment setting. Fluency-disrupting activities are then gradually introduced (e.g., listener loss, time pressure, greater linguistic demands). As the child's fluency becomes unstable, but prior to the point at which a child will produce fluency breaks, the clinician minimizes the disrupting activities. As a result of these procedures, the child will gradually become able to increase his tolerance and will become "toughened" to various forms of demands including communicative stress.

In order for the child to learn ways of changing the form of his stuttering, it is essential to identify both the desirable and the undesirable characteristics of his fluency breaks. One key for the child in making this distinction is for the clinician to use descriptive terms that the child can understand. Such terms should help the child differentiate the concepts of *hard, easy, smooth, gentle, stopping,* and *turtle* or *elephant* (slow) *speech* compared to *rabbit* (fast) *speech*. The concepts are usually learned more readily if combined with illustrative body movements. The clinician and the child can, for example, alternately tighten and relax various parts of their bodies (including the speech mechanisms), helping the child to differentiate between tightness and relaxation and giving the child a sense of control over the speech mechanisms. The clinician can make the experience of speaking enjoyable while giving the child a sense of power over his speech. This can be accomplished by producing speech or nonspeech sounds during solo, parallel, and tangential play with intermittent interaction between child and clinician (Conture, 1990; Peters & Guitar, 1991; Van Riper, 1973). As Conture (1990) suggests, games provide the opportunity to move into cooperative play and turn taking during verbalization. Thus, the clinician can direct the level of communicative demand and model the activities, as described by Ramig and Bennett (1995).

Some clinicians are undoubtedly concerned about using the "s-word," *stuttering*. Most writers (including myself) believe that referring to what the child is doing as stuttering is not a major issue during the treatment of young children. It is true that if we assign positive or negative value to the word, it tends to become more powerful. However, using the word *stuttering* in a normal conversational manner is not, in and of itself, likely to result in increased stuttering by the child. Whether the word *stuttering* is used or avoided, it is probably better to use behavioral terms that are more descriptive and meaningful to the child. Words such as *bumpy* and *easy speech* are less likely to carry with them negative values. As we discussed with fluency modification techniques, Ramig and Bennett (1995) also provide a list of suggestions for the clinician, parents, and teachers when using a stuttering modification approach with younger children. They indicate that the clinician should:

1. Explain the nature of the speech production system to the child and the parents thereby, providing him with greater understanding and the means of controlling his own system.

2. Illustrate the physical behaviors associated with his formulative and motoric fluency breaks, using terms that he can understand.

3. Show the child how to vary his speaking behaviors, adjusting his levels of tension and struggle. Making use of modeling and negative practice, the clinician and the child can explore ways of altering his fluency breaks. The child can gradually change the behaviors affiliated with tension and fragmentation and move toward easier, forward-moving fluency breaks. The child's speech does not have to become completely fluent, but simply easier and smoother. For example, Gregory (1989) suggests that after a child experiences a difficult and tense moment of stuttering, the clinician should direct him to produce the word again, this time reducing the tension by half. Conture's (1990) analogy of a garden hose with the possible levels of constriction that prevent the flow of water is a good way to make the child's speech production system less mysterious for him.

The clinician and the child can explore procedures for "opening the clogs in the hose" and creating a more open flow of sounds. The incorporation of fluency-initiating gestures at this point is a good example of how the two general strategies can be intertwined during treatment with young children.

4. With the child leading the way, the clinician can discuss strategies for responding to people and situations that arise in the child's world. Together, the clinician and the child (as well as parents and teachers) can role-play responses to teasing, participation in social and class activities, relaxation in preparation for stressful situations, changing negative into positive self-talk, using visualizations and positive affirmations, and responding to time pressures.

5. Help the child and his parents to prepare for the possibility of relapse by considering responses to possible increases in fear, avoidance behavior, struggle behavior, and fluency breaks. The clinician, the child, and his parents can discuss self-assessment procedures as well as prescribe possible responses.

6. Develop a schedule for the maintenance and use of both stuttering modification and fluency-maintaining skills in real-world contexts.

A central theme in stuttering-modification procedures with children is the contrasting of hard and easy speech. As described by Williams (1971), this distinction is the basis for giving the child the ability to take control of his speech system. The child learns that he is not helpless; rather, he has a choice about how to stutter and how to speak. There is a great deal that he can do to change his speaking pattern. The clinician can take the lead and demonstrate both forms of speech. It is not necessary to demonstrate extreme forms of stuttering, only some degree of mild tension and fragmentation in order to make the point. The child can then be instructed to identify the moments of hard and easy speech produced by the clinician. This can also be done with audio- or videotapes of other speakers and eventually with the client himself. As the child is able to consistently identify moments of hard and easy speech, the clinician can show the child how to gradually change moments of one into the other. Struggle behavior, including blocking the airflow at various levels of the vocal tract, can be created purposely. Varying degrees of these constrictions can be voluntarily created by both the clinician and the child. They can then be analyzed and altered in order to create greater airflow and smoother movements with easier transitions from one sound and syllable to another. The child can direct the clinician as she makes these adjustments during a variety of activities and speaking situations.

Parents can be shown how to highlight the child's moments of hard speech in a sensitive way and to reward easy speech as it occurs. The clinician cannot assume that parents will be able to do this without considerable observation and practice. Some parents will continue to be afraid of putting hard speech into their own mouths or to discuss these events even a little. As Conture (1990) indicates, some parents tend to reprimand, correct, nag, or badger the child regarding his speech, and they must be taught instead to assist in a gentle and appropriate manner.

Anything that will assist the child to produce speech with an open and flowing vocal tract will greatly facilitate fluency and help to alter the form of his stuttering. Conture's (1990) lily pad analogy, in which the child is instructed to "lightly touch" each sound or word as he lightly "talks across the lily pads" is a good example. The creation of greater airflow, as Conture (1990) explains in his garden hose analogy, and the use of software that provides feedback enabling the child to visualize appropriate respiration, airflow, phonation, and smooth speech production (Gobel, 1989) can be beneficial also. Van Riper's (1973) modifications of his pullout techniques, which are used with older clients (see Chapter 6), Williams's (1971) technique of reminding the child to "move on" during stuttering moments, and Conture's (1990) similar recommendations to the child to "change and move forward" are all useful adaptations of stuttering modification procedures. The child, by using such suggestions, can gradually learn to release the struggled speech behavior and make the necessary transitional gestures that will enable him to move to the next sound segment. Conture (1990) suggests the general rule of producing speech by using appropriate rate and physical tension to initiate speech and to move from the initial sound into the following sounds. As always, especially with children, it is better to model these suggestions rather than tell the child what to do.

Cognitive and Affective Considerations. As we've discussed, many authors believe that, even with young children, it is important to attend to the feelings and attitudes associated with the onset of stuttering behavior. There are levels of frustration and fear that need to be faced, not only by the child who is stuttering but also by his parents. By making speaking fun and enjoyable and helping the child to create a sense of power concerning his speech, you increase the chances of his long-term success following treatment. Such cognitive changes, along with procedures for desensitizing (as Van Riper, 1973, described), and toughening the child to teach him to tolerate fluency disrupters in his environment, are essential aspects of treatment. Fortunately, for many children, such activities are not complicated or long term.

FLUENCY AND OTHER COMMUNICATION DISORDERS

It has been noted by several investigators that many children with fluency disorders tend to have other communication problems as well. Most often noted is the relatively high co-occurrence of articulation and phonological problems (Blood & Seider, 1981; Conture, 1990; Daly, 1981; Louko, Edwards, & Conture, 1990; Schwartz & Conture, 1988; St. Louis & Hinzman, 1986;

Riley & Riley, 1979; Thompson, 1983; Williams & Silverman, 1968). Reviews of this literature have resulted in estimates suggesting that something on the order of approximately one-third of all children who stutter can be expected to also demonstrate articulation or phonological difficulties (Bloodstein, 1987; Conture, 1990). For example, Riley and Riley (1979) identified 33 percent of one hundred young stuttering children with articulation problems. In contrast to nonstuttering school-age control subjects, who typically demonstrate a difficulty in accurately producing speech sounds of 2 percent to 6.4 percent (Hull, Mieke, Timmons, & Willeford, 1971), well over half of children being seen for fluency intervention also have articulation disorders (Daly, 1981).

The co-occurrence of fluency disorders and language impairment is less well documented but has also been noted (Blood & Seider, 1981; Louko, Edwards, & Conture, 1990; Merits-Patterson & Reed, 1981; St. Louis & Hinzman, 1986; St. Louis, Murray, & Ashworth, 1991). Furthermore, the presence of coexisting disorders may not always be apparent at the outset of treatment. For example, a language impairment may only become evident after fluency has improved (Merits-Patterson & Reed, 1981). Although other voice or hearing problems have not been noted to occur with greater-than-typical frequency (Conture, 1990), these should be evaluated prior to the beginning of treatment.

Two Effects of Coexisting Problems

There are two basic issues the clinician must consider because of the possibility of coexisting communication problems. First, it has been observed by some clinical researchers that, on occasion, children who are being treated for language disorders become more disfluent as a consequence of treatment (Conture, 1990; Merits-Patterson & Reed, 1981; Meyers, Ghatak, & Woodford, 1990). Conture (1990) suggests that if a child is receiving treatment for severe articulation problems or unusual phonological problems, the possibility of stuttering onset may be increased. Treatment for articulation or language impairments also may precipitate fluency breaks if children are placed in treatment too early. That is, premature treatment may require the child to improve his articulation before he is capable of producing sounds correctly with relative ease and without excessive scanning or effort. As a result, treatment demands may exceed the child's still limited capacities for producing speech fluently. Conture (1990) notes that this may be most likely to occur for children who are approximately five to six years of age.

> We are inclined to speculate that increases in the length and complexity of verbally expressed languages increases the opportunities for instances of disfluency to emerge and is probably a natural byproduct of improved but still unstable expressive language skills. (p. 105)

Another therapeutic issue for children who are being treated for fluency and other impairments is the demonstrated "trading" relationships (Ratner,

1995) among the fluency, language, and phonological capabilities of the child. Such interaction has been suggested between fluency disorders and both language and phonological capacities (Crystal, 1987; Masterson, & Kamhi, 1992; Ratner & Sih, 1987; Stocker & Gerstman, 1983; Stocker & Usprich, 1976). This relationship has been particularly well documented for expressive syntax and fluency (Gaines, Runyan, & Meyers, 1991; Gordon, 1991; Gordon, Luper, & Peterson, 1986; Ratner & Sih, 1987; Stocker, 1980). The affiliation of a child's expressive and receptive capabilities is a major influence on clinical decision making for young children who stutter. That is, the clinician should introduce fluency skills at carefully graded levels of linguistic demand (Ratner, 1995; Stocker, 1980). According to Ratner:

> Imitation and modelling tasks designed to address syntactic or morphological deficits, shown to be most efficient clinically in inducing changes in expressive language performance[,] . . . may evoke fluency failure. Similarly, fluency practice, if structured in such a way that it does not address the demand it poses on a child's expressive language capacity, may not produce desired changes in fluency. (1995, p. 183).

As discussed in Chapter 2, such trade-off relationships and their resulting effect on a child's ability to produce fluent speech provide clinical support for a capacities and demands model (Adams, 1990; Starkweather & Gottwald, 1990). That is, at least for some young stuttering children, any task that requires a child to formulate complex ideas with greater levels of language demand may result in decreased fluency. In fact, that is what Weiss and Zebrowski (1992) found with eight child-parent pairs. When these young stuttering children (average age six years, eleven months) were asked to respond to questions requiring greater linguistic sophistication there was a greater occurrence of fluency breaks. That is, higher levels of language demand (Stocker & Usprich, 1976) resulted in significantly more disfluencies than lower-level parent requests. In addition, disfluent utterances were significantly longer and more complex than those produced fluently.

To Intervene or Not?

Although clinical decisions are made more complex with the presence of multiple problems, the answer to the question of whether to include in treatment a child who happens to have a fluency problem as well as other concomitant disorders is often "yes." Articulation and language problems require long-term treatment, and the clinician is unlikely to be able to wait until these problems are resolved before initiating treatment for fluency problems. Given the success that is likely for early intervention of fluency disorders, waiting may only complicate the problem. Conture (1990) provides some guidelines concerning whether a child should be seen for fluency intervention. He suggests that children with multiple problems should begin treatment as soon as possible if:

1. The child is producing two or more sound prolongations for every ten instances of stuttering.
2. The child breaks eye contact with the listener more than half the time during conversation.
3. The child exhibits concomitant speech sound articulation problems and especially if he produces phonological processes that are indicative of delays or deviations in phonological development.

Depending on the other associated problems, the clinician will have to decide whether the problems should be addressed sequentially or concurrently. Conture, Louko, and Edwards (1993) advocate a concurrent approach for children with both fluency and phonological problems, making use of a fluency-shaping protocol along with indirect phonological intervention. The clinician is cautioned, however, to avoid any overt correction of the child's speech. It is agreed by most authorities that children should not receive any direct feedback concerning the accuracy of their articulation, which would prevent possible communicative or emotional stress from impacting on the child's capacities. Obviously, each child will be very different, with unique capacities and responses to communication demands. Ratner (1993) indicates that subtle forms of feedback in the form of imitation, recasts, and selective emphasis on language structures that children are finding difficult may facilitate overall communication development. The clinician should feel free to model fluency-enhancing gestures in her own speech. Certainly, the child's response to linguistic as well as emotional demands must be carefully considered, both within and outside the treatment environment.

Ratner (1995) suggests that the blending of treatments (e.g., phonology and fluency) during a treatment session may work well for some children whose fluency system does not appear to be stressed by the requirements of feedback monitoring. However, if working on one aspect of speech or language production places stress on the child's ability to produce fluent speech, it may be better to sequence treatment, achieving a stable level in one area before tackling the other. This is a good example of the kind of clinical decision the experienced clinician must be entrusted to make. If fluency problems stem from problems of expressive language formulation, the clinician may choose to emphasize language intervention skills prior to fluency treatment. Obviously, as Ratner (1995) points out, an inappropriate justification for targeting language prior to, or in place of, fluency is the lack of confidence a clinician may have for conducting fluency therapy. Given the evidence concerning clinician attitudes about people who stutter and about treatment with this population of clients (see Chapter 1), this is a valid concern.

Finally, Ratner (1995) suggests some principles that clinicians can use for making clinical decisions for children with fluency and other concomitant problems:

1. The clinician should recognize that demands for phonological and grammatical processing compete with resources that permit fluent speech production.

2. The clinician should organize treatment hierarchically, proceeding from language and articulation activities that the child has established and stabilized to tasks that involve greater demands.

3. Even though it may slow progress in articulatory and linguistic growth, the clinician should structure intervention for children who stutter with minimum overt feedback.

4. The clinician, based on the child's individual capacities and responses to communicative demands, should determine whether a child's multiple impairments should be treated concurrently, sequentially, or cyclically. Furthermore, this strategy should be subject to change in the event that progress in one domain comes at the expense of regression in another.

Although children with multiple communication problems may require a greater amount of decision making by the clinician, all children, and indeed all clients, would probably benefit from the application of a similar policy. Intervention for all clients is likely to be most efficient when a careful analysis of the speaker's capacities and responses to demands are factored into the treatment strategy. Clients can, and should, be pushed to the upper ranges of their ability in order to help them to change the many features of their fluency disorder. The clinician working with young fluency-disordered children should be able to help the child to learn to *easily* produce difficult sounds or new grammatical structures without introducing the idea that they need be concerned or frightened or should struggle with their speech. It is possible to model a smooth and flowing manner of speech production while also giving the child a real sense of command over himself.

TRANSFER AND TERMINATION ISSUES

Prior to his dismissal from formal treatment, the clinician will want to determine how well the child has been able to transfer his new capabilities and techniques to the world outside the treatment setting. If the parents have been involved and if performance in extratreatment settings has been stressed from the outset, such transference is more likely to take place. Fortunately, as Conture (1991) points out, for many children the skills learned in the treatment setting transfer quite easily. The nature of change and progress during treatment is discussed in Chapter 8 in some detail. Peters and Guitar (1990) note that progress with younger children can be judged by such things as the improved use of techniques, decreased reliance on cuing by the clinician, increased control of fluency, taking risks, and decreased avoidance of speaking and speaking situations. As treatment progresses, there is a gradual shifting of the responsibility of increasing fluency from the clinician to the child and his parents. Group meetings are particularly helpful in this regard. The support and encouragement provided by parent groups does much to facilitate this change in responsibility.

Recommended criteria that the clinician may consider for the termination of formal treatment are provided by Gottwald and Starkweather (1995). Parents and teachers should feel confident about their ability to manage the child's improving fluency. These adults will need to assess and make independent decisions concerning how to alter fluency-disrupting stimuli such as time pressure and linguistic demands across a variety of social and educational settings. Parents need to be able to create an environment that corresponds to the child's capacity to maintain fluency. In addition, the young child should be normally fluent for his age. Some mild fluency breaks, particularly whole-word and phrase repetitions produced without effort, are unexceptional for three- to four-year-old children. Even fluency breaks produced with mild levels of tension may be acceptable if the clinician anticipates that the child will make continued improvement. Termination is also facilitated by a gradual phase-out of treatment that provides the clinician with the opportunity to monitor the child's progress. Ideally such monitoring should take place through age seven or eight, when basic skills underlying fluency are thought to be internalized. Finally, parents and teachers should be informed about the characteristics of relapse, made aware of the signs of incipient stuttering, and encouraged to contact the clinician if such indicators occur.

THE POSSIBILITY OF RELAPSE WITH CHILDREN

Unlike the situation for older speakers, the maintenance of the gains made during formal intervention is not usually a major problem with younger children. The available data indicates that once formal treatment has been successfully completed, the chance of regression is much less likely with children than it is with adolescents and adults who have been stuttering for much longer (Gottwald & Starkweather, 1995; Peters & Guitar, 1991; Starkweather, Gottwald, & Halfond, 1990). On the other hand, a comprehensive treatment program will include, at the very least, periodic checks for approximately two years following the end of formal treatment.

In a summary of the families seen from 1981 through 1990 at the Temple University Stuttering Prevention Center in Philadelphia, Gottwald and Starkweather (1995) indicate that:

Forty-eight of these families received individualized intervention services, ranging from parent counseling only to family counseling and direct therapy for the child. At the time these results were reported, three children and their families were still in therapy and seven families had withdrawn from the program for a variety of reasons. The remaining 45 youngsters and their families completed the program. All 45 children were speaking normally at the time of discharge. Follow-up telephone calls to each of the families 2 years following program completion revealed that fluency had been maintained according to parent report. (p. 124)

Starkweather (1995) estimates that the relapse rate following successful treatment for young children is approximately 2 percent.

Partial or even complete relapse can occur, of course, and one procedure that may prevent such regression may be the use of a "buddy system." This may be especially helpful for the child who is having difficult with motivation, carryover, or maintenance. When entering into new and difficult speaking situations outside the treatment setting, the presence of someone who understands the dynamics of the situation can have a powerful supporting effect. If the clinician or parent is not there, the presence of a speech buddy may be extremely beneficial. This strategy may be particularly useful with pre-adolescent or adolescent clients who tend to spend the vast majority of their time with people other than parents or clinicians.

SUGGESTIONS FOR THE CLASSROOM TEACHER

For school-age children, classroom teachers can also play a major role in facilitating therapeutic change (Ramig & Bennett, 1995). In some instances, the child's classroom teacher will have as much influence as the child's parents. In order for teachers to assume such a role, it is essential for them to have an appreciation of both the nature and treatment of stuttering. Of course, the character of the clinician-teacher relationship will depend somewhat on the model used for service delivery in the school. One possibility is a consultative model where the clinician works through the teacher and parents to help the child. A collaborative-consultative model has the clinician working with the child on an individual basis but also collaborating with the teacher and parents in planning appropriate activities in the child's daily world. A pullout model, where the children are taken out of the classroom and seen individually or in small groups by the clinician is probably the strategy that is least apt to create professional interaction as well as long-term change for the child (Gregory, 1995).

A most efficient first step for involving the classroom teacher is to present a workshop for teachers and related school personnel. Highly effective presentations can result from a basic discussion of one of the several informative videotapes available through such groups as the Stuttering Foundation of America or the National Stuttering Project (see Appendix B). Pamphlets, which are also available from these groups, can be distributed and questions concerning fluency and fluency disorders addressed. Nearly everyone is interested in stuttering, and it is usually relatively easy to draw an audience for these presentations.

Suggestions for the classroom teacher can be found in several sources (Cooper, 1979a; Dell, 1970; Van Riper, 1973, pp. 446–450). It is far better for the teacher to be proactive regarding a stuttering child in the classroom. Certainly this makes more sense than waiting for a child who stutters to appear in class and then seeking advice for how to best respond to the situation. Furthermore, with information provided by the clinician concerning the nature of both the surface and intrinsic features of stuttering, the teacher will be much more likely to recognize a child with a fluency disorder. As the classroom teacher understands the dynamics of the syndrome, especially patterns of avoidance, postponement, and escape behavior, he or she will be in a much better position to help.

As the goals and techniques of treatment are explained to the child's teacher, she or he is likely to become involved in treatment. As with parents, it is often better to show, rather than tell, this colleague what takes place during your treatment sessions with the child. Such demonstrations are especially important if a pullout, rather than a classroom intervention, program is used. As the classroom teacher recognizes that a child is choosing to participate in class in spite of some stuttering events, the teacher can reward that response (either during or following the event, and either verbally or nonverbally). When a child successfully uses a fluency-modification technique in the classroom, the teacher will recognize it and know how to respond. When a child alters his usual tense and fragmented speech into a more open and forward-moving pattern, the teacher can reward the accomplishment. Until the teacher is able to interpret these seemingly small events as victories, they will go unrecognized and unrewarded. As the teacher takes part in treatment with the child, the choice of how to respond to the child in the classroom, playground, or the school lunch room will be apparent. The teacher will be much more likely to discuss the problem with the child and be another important source of support and encouragement in the child's daily school environment.

The clinician should alert classroom teachers that one possible outcome of successful treatment is increased participation, increased speaking, and, possibly, an increase in the occurrence of fluency breaks. As the child becomes successful at decreasing his avoidance behaviors and increasing speech assertiveness and risk taking, one possible result may be greater participation in the classroom. Prior to treatment, the child may have been an "ideal" student, sitting quietly. Following successful treatment he may start to talk to his friends and, on occasion, stutter more as a result of his increased involvement in classroom activities.

Perhaps one of the most important concepts the clinician can impart to the classroom teacher is the notion that, unless she is nearly completely insensitive, she is not likely to unintentionally harm the child who stutters. The clinician can provide a great service to teachers by informing them of this fact. Yes, it is possible for an inappropriate insensitive teacher to make things somewhat worse for the child who stutterers. Clearly such people do exist, as reflected by reports of that sort in the National Stuttering Project publication, *Letting Go*. More often than not, however, classroom teachers are well intentioned and need to be allowed to respond naturally without fear of somehow damaging "this fragile child who stutters."

Many suggestions provided to parents can be applied, with slight modification, to the classroom teacher as well. For example, although there may be some exceptions, children who stutter should generally not be permitted to escape from school assignments and responsibilities. Just as the other children are required to take their turn, the child who happens to stutter must also take his turn in reciting, reading, and answering questions. To allow a child to escape these responsibilities may foster more harassment from his peers than the fact that he sometimes stutters. Some children who are fluent also would, if they could, choose not to have to face the trials of class participation. These decisions, of course, vary with the child and the circumstances, and it would be inappropriate to say that a child must always be required to take part in every speaking situation. However, the exceptions should be rare. Even children who stutter severely are able to take part in class presentations or plays. When the teacher understands that children who stutter are unlikely to stutter when playing a role, speaking with a dialect, singing, or speaking in unison with other children, the teacher is apt to have the child participate. At the very least, the child could have a nonspeaking part or play a character that makes mechanical or animal sounds.

As the teacher begins to appreciate the effect of time pressure on fluency, she or he may decide, on occasion, to call on the child unexpectedly or early in the class, when he is less likely to stutter. The child can then relax a bit and attend to the rest of the class. By understanding the dynamics of fluency-enhancing or -disrupting stimuli for a particular child, the teacher may choose to call on him when the anticipated response is a short—perhaps one-word—answer. Of course, the teacher can reward the child for not avoiding the opportunity to participate. With the assistance of the clinician, the teacher can talk privately with the child before or after class so there can be an understanding about what will or did occur. Stuttering can be a serious topic, but the teacher can become desensitized and show the child that it is possible to openly and easily discuss the problem.

Like parents, teachers can be shown the powerful effects of listener loss on the child's fluency. The ability of the teacher to remain calm, even during a moment of severe stuttering, communicates much to the child. Nonverbal indicators of anxiety and avoidance, such as becoming tense or rigid, turning away, or breaking eye contact, can be monitored and changed with some practice. Voluntary stuttering during role-playing activities with the clinician or other teachers and desensitization activities using videotapes also can be very helpful. Generally, but again with some few exceptions, the teacher should not help the child say a word when he is experiencing an extended long block. There may be some occasions when there is no other choice but to help the child, but this should be a rare event.

Certainly the teacher should not let other children interrupt a child while he is stuttering. Similarly, it is never beneficial for the teacher to suggest to the child that he stop and think about what he is going to say. Such comments simply show the naivete of the listener concerning the nature of stuttering. A better response is for the teacher to restate to the class what the child has said. That is, even though the child may have struggled through his comments, the teacher can increase the value of what the child said by paraphrasing his words. Such a restating of the child's words gives them increased importance and allows the other children in the class to appreciate the content of the child's response. It may take some practice to do this gracefully, but providing such a response is clearly much better than reacting with silence and pretending that nothing has occurred or giving the impression that what the child has said is unimportant. Such an open and forthright response by the teacher also carries a strong statement of acceptance of the child and what he said.

Perhaps most important, the classroom teacher can become an advocate for the child. If classroom teachers react negatively to a child who stutters it is most likely due to a lack of understanding. By showing understanding, being available to the child, and rewarding what she or he recognizes as progress in the direction of behavioral and attitude change, the teacher, like the parent, can be a powerful force for decreasing the handicapping impact of stuttering and for preventing the maintenance and further development of the syndrome.

A comment about teasing by other children is in order. Obviously, such activities in the classroom should be off-limits. However, there will be situations where the teacher will not be able to prevent this behavior by other children, and, in some cases, it will occur to some degree. Certainly the teacher or parent may discuss the injustice of such behavior with those involved, but of course, this may not help, and in fact, it may increase the problem in some cases. In some instances, educating the children in the class about stuttering may be helpful. Having an adult who has undergone successful treatment speak to the class may be a good option. Volunteers for such discussions may be located at nearby clinics or local chapters of self-help groups. Silverman (1996) suggests that the classroom teacher can help the child to bring the problem out into the open by having him discuss information about stuttering and perhaps describing the accomplishments of the many highly successful and famous people who have stuttered. How to best proceed will depend on the dynamics of the situation, including the child's personality characteristics and response to various suggestions.

Finally, role-playing with the children who are involved in teasing the child or, at the very least, with the clinician and the child can provide a good way to desensitize him. This may be the only option if others involved in the situation refuse to cooperate. Role-playing activities (see also Chapter 6) will also provide the opportunity for the child to ventilate his frustration and anger.

For example, the clinician and the child can take turns giving and receiving specific taunts and insulting comments. Each can gradually become desensitized to the expected comments and discuss alternative responses. The child can practice a series of verbal and nonverbal responses to teasing. Depending on the particular child, a humorous response may be considered as an alternative reaction. The child may be able to defuse or redirect the sting of the comments by acknowledging the obvious and directing the comments of others back to them. For example, the child may say: "Yes, as a matter of fact I do stutter. But what you said was stupid and mean." In addition, depending on the circumstances and possibly the size of the children involved, the child may want to add, "And tomorrow I might no longer stutter but you may still be stupid and mean." Alternately, in response to other children imitating a child's moment of stuttering, he may say something like: "Look, if you're going to stutter you ought to learn how to do it correctly. Prolong the first sound like this and add a little more tension. If you get really good at it and you're brave enough, try it with me in class tomorrow."

Last, it is important to recognize that the clinician may choose to make referrals to other professionals such as reading specialists, physicians, psychologists, social workers, and audiologists. As Conture (1990) points out, the clinician is often the first person to recognize the possibility of other problems.

EXAMPLES OF FLUENCY PROGRAMS

Although representative, the following list is far from exhaustive, for there are many excellent programs being conducted by experienced and highly qualified clinicians. The purpose of this listing is to indicate the general principles that are employed in treating children. Further descriptions of these and other programs for children (as well as adults) may also be found in Bloodstein (1993, pp. 157–165) and Ramig and Bennett (1995).

Programs for Younger Children

The Fluency Development System for Young Children (TFDS). Developed by Meyers and Woodford (1992), this is a cognitive, fluency-shaping approach. The program includes procedures for assessment and intervention that are comprehensive but easy to follow. Child-centered activities follow "fluency rules" that emphasize slow versus fast speech, smooth versus bumpy speech, and turn taking. Children become desensitized to time pressure and difficult speaking situations. In addition, there is a parent education and counseling scheme, which includes thirteen behavioral exercises.

The Stuttering Intervention Program (SIP). The SIP is a program developed by Pindzola (1987) for young children age three through nine (grade three). The program consists of assessment procedures, parent counseling, and intervention procedures. Also included is a protocol for differentiating incipient stuttering and normal fluency breaks. This fluency-shaping program includes formatted individualized educational plans and informational handouts for both parents and teachers.

Systematic Fluency Training for Young Children. This program was created by Shine (1980) for young children between the ages of three and nine. It is a highly structured program that includes both assessment and intervention strategies. Using a fluency-shaping approach, it makes use of picture identification, a storybook, picture matching, and spontaneous speech. Parental involvement is emphasized.

Easy Does It—One. This program was developed by Heinze and Johnson (1985) as a fluency-shaping program for preschool children through grade two. The program consists of five phases: (a) experiencing fluency, (b) establishing fluency, (c) desensitizing to fluency disrupters, (d) transferring fluency, and (e) maintaining fluency. During each stage, parents are provided with activities for use in the home.

Programs for Older Children

Personalized Fluency Control Therapy (PFC). Developed by Cooper and Cooper (1985b), this program provides the clinician with procedures for directly modifying the child's stuttering using fluency-initiating gestures. Each gesture or technique is associated with a character in order to help the children conceptualize the nature of fluency and specific modification techniques. Changes in the child's affective, cognitive, and behavioral features are an integral part of the program.

The Successful Stuttering Management Program (SSMP). Developed by Breitenfeldt and Lorenz (1989), this is a comprehensive stuttering-modification approach designed for older adolescents and adults. Although the program is designed as an intensive treatment, many of the procedures can be used in a less intensive environment. The program includes both assessment and intervention phases that are well organized and easy to follow. The notebook that accompanies this program contains session-by-session outlines (including assignments) that focus on affective, cognitive, and behavioral features of stuttering experiences. Suggestions for transfer and maintenance activities are included.

Easy Does It—Two. Created by Heinze and Johnson (1987), this eclectic approach makes use of both fluency and stuttering modification principles. It is designed for children ages seven through thirteen. The program consists of six stages stressing: (a) preparing for fluency, (b) distinguishing fluency from stuttering, (c) establishing fluency, (d) desensitizing to fluency disrupters, (e) transferring fluency, and (f) maintaining fluency.

Gradual Increase in Length and Complexity of Utterance (GILCU). Developed by Bruce Ryan and Barbara Van Kirk (1974), GILCU is a programmed, behavioral, fluency-shaping model. It was one of the earliest programs in behavioral treatment to be widely used. The program makes use of operant-conditioning principles using verbal reward for fluency and verbal punishment for stuttering. The program is best used with the younger child who has not developed many cognitive and attitudinal features. The program takes the child through the three phases of establishment, transfer, and maintenance, with gradually increasing length and complexity of child utterances (GILCU) as the child proceeds from reading, monologue, and conversation. When necessary, fluency is established using delayed auditory feedback, with the child being instructed to speak in a monotone, slur his articulation, and prolong sounds. Transfer activities take the child from treatment to a variety of extratreatment settings. Follow-up evaluations take place at posttreatment intervals of two weeks and monthly intervals of one, three, six, and twelve months. If a child exceeds a specific threshold of fluency breaks during these evaluations, he is cycled back through the program.

Extended Length of Utterance (ELU). Developed by Costello (1983), this is also a fluency-shaping program that makes use of operant and learning principles. The program controls for linguistic complexity as the child is taken through establishment, transfer, and maintenance procedures.

The Fluency Rules Program (FRP). Developed by Runyan and Runyan (1986), this is a fluency-shaping program that has been designed for use in a school environment. The program incorporates seven rules for fluent speech production, which include (a) speaking slowly, (b) learning to breathe for speech, (c) touching the "speech helpers" together lightly, (d) using only the speech helpers to talk, (e) keeping the speech helpers moving, (f) keeping "Mr. Voice Box" running smoothly, and (g) saying a word only once. The linguistic demands of the speaking tasks are considered. Children are taken through stages of self-monitoring, transfer, and maintenance.

Speak More Fluently, Stutter More Fluently. Developed by Gregory (1991), this program uses fluency-shaping procedures with school-age children. The program emphasizes relaxed speech production with additional modification of any remaining stuttering behaviors. The fluency-shaping procedures stressed include the use of smooth, slower-than-normal transitions on the first two sounds of a word or utterance and an easy initiation of phonation with smooth articulatory movement during the utterance. Emphasis is also placed on the child maintaining normal rate, intensity, and inflection. The program incorporates learning principles and a variable lesson plan format, which can be used to individualize the treatment for each child.

Cafet-for-Kids. Developed by Goebel (1989), this program involves eclectic fluency and is patterned after the CAFET program for adults. The program makes use of a computer-assisted self-monitoring system (CAFET) that allows the child to regulate and change the usual fluency-enhancing targets such as a full inspiratory breath coupled with a slow exhalation of air. The computer program also provides for visual reinforcement as children achieve treatment goals.

CONCLUSION

Although treatment is often highly successful with young children who stutter, it will take the involvement of the child's parents and teachers. Stuttering is generally less complex with younger clients, and the difficulties of transfer, maintenance, and relapse usually take considerably less time and effort than with older speakers. Nevertheless, the clinician faces major decisions concerning the directness of intervention, the overall strategy of treatment, and when and how to intervene if additional communication problems are present. The clinician will play a significant role in educating and counseling the client's parents in order to lessen the guilt and misinformation that may have grown up around the problem. As parents gain greater understanding and control of the developmental aspects of stuttering, they will more likely become a powerful force in facilitating their child's fluency. By considering both the child's capacities for speech production and the demands placed on him, the parents and the clinician can enhance his ability to achieve fluency in a variety of speaking situations, both inside and outside the treatment setting. Classroom teachers also play a major role as they come to understand the dynamics of this communication problem and the nature of the treatment process. The clinician can provide valuable information that will increase the ability of the classroom teachers to identify fluency problems and assist the child in participating in daily classroom activities.

RECOMMENDED READINGS

Dell, C. (1970). *Treating the school age stutter: A guide for clinicians* (Publication No. 14). Memphis, TN: Speech Foundation of America.

Letting Go, A publication of the National Stuttering Project, Anaheim Hills, CA. See Appendix B for address and related information.

Starkweather, C. W., Gottwald, S. R., & Halfond, M. M. (1990). *Stuttering prevention: A clinical method.* Englewood Cliffs, NJ: Prentice-Hall.

Van Riper, C. (1973). *The treatment of stuttering* (2nd ed.). Englewood Cliffs, NJ: Prentice-Hall. See Ch. 14, pp. 371–425 (on the treatment of the beginning stutterer).

CHAPTER 6

Treatment for Adolescents and Adults

INTRODUCTION

Earlier in this text we discussed the nature of stuttering onset and development. Although these previous chapters did not discuss the specifics of treatment, it should be apparent that understanding stuttering behavior, and particularly the characteristics of the person who is doing the stuttering, is essential for establishing successful intervention. Understanding the intrinsic nature of the person who is asking for help is fundamental to making wise clinical decisions. Silverman puts it well when he says, "The better able you are to understand the problems your clients will encounter as they try to change, the better able you will be to help them do so" (1996, p. 170).

It is good to begin with a note of optimism regarding treatment for adolescents and adults who stutter, for there is plenty of literature that is confusing or not so encouraging. Because of the volume of information and the many uncertainties about the important issues of etiology, treatment, and relapse, the literature can be discouraging for clinicians interested in helping speakers with fluency disorders. It is no secret that many clinicians are unsure of general strategies and specific techniques to employ with clients who come to us with fluency disorders. Students graduating with a master's degree are no longer required to receive specific training in fluency disorders.

They are required, however, to receive experience with a wide variety of communication disorders (e.g., language and learning disabilities, aphasia, motor-speech problems, dysphagia, neurogenics, augmentative communication, and multicultural aspects of diagnostics and treatment). Fluency disorders, an area that for many years was at the core of the academic and clinical experience of students, is often omitted from the student's program or given far less than adequate emphasis. As a result, many clinicians actively avoid, or at the very least, are anxious about, the possibility of working with children and adults with fluency disorders (Conture, 1990; Silverman, 1992). Over the years I have spoken with students who had been told by past instructors that treatment for fluency disorders was rarely successful and that the student would be well advised to concentrate on those clients who were more likely to make progress.

THE LIKELIHOOD OF SUCCESS

Successful treatment for fluency disorders must take place with an acceptance on the part of the clinician that the problem is complex. This is also a communication problem that takes time—often years—to change, especially for adults who have been stuttering for decades. On the other hand, it is also important to appreciate that this syndrome is probably no more enigmatic than many other problems that humans can have. Andrews, Guitar, and Howie (1980) provide one of the few positive comments suggesting that stuttering, although complex, is reasonably well understood and not so terribly difficult to treat. Using a mathematical technique called meta-analysis, these authors compared the results of forty-two treatment investigations and found treatment for stuttering to be effective and stable over time. In addition, Howie, Tanner, and Andrews (1981) followed thirty-six adult stutterers for up to eighteen months posttreatment and found that adult clients have a 70 percent chance of gaining substantially improved speech as well as increased speaking confidence.

Another note of optimism is that working with children and adults who stutter is enjoyable. With few exceptions, fluency treatment results in varying degrees of positive change in the client's perspective of the problem, level of fluency, and in some cases, general approach to life and relationships. Just as most athletic activities are much more than the sum of many individual skills, the process of treatment is much more than the application of techniques to be mastered. As a matter of fact, it may be argued that the consequences of overemphasizing therapeutic microskills leads to ineffective treatment. As Rogers (1980) contends, treatment for human behavioral problems is a *fully human endeavor*.

A PHILOSOPHICAL PERSPECTIVE

The process of growth goes well beyond treatment techniques and behavioral changes. Important cognitive and affective changes must also occur. On occasion, as the client grows the clinician grows also, for the most effective clinicians are nearly always learning. They are making real-time decisions about the needs of the client, and many times these needs are not apparent. Thus, while the treatment process for fluency disorders can be complex, it is often dynamic and exciting.

The success of treatment requires commitment and motivation by the client. Although Peck (1978) is reflecting on the nature of psychotherapy in his book, *The Road Less Traveled,* his comments easily apply to any treatment that requires behavioral as well as cognitive change. He suggests that, of the choices one may have in dealing with a problem, treatment is usually the more difficult path. This is so, he argues, because each of us is always working against entropy, as manifested within the individual in the form of laziness. Laziness takes the form of fear associated with changing one's view of reality and the resulting changes in the status quo. Peck indicates that as many as nine out of ten patients who begin psychotherapy (or any other therapy) stop long before the clinician believes that the process has been completed. Often, after the clients experience a degree of success and a corresponding lessening of the problem, the cost-benefit ratio decreases and further change is no longer worth the effort. Unfortunately, this is also the case for clients with fluency disorders.

It is also worth noting that there are some influential forces against which the clinician and the client must work during treatment. For example, there are old ways of seeing the problem and oneself. In order to change, there may be a period of holding on to the old perceptions and the old self. This is more likely, of course, with adults. We show them new ways of viewing which, although often attractive, also indicate that the old ways are in error. Several authors (Emerick, 1988; Hayhow & Levy, 1989; Peck, 1978) acknowledge that the loss of the old belief system is a blow to the client. For example, Kuhlman (1984) suggests that a "mourning process" is necessary for the loss of the old belief system. New insights about the shortcomings of the old system of beliefs are a blow to a client's narcissism or self-esteem. This effect is not always a major problem during treatment, but it is likely to occur to some degree and thus to provide some resistance to change.

THE TREATMENT OF CHOICE

When reading through the literature on treatment efficacy, it is possible for the clinician to get the feeling that what is being contrasted is the dogma of political or even religious positions. Each writer invites the reader to take a stand concerning the treatment of this problem. To be sure, the logic and techniques associated with most intervention strategies provide the clinician with a framework and a sense of direction about the syndrome and its treatment. Each strategy comes with its own doctrine. Each of these approaches can provide something of value for the clinician and her client, depending on such variables as the needs of the client, the stage of treatment, and the talent and experience of the clinician.

Most treatment strategies are reasonably straightforward and relatively easy to understand. This is not, after all, rocket science. However, while the concepts themselves are not difficult to understand, it is considerably more difficult to put them to use with a client. It is one thing to be able to remember textbook information for an examination and quite another to respond to a person with an appropriate and perceptive clinical decision *during* treatment. Despite what may be written in a text or treatment manual, the most appropriate clinical choice is not always obvious, even to the experienced clinician. Whatever the structure of the treatment program, the process of change is far more than the use of the dogma of a treatment method and associated criteria. Real intervention for human communication problems is dynamic. At its finest, treatment is the clinician's astute and precise response to the *person* who has come for help. These responses become more likely as treatment progresses and the clinician becomes calibrated to the client. Depending on the client, the clinician may use a variety of techniques and possibly more than one overall treatment strategy. Even if a single overall strategy is used, the application will never be quite the same with each client, for individuals often respond differently to identical techniques.

LEADING FROM BEHIND

Conducting treatment with fluency disorders is similar to many other relationships, both therapeutic and otherwise. Certainly, as clinicians, we must have a clear direction about where treatment is leading. However, it is also true that if we too closely control the relationship, we may narrow the possibilities for change and growth. Unquestionably, the clinician must have an overall plan and a direction for treatment and must be familiar with many associated treatment techniques. However, we cannot control all aspects of the other person and make him into our own image of him. Our goal is to help him to self-manage his handicap, and we can direct that process. However, sometimes it is clear that we have to lead from behind, following the client where he needs to go and helping him to get there. We can assist him in developing new views of himself and new options concerning his fluency. With the right timing in response to changes by the client, we can help him to make better choices and to become less handicapped. We can also acknowledge that while we provide direction, insight, and information, the person who must ultimately take the lead in repairing the problem is the client.

The purpose of this chapter is to discuss the direction and logic of treatment as well as to introduce specific treatment techniques for adolescents and adults with fluency disorders. The clinician must know the choices that are available in terms of overall treatment strategies and associated applications. However, the mark of an experienced clinician is not knowing what strategies or techniques to use. Every clinician should have that information. The mark of an effective clinician is reflected in her clinical insight about *why* and *when* to employ it.

THE GOALS OF TREATMENT

Of course it is necessary to have a good idea where we want to go during treatment. One of the first objectives during the initial treatment sessions is to demonstrate our sense of direction to the client by providing a map of the journey (see Cooper, 1985, and Maxwell, 1982, for excellent examples of pretreatment orientation statements). It is important for the client to have a clear understanding of the treatment process, and success is more likely to occur if both the client and the clinician share a similar view. At the outset of treatment the client's concept of his fluency disorder itself is apt to be ambiguous. The clinician who is able to help the client decrease the mystery and understand the lawfulness of the stuttering syndrome provides a valuable service to the client. Before the client can begin to accurately monitor and self-manage himself and his speech, he must begin to appreciate the nature of the problem in general and the dynamics of his own, specific response to his situation.

Levels of Fluency

Speakers that are regarded as normally fluent demonstrate a wide range of fluency across different situations. As discussed in Chapter 3, this range of fluency is greatest in speakers who stutter. When considering the goals of treatment, authors have found it useful to distinguish at least three levels of fluency (Peters & Guitar, 1991).

Spontaneous fluency can be thought of as ideally normal speech. The speech is smooth and may contain only sporadic fluency breaks, which are formulative in nature. Speech flows easily with little apparent effort, and virtually no attention is paid to how the speech is produced. The speaker as well as the listener are able to attend to the message, and the speaker's fluency does not detract from the information being delivered. Although relatively rare, it is possible for some clients who stutter, even adult clients, to eventually achieve this level of spontaneous fluency in all speaking situations.

Controlled fluency is nearly normal speech production but with the price of increased effort on the part of the speaker. Although the speaker must attend to his manner of speaking in order to maintain fluency, the speech moves forward with few obvious fluency breaks. There is a price to be paid in the form of vigilance and self-management of those fluency breaks, which could otherwise go out of control. This effort, to the degree that it is perceived by the listener, may detract somewhat from the message. Thus, the method and the message of speaking may carry nearly equal weight. Depending on the ability of the speaker to apply techniques that facilitate the smooth coordination of respiration, phonation, and articulation, this type of fluency may be perceived as *Unstable speech*, as discussed in Chapter 3. In many ways, this type of fluency is similar to that of a normal speaker who is placed in a speaking situation that contains a high level of communicative or emotional stress.

Acceptable fluency takes the level of monitoring and self-management of the speaker to another stage. Now the effort to maintain fluency is increased and the method of producing speech may be slightly more obvious than the content of the message. Even though stuttering events are occurring, the speaker is actively changing the form of these events. This is far less than ideal fluency but much preferred to the client's old, automatic, reflexive form of stuttering. Although stuttering is taking place, because these events are undergoing modification or smoothing it is possible for the speaker and the listener to achieve a high degree of satisfaction and contentment. Although more research is needed, there is some suggestion in the literature that people who do something about their problems are regarded more positively than those who do not (Blood & Blood, 1982; Collins & Blood, 1990; Hastorf, Windfogel, & Cassman, 1979; Silverman, 1988a). Most important, however, it is possible for the speaker, despite the presence of some stuttering, to make decisions that result in a significant decrease in the handicap of the fluency disorder.

Achieving Spontaneous Fluency

Even for the most severe clients, the quickest way to reduce the frequency of stuttering is to have the speaker use a number of techniques or devices that result in nearly instantaneous fluency. It is well known that immediate, if temporary, fluency can be achieved by having most clients sing, read, or speak in unison with another person; speak in a loud or whispered voice, use a dialect or bouncy intonation, or speak while rhythmically moving a finger, arm, or leg. In addition, devices that provide for auditory masking of the speaker's voice production, a pacing tone, such as a metronome, or an audio delay in the speaker's speech also tend to result in less frequent, or at least less severe, stuttering events. The fluency-enhancing effects of these activities have been attributed to both the rhythmic effects (Van Riper, 1973) and the modification of phonation (Wingate, 1969).

These fluency-enhancing activities can provide highly dramatic results, and such instantaneous improvements tend to have the effect of making anyone who uses them an "expert" on how to help people who stutter. Although many early stuttering and stammering schools were built around some of these efforts, the effects on the speaker's fluency are generally short-lived (Silverman, 1976). In instances where the speaker has been unable to achieve lasting benefit from other treatment methods, such devices have been advocated. For chronic stutterers (Cooper, 1986a) such devices may provide the only way to effectively communicate. Although these devices are helpful, it is usually best if the speaker can systematically wean himself from their use.

The achievement of *spontaneous* fluency is often the primary outcome many of our clients ask of us. However, should the achievement of spontaneous fluency be held as the only criterion for successful treatment? Spontaneous fluency is more likely to be a reasonable goal for young children. Something approaching complete fluency is also attainable for the rare adult who, as a result of emotional trauma, has experienced a sudden onset of stuttering in adulthood. As the underlying or associated problems becomes resolved, these speakers may be able to achieve their previous levels of fluency.

High levels of posttreatment fluency may also occur for adults who stutter if the speaker is taking part in an intensive, residential program. However, because of logistic or financial reasons, that is not where many clients find help. In addition, the difficult transition from the focused and supportive clinical environment of an intensive program back to the client's home and work environments usually has an adverse effect on the gains made during formal treatment. It has been suggested that rapid and dramatic improvements that can occur in an intensive program may result in a fluent speaker who is unsure what he did to accomplish change (Boberg, 1986; see p. 491). Prins (1970) indicated that intensive, residential programs may produce *disfluency overkill* and provide the client with the notion that stuttering will not occur as long as he follows the techniques he has mastered. Kamhi (1982) cautions clinicians who suggest to clients that the use of fluency-shaping techniques will result in error-free speech on all occasions. Perhaps the best statement in this regard was Sheehan's (1980) comment that producing stutter-free speech is no more realistic than playing error-free baseball. He reasoned that because the person possesses the capacity to function in an error-free manner it does not follow that this will always be the case.

Thus, for most adults who have stuttered since childhood, some fluency breaks are the rule. The question is not so much whether the client will stutter, especially in more difficult speaking situations. In may instances, he will. The more basic question is *how* he is going to stutter and what he is going to do about each stuttering event. As Van Riper often stated, the speaker may not always have much of a choice about when he is going to stutter, but he certainly can have a choice about how he is going to stutter (Van Riper, 1990).

This is not to say that it is impossible to achieve fluency levels approaching 100 percent both within and outside the treatment setting. However, it is not necessarily realistic to expect such levels of fluency before dismissing the client from treatment. Using a stringent criterion of 100 percent fluency is problematic for other reasons. First of all, this measure of success places far too much emphasis on a single surface feature of the syndrome: the frequency of stuttering. Decreasing the occurrence of overt stuttering events is clearly one of the things clinicians can target during treatment. For many others, however, it provides a compressed view of progress and success.

It is not surprising that the surface features of the stuttering syndrome will be the first to change. A client will often demonstrate rapid improvement in his level of fluency prior to or during the initial days or weeks of treatment.

Much of this change is a result of the client acknowledging his problem and adapting to the clinician, the treatment setting, and the client's understanding of his role during treatment. The client's fluency improves as he understands what is expected of him and what challenges he is asked to meet. Certainly, an increase in fluency is reflective of change. However, it may not necessarily indicate progress. That is, the increased fluency in the treatment setting may have little relationship to the client's level of fluency in his daily environment. Even complete fluency in a clinical environment can provide an unrealistic indication about the probability of such success in extratreatment speaking situations. It is one thing to hit ten out of ten shots when playing basketball alone, but the real question is how many shots will be successful during competitive game conditions, when the pressure is great and performance counts.

As obvious as overt fluency breaks may be and as much as they get in the way, there is much more to the syndrome of stuttering than these surface events. It is tempting to focus the majority of the diagnostic and treatment efforts on the surface features while failing to consider changes in the intrinsic features of the syndrome, which are nonetheless important, both for a comprehensive diagnosis and for lasting therapeutic change. Most authors suggest that, at least with adolescents and adults, a truly comprehensive treatment strategy should be multidimensional (Hillis, 1993; Prins, 1970; Van Riper, 1973). That is, the criterion of success in treatment is considerably broader than a relatively simplistic measure of the number of fluency breaks. Assuming that the syndrome of stuttering involves, not only surface behaviors, but also attitudinal and cognitive features, it will be necessary to promote changes across these features as well.

Although spontaneous fluency is both a reasonable and an attainable goal for some clients, many people tire of treatment before such levels of fluency are reached. They reach the point where they are less handicapped and the fluency breaks, although still present, no longer present a large threat to the quality of life. In addition, there are some clients, especially those described in Chapter 4 as chronic stutterers, who are unable to make lasting progress toward high levels of fluency. Even speakers with frequent fluency breaks can learn to revise features of their stuttering and adjust to listener reactions in order to become less handicapped.

VARIABLES IN CHOOSING A TREATMENT

There are several basic treatment characteristics that are influenced by such things as the clinical setting and the client's needs and capabilities. These characteristics often require the clinician to make decisions about the form that treatment will take. In some instances, the choices are already made for the clinician according to the nature of the treatment setting or the options that are available because of such issues as time and expense (Starkweather, St. Louis, Blood, Peters, & Westbrook, 1994).

The Timing and Duration of Treatment

There is considerable variation here, ranging from intensive, residential programs lasting six or more hours each day or one or more weeks to treatment in public schools, which may take place as little as one hour or less each week. Generally, adolescents and adults who stutter require a longer time in treatment. Preschool clients require a shorter time and often make faster progress. Treatment that is less intensive disrupts the client's everyday life less, but the change involved can be slow and the client may become discouraged. On the other hand, intensive treatment often results in more rapid change (Prins, 1970), with the likelihood of greater problems when it comes time to transfer the gains made in the clinical setting to the speaker's everyday life. The duration of treatment also can be influenced by such factors as the complexity of the fluency disorder, other coexisting communication problems, and especially, the client's motivation. For adult speakers, formal treatment lasting one year with at least one individual and one group meeting each week seems to be regarded as a minimum (Maxwell, 1982; Van Riper, 1973).

The Complexity of Treatment

A client's degree of handicap across the social, educational, and vocational aspects of his life will be a major factor in determining the course and length of intervention. Furthermore, the client's personality and emotional characteristics such as defensive behaviors, coping strategies, resistance to change, anxiety, inhibited behavior, or even, on occasion, depression or sociopathic behavior can also increase the length and complexity of treatment. In such instances, treatment may require the use of many strategies and techniques as well as other professional clinicians in areas such as counseling, psychology, or psychiatry.

The Cost of Treatment

This important aspect of treatment also varies widely. Because of the typical length of treatment, the cost of successful treatment can quickly become prohibitive for many clients. Fees for diagnosis and treatment are generally lower when there are restrictions on the intensity of service, as in some training programs. Service in these settings can be secondary to the academic and clinical training requirements of the program. The level of service can also be compromised somewhat in public or private school settings, where caseload requirements may vary widely.

The Treatment Setting

The treatment that is provided is often determined in large measure by the setting. In this regard, St. Louis and Westbrook (1987) provide an insightful comment explaining that the choice of treatment may not be made with the client as the primary consideration.

> It seems plausible that typical delivery models for stuttering therapy evolved as much to suit clinicians' tastes, administrators' desires, school, university, or hospital schedules, or physicians' prescriptions as they did to provide the maximum benefit to stutterers. (1987, p. 250)

The treatment strategies and techniques the clinician selects may or may not coincide with the available environment. That is, the clinician may want to schedule the client for several sessions each week, but this may not be possible due to the logistics of the client's work schedule and distance from the treatment center. The clinician may consider parent participation to be critical for success, but the parents may be employed in one or more jobs and unable or unwilling to attend sessions. Individual treatment may be necessary, but yet the caseload in the clinical facility (particularly in the public schools) will only allow for group treatment, sometimes with clients who possess a variety of other communication problems.

In addition, the opportunity for monitored practice outside the clinic or school setting is essential. Often, however, because of logistic, legal, insurance, or time constraints, the clinician may be unable to go with the child or adult to more realistic speaking situations in offices, restaurants, or shopping malls. This is an important feature, for as the American Speech-Language-Hearing Association *Guidelines for Practice in Stuttering Treatment* (Starkweather, St. Louis, Blood, Peters, & Westbrook, 1994) suggests, treatment settings that fail to create such experiences also may fail to provide realistic indications of change or progress. At the very least, the clinician should create opportunities to monitor the client's performance in the form of direct observation, interviews with the client following practice sessions, or monitoring with audio- or videorecordings of extra-treatment practice. The logistics of distance, cost, and location of the treatment setting may prevent many desired features of treatment from occurring, and often this cannot be helped. At the very least, however, the client should be made aware of any important limitations of treatment.

TREATMENT STRATEGIES

The first decision for the clinician when initiating treatment is the choice of a general intervention strategy. There are many paths for the clinician to follow, each with something to offer. We will begin by simplifying the situation and discussing the most popular paths currently being taken: fluency modification and stuttering modification. We will also discuss a third, less frequently used, strategy, which may be called cognitive restructuring. To take the possibilities a bit further, the *Guidelines for Practice* referred to above indicates a total of ten treatment goals involving a variety of treatment choices. Clinicians should be familiar with each of these goals.

The essential difference between fluency modification, stuttering modification, and cognitive restructuring is best illustrated by considering the relative emphasis placed on the surface and intrinsic features of the syndrome. Fluency-shaping approaches tend to focus on the surface features of the syndrome. That is, the physical attributes of stuttering in terms of the normal or dysfunctional use of the respiratory, phonatory, and articulatory systems are central to the treatment process. This approach might be thought of as *physical therapy for the speech production system*. The primary goal with this treatment strategy is to modify the surface features of the syndrome and not (as Emerick, 1988, explains) to deal directly with such intrinsic features as the client's cognitions about loss of control or attitudes of fear or anxiety associated with stuttering. A basic assumption of the fluency-modification strategy is that once the client has learned new ways of producing fluent speech, he will eventually show a corresponding change in the cognitive and affective features of his problem. Relatively little counseling, in a traditional sense, takes place.

The stuttering-modification strategy is, by nature, more cognitive in nature in that the treatment requires the client not only to evaluate and change behavioral characteristics, but to self-monitor and self-manage cognitive and attitudinal features of the syndrome as well. Informal counseling, in some form, is typically an integral part of this approach.

With the third generic path, cognitive restructuring, the intrinsic features of the syndrome become the major focus of treatment. With this approach, relatively less effort is directed toward the direct modification of surface behaviors. The primary goal is to change the way in which the client considers himself and his stuttering and how he interprets the events of stuttering. By becoming more assertive and decreasing avoidance behavior, the speaker is often able to make significant changes in the handicapping effect of his fluency disorder. Rather than fighting his speech blocks, he may be asked to stutter more openly. Although the frequency of stuttering moments will stay the same or even increase, the quality of the fluency will improve. In addition, and most important, the quality of the client's communication as well as his lifestyle will often change for the better.

Rational-emotive therapy (RET) (Ellis, 1977) may be the best known of the cognitive psychotherapies (Emerick, 1988). The basic premise of this approach is that a person's belief systems are not always logical, rational, or realistic. Thus, a restructuring of a client's internal verbal statements (and, hence, his belief systems) may result in a corresponding reorganization of the individual's problem. Although there are relatively few practicing clinicians who have advocated this approach exclusively for the treatment of stuttering (Fransella, 1972; Hayhow & Levy, 1989; Johnson, 1946; Williams, 1979), there is much to be gained by incorporating some of the techniques associated with this strategy into the process of treatment, particularly for many adults who stutter.

Although there are obvious differences between these three generic treatment strategies, they are far from mutually exclusive. For example, the consistent contact between the clinician and the client that is required during any treatment approach is, by nature, interpersonal and offers the likelihood of some form of supportive counseling. In addition, during the later stages of stuttering-modification treatment, many of the fluency-initiating techniques used during fluency modification coincide with and complement the stabilization and maintenance activities. Each of these treatment strategies requires the client to monitor and self-manage many aspects of his surface and intrinsic behaviors. Each strategy dictates that the speaker systematically learn and practice techniques, first within the treatment setting and then, gradually, outside the security of the clinic, in real-world speaking situations. Each method places great emphasis on the client taking primary responsibility for his own self-management. By beginning from somewhat different perspectives, each approach can result in increased fluency as well as increased assertiveness and risk-taking behavior. Finally, each approach can result in a significant reduction of the client's handicap associated with his fluency disorder.

Which of these approaches is currently preferred by professional clinicians? St. Louis and Westbrook (1987) reported the results of a survey of thirty treatment intervention studies that were published from 1980 through 1986. These authors found that the reported treatment of choice for the majority of adult stutterers was a form of prolonged speech- or rate-control procedure, both forms of fluency modification. Furthermore, St. Louis and Westbrook pointed out that few of the authors of the studies listed activities such as the modification of stuttering moments, client counseling, or desensitization as a significant part of treatment.

Whether these published manuscripts describing intervention accurately reflect the treatment approaches that were being used in the many clinical centers throughout the country is open to question. Whether or not stuttering modification, counseling, and desensitization techniques are highlighted as the major focus of treatment, there is little question that such aspects of treatment are used in some form. The very nature of a clinician working closely with an individual and guiding him through the many components of treatment provides the client with a degree of support and insight about his problem. Therapy, by definition, is always personal, for treatment involves one person assisting another in order to define and manage the problem (Emerick, 1988). Any systematic analysis and subsequent self-management of attitudes and speech behaviors will provide a degree of desensitization during treatment. Whether or not counseling is identified as a basic or formal goal of treatment, in some form it is taking place if the client is being listened to, encouraged, motivated, and challenged. If, on the other hand, the only changes that are emphasized during treatment have to do with the client's speech rate and the related improvement in fluency, it may explain the reasonably high occurrence of relapse with this treatment strategy (Silverman, 1981). Moreover, if, following treatment, the client's speech sounds and feels unnatural and lacks spontaneity, the long-term effects of these changes are not likely to last (Boberg, 1986; Kalinowski, Nobel, Armson, & Stuart, 1994). As the field of fluency disorders matures, there is the possibility that clinicians are more likely to prefer a treatment approach that is eclectic, one that incorporates elements from each of these three generic strategies according to the capacities and needs of the client.

SOME SPECIFICS OF FLUENCY-MODIFICATION STRATEGIES

It is not usually difficult to invoke fluency in even the most severely stuttering speakers. Bloodstein (1949, 1950) researched a variety of conditions where stuttering was reduced or absent. He found that there were as many as 115 conditions that decreased stuttering markedly. Such circumstances included activities such as speaking alone or during a relaxed state, speaking in unison with others, talking to an animal or an infant or in time to rhythmic stimulus, singing, using a dialect, talking and simultaneously writing, or speaking during auditory masking, in a slow, prolonged manner, under delayed auditory feedback, or while shadowing another speaker. Many of these fluency-producing activities involve combinations of altered vocalization (Wingate, 1969) or enhancement of the speaking rhythm (Van Riper, 1973).

Originally, fluency-modification approaches, because they were based on behavior modification, placed little emphasis on the intrinsic features of the stuttering syndrome. Although this has changed somewhat in recent years, the major focus of these approaches continues to be on managing the surface features and achieving a high level of fluent, as well as natural-sounding, speech.

Fluency-modification approaches are also referred to in the literature as fluency shaping. Many of the actual techniques used with this approach are similar to fluency-enhancing procedures that have been noted for many years to elicit fluent speech, including producing slowed, rate-controlled, or prolonged speech. With the addition of operant-conditioning and programming principles in the past several decades, these techniques provide a systematic approach to fluency enhancement.

The essence of this approach is the establishment of fluent speech in a controlled clinical setting. Once fluent speech is attained, it is shaped and expanded so that the speaker can gradually maintain fluency in conversational speaking situations both within and outside the clinical setting. Although clinicians using a fluency-modification approach typically do not directly deal with the speakers's attitude, fear, and avoidance behavior, treatment often results in more assertive attitudes and a reduction of avoidance behavior as the client increases his fluency. Examples of such fluency-shaping programs are described by Perkins (1973), Ryan (1980), and Webster (1974).

Because, as mentioned previously, fluency-modification treatments tend to be behavioral and highly structured, they can be easier to teach than stuttering modification or, especially, cognitive restructuring strategies. However, as Conture (1990) points out, being able to modify aspects of fluent or stuttering behavior does not mean that we are necessarily changing all, or even the most, critical aspects of the syndrome. After many years of conducting behavioral studies in fluency disorders, Siegel (1970) provided a perceptive review of the problems and unresolved issues inherent in the behavioral-modification approach. More recently, Prins and Hubbard (1988) pointed out some of the potential problems associated with this strategy. After more than four decades of intense research, behavior-modification strategies have not come any closer than the more traditional stuttering-modification approach to solving the problem of stuttering. There is no question, however, that behavior modification techniques have provided valuable insight about the techniques that clinicians can use to modify many of the surface features of the disorder.

One of the best examples of a fluency-modification program is the Precision Fluency Shaping Program (PFSP) developed by Webster (1975). Stuttering is viewed as a physical phenomenon, and there is little or no discussion of emotional or affective features of the syndrome. If the speaker follows the rules of speech mechanics, his speech will be fluent; if he violates these rules, his speech will not be fluent. As incorrect and distorted muscle movements are altered, the speaker is able to achieve fluent speech. The client is carefully taken through five gradations of muscle movements associated with, first, less complex and, then, more complex sound sequences. Clients are informed about the basic classes of sounds in English and the associated vocal tract features associated with each sound. Clients are taught specific new muscle movements associated with each sound and class of sounds. Muscle movement targets related to respiration, phonation, and articulation are provided to the client along with the opportunity to practice the new movement skills. The ability to self-monitor the accuracy of their new skills is emphasized. Clients are provided with systematic opportunities to feel and control their new skills in a wide variety of treatment and extratreatment settings. Eventually, the client becomes completely responsible for self-managing his speech.

A concise description of a typical fluency-modification approach is provided by deNil and Kroll (1995).

> The basic premise of this approach is that stuttering is a physical behavior that can be modified by systematic exposure to a series of rules for fluent speech. The specific and observable behaviors of speech that are reconstructed include those related to speech rate, respiration, voice onset, and articulation. Clients are provided with specific instructional sets for individual response units initially taught in isolation. These responses are then transferred gradually to more complex sequences and ultimately to conversational speech. During the first sixty hours of the program, clients work at establishing fluent speech skills both during individual and group learning sessions. Target behaviors are established by strict adherence to detailed and sequenced exercises under close clinician supervision. The final third of the treatment procedure involves the transfer of newly acquired fluency skills to everyday settings. Transfer activities are structured such that clients progress gradually from simple, one message questions to complex conversational dialogues in

natural settings. Following the three week intensive program, clients are scheduled for a one-year follow-up program consisting of weekly group sessions for the first month, followed by groups sessions every other week for the next two months, and monthly group sessions for the remainder of the year. Each year, a refresher course, which is open to all former participants in the program, is organized.

SOME SPECIFICS OF STUTTERING-MODIFICATION STRATEGIES

The stuttering-modification strategy is also referred to as the traditional, Van Riperian, or nonavoidance approach. It is based on the concept that a large part of the problem is the speaker's struggle and avoidance of the core moment of stuttering. Whatever the reason for the motoric break in the first place, there is no question that the problem becomes dramatically expanded when speakers begin avoiding feared sounds, words, and situations and increase their struggle, fear, and tension associated with the stuttering moment.

A primary focus of the stuttering-modification strategy involves the reduction and management of fear and avoidance, typically via desensitization and assertiveness training. In addition, treatment focuses on modifying the surface features of the stuttering into intentional, open, smooth, and relaxed forms, which are intended to replace the old, out-of-control, and reflexive stuttering. The result of this treatment can be a form of easy, less handicapping, even acceptable stuttering. In contrast to a common misconception concerning this treatment strategy, clients are not just trained to be "happy stutterers." In some instances, clients can achieve speech that is completely and spontaneously fluent. If not, at least the speaker learns to exert control over previously uncontrolled stuttering moments and to make decisions that are less influenced by the possibility of stuttering. Examples of this approach can be found in Luper and Mulder (1964), Sheehan, (1970), Van Riper (1973), and Williams (1971).

Stuttering-modification strategies also have as a goal the achievement of fluency, but with greater emphasis on the client's self-perception of the stuttering experience. That is, while the attainment of fluency is one indicator of progress, the nature of the fluency breaks are also taken into account. Progress is noted as the types of the stuttering events change from higher levels of tension and fragmentation of syllables and words to fluency breaks that are characterized by less effort and increased smoothness. As stuttering events are systematically identified, varied, and modified, the speaker is able to incorporate the various techniques in conversational speech during treatment as well as in extratreatment speaking situations.

Stuttering-modification approaches tend to be somewhat eclectic and therefore somewhat difficult for the new clinician to conceptualize and learn. While being able to observe a model clinician is always helpful when learning any treatment approach, it is especially important when learning treatments that involve the modification of affective and cognitive features of stuttering. The more eclectic the approach, the less opportunity the clinician has to "go by the book" or treatment manual. Stuttering-modification approaches tend to be somewhat more counseling-based and require greater adjustment of the treatment to the individual client. Again, while not usually directly addressed, cognitive and affective changes may also occur during fluency-modification programs as clients begin to consider new ways of thinking about themselves.

Change often occurs rapidly during the first few treatment sessions. At the outset, the client is inclined to be highly motivated, and there are many interesting, even exciting, things to learn about this fluency disorder. The clinician has the opportunity to introduce the lawful aspects of the problem in general and for this client in particular. She can demonstrate that she is unafraid, interested, and excited about exploring how this person manifests the problem in his unique way. The clinician cannot fake an open and interested approach; it must be genuine (see Chapters 1 and 7 concerning clinician characteristics).

The stuttering-modification strategy, as described by Van Riper (1982), takes the client through the stages of Identification, Desensitization, Variation, Modification, and Stabilization.

Identification

Clients are first asked to identify both the surface and intrinsic features of their stuttering. They are asked to identify, analyze, and confront the specifics of their individual patterns of stuttering. With the assistance of the clinician, clients can make a list of "Things I do *when* I stutter" to identify the surface features of their stuttering. These are behaviors that can be observed in a mirror, recorded, and identified on video- and audiotapes. Another list, termed "Things I do *because* I stutter," can include the less obvious, intrinsic features of the syndrome such as avoidances, anxieties, feelings of fear and helplessness, and the decisions and choices the speaker makes because of the *possibility* of stuttering. The identification of features that occur frequently during treatment is often a good place to begin simply because there are multiple occurrences. Features that are particularly abnormal or distracting may result in increased motivation on the part of the client.

Although the clinician will obviously lead the way during the initial stages of identifying the client's stuttering characteristics, it is important for the client to make this list and write down these features of his stuttering. It is very likely the first time he has been asked to assume the responsibility for this behavior and these feelings. By writing down and analyzing these surface and intrinsic features, he is taking the first step toward self-management of the many aspects of his fluency disorder.

Desensitization

The process of identification naturally leads the client toward becoming desensitized to both the overt (surface) and covert (intrinsic) features of his stuttering. It is difficult to critically identify and analyze one's behavior and attitudes without achieving at least some distance and objectivity. Some clients continue to be overwhelmed by the stuttering experience and take considerably longer to reduce their anxiety as they are in the midst of their own stuttering. If the clinician can model a reasonable level of calm during stuttering, the client will be more likely to adopt the same attitude. As the client learns that it is indeed possible to stutter without losing complete control, he will begin to realize that he has some choices that were not apparent before. For example, he has the ability to alter selected features of his stuttering syndrome. He will come to appreciate that he is able to reduce his anxiety during the stuttering event and to realize that some variation of this event is possible. His anxiety does not have to be nil during stuttering, but as he is able to reduce his fear to a manageable level, he will have the chance to accurately identify and analyze his behavior. He will also set the stage for making some variations to his surface behaviors as well as beginning to alter some of the cognitive aspects of his disorder. He may even begin making choices to decrease his avoidance of situations, sounds, and words.

Variation

As the client becomes able to identify specific behaviors and attitudes and to decrease his automatic reaction of fear and anxiety associated with the moment of stuttering, he will slowly achieve the ability to make some changes in the features of his stuttering, which are no longer things that happen to him but rather aspects of his speech that he is producing, things that he can identify and change. Of course, going from his old, reflexive, and automatic response of stuttering to perfectly fluent speech is an enormous leap and not one that he should be expected to accomplish early in treatment. He has a much greater chance of success if he is asked to simply alter or vary some feature of his stuttering. A small step forward is all that is necessary, or expected, at the outset. Moreover, success is apt to be intermittent. As with identification, secondary or surface behaviors (eye blinks, junk words, postponement devices) that occur frequently and are especially distracting or unappealing are ideal features on which to concentrate. The client is not asked to stop performing these features, but rather to vary them in some preplanned manner. That is, the client may select the feature of producing a series of "ahs" prior to a feared word. Rather than attempting to cease production of the "ah" as a postponement or timing device as he anticipates a feared word, he could choose to systematically vary the rate, intensity, number, or vowel segment (e.g., "eh," "oh," or "uh," instead of "ah"). As long as he achieves some measure of control as evidenced by his ability to vary his old automatic utterance of "ah," he is successful. Of course, this may result in a decrease in his overall fluency, but the critical issue here is that he has achieved a level of control over his speech that he had not experienced before. The variation of his previously uncontrolled behavior will set the stage for the client to further modify his stuttering moments in even more specific and better ways.

Modification

During this stage the surface features of the client's stuttering that have been identified are further altered. The client is now asked to begin varying some of his behaviors in even more specific and appropriate ways. These changes are, in a sense, closer to the core of the stuttering moment. The goal is to replace the old, out-of-control fluency break with a new, smoother utterance which he can completely control.

By approaching the stuttering event from after the fact, the client is first asked to perform a postevent modification. That is, immediately following the client's production of a stuttered word, he is asked to stop and pause for approximately three seconds. Undoubtedly, this pause acts as a form of mild punishment, for the speaker can no longer continue with his message to the listener. Furthermore, the pause highlights the behavior that he just produced. While all clients tend to have difficulty with this task during reading or, especially, conversational speech, those speakers who have not achieved a reasonable degree of desensitization will find this task especially difficult. As with most people who stutter, they are somewhat driven to complete the message, and any stoppage both increases the time pressure to communicate and creates the hurdle of having to reinitiate speech.

As the client is able to recognize the stuttering moment and consistently pause following the event, he can now perform an analysis of his stuttered behavior. Following the clinician's lead, he can do this by pantomiming the stuttered word and examining the physical features of his behavior. He can ask himself how and where he may be cutting off his airflow or voicing. As he rehearses his just-stuttered speech, he can identify points of constriction in the vocal tract, postural fixations he may be using, and inappropriate use of his respiratory or phonatory systems. Once this is accomplished, he is rewarded by being allowed to continue with his message.

Once the client becomes consistently able to stop and accurately analyze his stuttered speech, he will progress to the point where, following a real stuttering moment, he will routinely stop and silently practice a new, smoother, and more open way of stuttering on the word. Although he could easily pantomime a completely fluent version of the word, the task here is to produce a smooth form of "fluent stuttering." This is usually done during reading, monologue, and conversation, both inside and outside the treatment setting. Following his pantomiming of the new fluent form of stuttering, the client is requested to stop after each stuttered word for a moment and this time produce the new form of fluent stuttering out loud. Again, it is important to note that although the client could likely say the word again completely fluently, the purpose here is not to be fluent but to replace the old, automatic stuttering with a new form of fluent stuttering.

It is important to point out that the client is not canceling in order to be fluent. After all, the addition of yet another moment of (fluent) stuttering following a real stuttering event will result in speech that is even less fluent. However, what is occurring is that the client is not canceling the stuttering so much as eliminating the loss of control associated with that stuttering event. The sense of power and control that the client is able to achieve with this (*cancellation*) technique is important for the client to appreciate. Each moment of stuttering, while it may be undesirable, is an opportunity to take charge of the stuttering—a chance at bat. At the outset of treatment, stuttering is scoring run after run while the speaker has not rounded the bases once. Once the speaker begins to achieve control of a large majority of his stuttering moments (something approaching 80%), there is often a flow of fluency and, more important, a dramatic increase in the speaker's confidence about repairing the situation. The analogy of rolling back to the surface after an error in paddling a kayak, as detailed in Chapter 8, is an especially good way to describe this experience.

The fluency that results from this repair technique is earned fluency to be sure, but it is extremely tenuous. On occasion, especially if additional desensitization to stuttering needs to be done, a speaker will be unable to successfully cancel the stuttered word. That is, as he begins to replace the old stuttering with a smoother, controlled version of stuttering, he will lose control and revert back to his old, automatic, and helpless stuttering. If this happens, the client should attempt the cancellation of the stuttered word again until he regains control of the fluent stuttering. Success is defined by being in charge of the word. The client can signal to the clinician with his finger whether he is in control of his stuttering. On occasion, it may take several cycles of regaining and losing control before he is able to be completely in charge of the stuttered word. In any case, he should not leave that word and go on to the next one until he has taken charge of that word by successfully canceling it.

The next step in the modification of the stuttered event is the paraevent modification, often called the *pullout*. Now, the client, rather than waiting until he makes it all the way through a stuttered word, will grab the word and begin to "slide out of it" by enhancing his airflow, altering his vocal tract with articulatory postures, and generally stuttering smoothly through the word. Clients often find that this technique of pulling out of a stuttered moment is a natural progression from the cancellation technique and may begin doing this spontaneously. The pullout is less obvious than the cancellation, and listener reactions tend to be more favorable. Thus, clients will want to stop using the cancellation technique. Nevertheless, even though the speaker may gradually improve in accuracy using the paraevent modification, it is important to continue practicing the postevent or cancellation technique as well, as there will undoubtedly be many stressful occasions when the speaker will not be able to catch and modify his speech using a pullout. The last line of defense, the final opportunity to catch and take charge of a moment of stuttering, will be the cancellation technique.

The final step in the modification sequence is the preevent modification or *preparatory set*. As the speaker anticipates an upcoming moment of stuttering and, of course, chooses not to avoid the word, he is able to approach it with a smooth form of stuttering. Many of the fluency-initiating gestures incorporated in the fluency-shaping techniques (full breath, air flow, gradual onset of constant phonation, light articulatory contacts) are helpful in achieving a smooth preparatory set. Furthermore, if a client's speech contains many, very brief fluency breaks that he has difficulty identifying, the preparatory set is one way to eliminate them.

Stabilization

During this stage, the newly learned modification skills are practiced under more stressful conditions and made resistant to stress and communicative pressure. In order to withstand the pressures of the real world, these techniques must be overlearned or they will fall apart when the pressure becomes too great. Techniques of heightening proprioceptive feedback by using auditory masking or delayed auditory feedback can be used to increase the ability to monitor production by proprioception. The client can bring forth and resist the old fears and anxieties. He can slowly learn to withstand the old, negative self-talk that he has played in his head many times in the past. The new patterns of speaking and thinking need to be tested in the difficult waters of the real world in some systematic way, gradually working through hierarchies of increasing difficulty. Telephone calls, public speaking, and social introductions are examples of particularly difficult speaking situations, which often need to be systematically confronted. Much of this stabilization takes place outside treatment and will continue long after formal treatment is concluded. The speaker must continue to push the envelope and challenge himself with new speaking adventures. This is also likely to be a good time to practice voluntary stuttering, particularly if others put pressure on him for unrealistic or perfect fluency.

COGNITIVE RESTRUCTURING

To some degree, regardless of the overall strategy of treatment, for long-term success to occur for the client, he must develop fresh ways of thinking about himself and his problem. This aspect of treatment does not always need to be dealt with directly for success to occur, as is the case in a behavioral modification approach, which does not emphasize changing the intrinsic features of the syndrome. However, the new ways of speaking and thinking will seem strange to the client, possibly making him feel that he is standing out even more than he has in the past. Such cognitive changes may be particularly important as the treatment reaches the transfer and maintenance phases. The client who retains self-defeating mental images and negative thoughts and beliefs about speech and his ability to manage it is much less apt to succeed once he is on his own.

Emerick (1988) suggests that clients who have an analytical and introspective orientation respond the most favorably to cognitive-restructuring approaches. According to Emerick, the cognitive aspects of treatment involve at least four main phases. Phase 1 focuses on educating the client about the overall approach of the treatment. The suggested changes in orientation to himself and his problem can pose a threat, which, Emerick says, should be viewed as a challenge. Threat or not, the clinician must often challenge the client if change is going to occur.

Phase 2 involves having the client identify his self-defeating thought patterns by analyzing his thoughts before, during, and after speaking situations and stuttering events. He is asked to identify his mental constructs about the event, keep a log of his emotions and thoughts, and indicate the outcome of situations. He then categorizes his responses in terms of dependency/helplessness ("I know I will relapse when therapy is over"), irresponsibility ("I just cannot control my feelings"), dichotomizing ("There are good listeners and bad listeners"), catastrophizing ("I know I will fall apart if I am asked to introduce myself") and fantasy ("Most of my problems would be solved if I didn't stutter").

Phase 3 is one of reality testing. The client's task is now to evaluate his mental constructs by asking (a) Does the construct deal with the reality of the situation? (b) Does this construct make unreasonable demands on me? and (c) Does the construct help me accomplish the treatment goals? In addition, the client also contrasts possible negative imagery with positive, self-enhancing imagery. As Emerick says, "It is difficult to think of failing in a speaking situation while at the same time concentrating on positive thoughts" (1988, p. 262). The old, negative cognitions must become cues for the client to tell himself, "Stop." At this point, the clinician can role-play for the client, alternating between the negative and positive self-statements. This is often an ideal activity during group treatment sessions.

The final and fourth phase involves having the client substitute self-enhancing language for the traditional negative thoughts. The new, positive affirmations may not always be completely true (e.g., "This may be a difficult situation, but I can deal with it"). Nonetheless, imaging success brings the possibility of success that much closer (Daly, 1994).

Clients can, of course, have problems with some of the above-mentioned activities, especially when they see stuttering as something that happens to them rather than something they do (a fairly common perception). According to Emerick (1988), such clients have great difficulty stopping the old negative cognitions. An even greater problem is posed by those clients who are unable to recognize the inaccuracy of their cognitions. Some clients believe that the way they are processing reality is the normal, correct, and most acceptable way. The client may agree intellectually that there are several ways to view something but still privately believe that his view is the most accurate.

A good example of a program that emphasizes cognitive restructuring along with a stuttering-modification approach is described by Maxwell (1982). The approach is educational rather than curative, with a primary goal of teaching the client better ways of managing his speech. Clients typically attend the treatment program for one individual and one group session each week for approximately one and a half years. Maxwell (1982) summarizes the program in the following steps:

1. *Information giving:* in this initial stage, the client receives verbal preparation and instructions. The purpose of this stage is to provide the client with a map of the treatment process. The client also receives a verbal or written summary of the treatment plan.

2. *Cognitive appraisal:* the client summarizes, in his own words, the objectives and methods of the treatment plan and how the plan will meet his needs. This process establishes a common perception of the treatment process for the client and clinician.

3. *Thought reversal:* the client begins to reduce and eliminate negative cognitions. Essential to this process is the technique of "thought stopping" when negative self-talk occurs. This requires the client to tell himself (initially out loud) to "stop" using the negative ways of thinking about himself and his speech. Later, this stopping process is done silently. The primary goal is for the client to begin disengaging from undesired thoughts and images. Near the end of this stage, the client begins taking steps to utilize positive and productive cognitions. These activities take place within the treatment setting.

4. *Vicarious observation:* once the client is able to experience some success at disengaging negative (and often self-fulfilling) cognitions, the clinician begins to model positive cognitions. As the client observes the clinician succeed and cope with challenges in her own life, the client's self-efficacy will be enhanced. Such modeling increases the client's hope that he, too, can perform as he desires, despite any setbacks.

5. *Speech modification:* in this initial stage of behavioral change, the client begins to improve his information-processing, decision-making, and problem-solving abilities. Maxwell points out that clients typically are not accurate self-observers. However, even before the client is able to successfully modify specific stuttering events, the fact that he is able to accurately self-monitor his behavior tends to have a positive treatment effect in terms of reduced avoidance and possibly even increased fluency (Cooper, Cady, & Robbins, 1970; Daly & Kimbarow, 1978; Wingate, 1959). Many aspects of the Identification and Termination steps as described by Maxwell are similar to the variation and modification stages

of treatment as described by Van Riper (1973). Rather than thinking about his speech as something that happens to him, the client eventually begins to understand the lawfulness of his syndrome. An essential aspect of this modification stage of treatment involves the client describing what he does with his speech production mechanism. With more accurate monitoring of his behavior, the speaker begins to see the lawfulness of his behavior and will be more likely to understand and predict his behavior.

6. *Identification:* the client becomes proficient at identifying specific moments of stuttering, beginning with ten-minute segments using short words, and progressing to reading and conversation.

7. *Termination:* the client terminates the old form of stuttering by following a moment of stuttering with a silent pause. The client then gradually replaces the fluency break with cognitive and behavioral skills that are more appropriate. This is accomplished first following (as in a cancella-tion), then during (as in a pullout), and finally before (as in a preparatory set) the stuttering moment. The client uses imagery to see, hear, and feel a new motor plan consisting of fluency-enhancing targets. The client is also asked to identify and modify avoidance or substitution behaviors.

8. *Cognitive restructuring:* as during the third stage of this treatment, the client is asked to "identify maladaptive speech-related emotions, and self-defeating cognitions on which these are based" (Maxwell, 1982, p. 415). This time, however, the client is asked to restructure his thought in more stressful extratreatment speaking situations.

9. *Coping skills:* the client begins to use positive self-statements and to model imagery techniques to revise negative aspects of his covert verbal behavior. With the clinician's modeling, the client reorganizes monologues in preparation for actual speaking tasks. Group sessions using role-playing activities are recommended here. Maxwell provides a clear example of how a client can alter his thought process about giving an oral report to an art history class. The first paragraph indicates the client's initial thoughts about this task.

Oh, Lord, here I am in class with all of these people and soon I'm going to have to talk. What if my controls don't work? What if I fall on my face—make a fool of myself? Then, they'll think I'm stupid. Maybe I ought to quietly get up and walk out of here. Maybe there won't be time to get to my report. If I stutter, will they laugh or feel pity? (1982, p. 417)

Following analysis of the nonproductive content of that self-message, the clinician then models a revision of more positive internal monologue as in this example.

I am now in class with other students like me discussing the subject of art history. Soon I will be asked to speak on a topic that I know well. I have interesting information to share. When I speak, I plan to use to the best of my ability the controls that I've learned to use well in therapy. What I want to convey is the strong interest I have in my topic. I'll remember to smile, maintain eye contact with my listeners, and try to be open and friendly. (Maxwell, 1982, p. 417)

10. *Self-management:* during this final stage of treatment, the client takes ever greater responsibility for setting his own goals and self-management of the cognitive and behavioral features of his speech. From the outset there must be the recognition that the "majority of therapeutic work takes place between, rather than during, therapy sessions" (Maxwell, 1982, p. 418; see also Kanfer, 1975). The time for dismissal from formal treatment approaches as the client becomes able to self-manage without the assistance of the clinician. Related to the above-mentioned activities are the recommendations of Daly (1992, pp. 135–136) for using positive affirmations for reinforcing and enhancing cognitive changes.

GROUP TREATMENT

One of earliest uses of group treatment in the field of communication disorders was the work of Backus (1947), who advocated the use of speech in social situations beyond the usual speech production drills popular at the time (Backus, 1957). The popularity of group treatment for adults increased as a result of World War II. The many men in need of treatment for various psychological and medical problems, in combination with the relative shortage of clinicians, resulted in group meetings taking the place of individual treatment. The decades of the 1970s and 1980s saw some decline in group treatment due to the popularity of behavioral-modification approaches that emphasized individual treatment (Conture, 1990).

The experiences provided by group interaction are a valuable part of a comprehensive treatment program. Luterman (1991) suggests that there are two basic types of groups: therapy groups and counseling groups. Group meetings for clients with fluency disorders typically serve both functions. The group setting provides opportunities for enhancing as well as maintaining change in both the surface and intrinsic aspects of the syndrome. Unless there happens to be a local support group chapter, the group treatment meeting will be the only way for the client to understand that he is not alone. The group provides a social setting where the client can discuss his problem openly. The group enables him to continue becoming desensitized to stuttering in general as well as his own stuttering in particular. As Conture (1990) points out, such groups can provide social and speaking opportunities for some people who might otherwise go for days or weeks without communicating with others. This group setting is also likely to be the only place where the speaker is permitted to stutter without being penalized. The members of the group can provide an important source of motivation and courage to keep members connected to the overall treatment process.

There are other advantages of group contact. The structure provided by a group setting provides the client with the opportunity to practice the techniques learned during individual treatment sessions. Group interaction provides the clinician with an opportunity to monitor the client's progress in a social context (Conture, 1990). When the treatment is taking place in an academic program, the group setting provides an opportunity for student clinicians to observe a broad range of behavior and to note the dynamics of progress in other clients. If the goal of treatment is to help the speaker to change both the fluency of his speech as well as his understanding of himself and his interaction with others, group treatment is essential. Furthermore, group activities are a natural extension of individual treatment (Levy, 1983). It is clear that group treatment permits a greater variety of treatment choices and a more comprehensive treatment approach than would be possible with individual treatment alone.

Determining Group Membership

The selection of those who will take part in the group is a first step in assuring the success of the group. Each individual participant must be committed and motivated and willing to contribute to the group process. Group treatment is not appealing to all clients, and it can be difficult to get adults who stutter to commit to a group setting. Silverman and Zimmer (1982) found, for example, that women who seek treatment tend to prefer individual rather than group settings. On occasion, some individuals will express the fear that their problem will become more severe by being exposed to others who stutter. For anyone with a long history of stuttering, even an informal group can be particularly aversive and carry with it the threat of severe social penalty. Thus, simply getting a client to attend his first group meeting can be a major success. However, almost without exception, once a reluctant client takes part or observes his first meeting, he will begin to change his mind. Most people are attracted by the interest, support, and energy provided by the other participants.

The initial decision about who to include in a treatment group is critical. Once included, it will be difficult to remove an individual. As Luterman suggests, individuals must have "a willingness to examine their lives and to share their insights with the group" (1979, p. 199). Furthermore, the group will be more likely to be dynamic and self-directed if the members are motivated and share a common interest for introspection and contributing to the success of others in attendance (Luterman, 1979). It makes little sense to attempt to include a client who strongly resists group contact. It may be possible to change his view of the experience through observation via a one-way mirror or by viewing videotapes of group meetings. However, individuals who tend to be argumentative, who consistently attempt to dominate group discussions, or who consistently withdraw from participation are generally not good candidates for group sessions.

Advantages of Group Treatment

Luterman (1991) indicated several characteristics of group treatment that are beneficial.

The instillation of hope: as other members of the group are able to make positive changes in their speech and ways of viewing their situation, the client can increase his belief that he is also capable of such success. The client can often gain momentum from others in the group who are becoming more assertive and taking risks. Much like being a member of an athletic team, group participation often motivates a client to extend himself beyond his original notions of what is possible.

The promotion of universality: by being a member of a group of individuals who share a common problem, the client comes to recognize that he is not alone. The group provides a means for coping with feelings of isolation and loneliness. The group setting also provides the client with the opportunity to practice recently learned modification techniques in a more realistic setting than alone with the clinician. Speaking in a group situation is a good initial step in generalizing the newly acquired and tenuous techniques to a social, albeit clinical, situation. Using the fluency- or stuttering-modification techniques in a group setting can also provide one means of reducing the client's dependence on his clinician.

The imparting of information: information is provided, not only by the group leader as in individual treatment, but also by the other group members and, in some cases, other clinicians. All members of the group are able to provide examples and advice based on their own, unique experiences, whether or not they stutter. The inclusion of other clinicians, spouses, or friends provides the opportunity for individuals who stutter to understand, many for the first time, that nonstuttering speakers share many of the same fears about speaking in public or formal situations and about risk taking in general.

The provision of altruism: each group member provides, not only information to other members, but also support, reassurance, and insight. Furthermore, as the group members are helping others, they also tend to experience an increase in their own self-esteem.

The enhancement of group cohesiveness: as with most small groups, the treatment group develops its own history and evolves through the stages of "forming," "storming," "norming," and "performing" (Tuckman, 1965). That is, group members discover and adjust to the group protocol, find out how to identify roles and resolve conflicts, become committed to working with each other, and eventually focus on group objectives and goals. As this process occurs, the group as a whole gradually becomes more self-directed and individual members experience an increased desire to maintain their role in the group and look forward to group meetings. As group unity increases, group activities will be more likely to facilitate growth and change of individual members.

The possibility of catharsis: the group provides a safe place for individual members to release and share feelings and attitudes concerning their own problems. As opinions and views are expressed, there is often a release from the control these feelings have had over the individual. This can be especially obvious during certain aspects of treatment for fluency disorders as members become desensitized to their long history of fear associated with fluency failure. The group provides a safe place to ventilate feelings of fluency and social failure associated with stuttering. Participants are able to let go of these past experiences by achieving distance and greater objectivity, and perhaps even allowing humor to be associated with past events.

The development of existential issues: the group can provide the opportunity for individual clients and clinicians to deal with questions concerning anxiety associated with daily living such as feelings of loneliness, dependency, and meaninglessness. The discussions can help reduce anxiety and allow the members to improve the quality of their decision making, including the many interpersonal aspects of their lives.

Of course, group treatment sessions also provide an ideal way to gradually phase individuals out of the more intensive individual treatment schedules. Following the conclusion of formal treatment, clients can return again to the group meetings as they experience signs of relapse (Levy, 1983) or simply feel the need for a booster session.

Potential Problems

As might be expected, there are apt to be a variety of problems with attendance and schedules. Group meetings are not always possible to schedule, and even when they are, it is often difficult to maintain consistent participation by all members. In some settings it can be a major hurdle simply to find a time and a place to meet. Often, it is difficult to gather together enough clients to form a group of a critical and consistent mass. Conture (1990) recommends a group size of approximately seven members, while Luterman (1991) suggests an upper limit of eight to fifteen members. A general rule might be that the group should be large enough for a variety of interactions but small enough that members have opportunity to know and trust one another. If clinicians are included (something that is highly recommended for student clinicians), the group can easily become too large. One solution is to break up the larger group into smaller subsets so that all members have the opportunity to participate. At the conclusion of the session, all members can gather together for summary comments.

Achieving diversity among the members is not usually a problem. In most instances clients will be at different levels of change or in treatment for varying lengths of time. Just as a mix of social and educational backgrounds provides variety, this provides a broadened experience for clients as well as students who are attending.

Obviously, group members will bring a variety of personalities and experiences to the meetings. As Sheehan (1970b) suggested, a group is only as good as its membership. The group will be less effective if one or more members tend to try and dominate or if members are reluctant to contribute to the group activities or discussions. Some participants may give feedback that is less than constructive, and, in some cases, members can become dependent on the group as their basic means of socializing (Levy, 1983).

Group leaders can also be a source of problems. The leader serves a critical role, for she provides direction and consistency for the group. However, she must be flexible and facilitate the growth of each participant. If the leader promotes a highly structured group in which she directs all activities, the result may be passive participation by the members. Clients will be less likely to initiate interaction and assume responsibility (Luterman, 1991). On the other hand, groups that lack the necessary leadership tend not to be task oriented and often lack a direction and purpose for the group meetings. As indicated by Levy (1983), this is especially apt to occur if the leader is unable to convey her understanding of the stuttering experience and therefore lacks credibility.

The Effective Group Leader

The effective group leader is able to establish credibility during the initial group meetings. This can be accomplished by demonstrating both a knowledge of stuttering and stutterers as well as a genuine interest in the members of the group. Just as the characteristics discussed in Chapter 1 describe the actions of an ideal clinician during the individual treatment, these same features indicate that empathy, warmth, and genuineness are necessary requirements of an effective group leader. Furthermore, the leader should be flexible; she should be able to sufficiently structure the group so that members have a sense of direction but also be prepared to discard prearranged plans when necessary. That is, the leader must provide a sense of mission to the group but at the same time be able to respond to the needs of individual group participants. Just as in individual treatment, the clinician is likely to be somewhat more directive during the early group meetings. Once the norms of the group become established and the purpose and direction of the group have been defined, the group leader will be less instructive so that there will be more opportunity for the members to be self-directive and interact with one another (Luterman, 1991).

Establishing Group Norms

Since the goal of the group is to have the individual members interact with one another, it is usually not helpful for the group leader to simply ask or answer questions. In order for the group to become self-directive, the leader must promote the concept that the members should take responsibility for the activities and topics. Another norm or characteristic of the group is one of self-disclosure. The leader and other clinicians can model such disclosure so that the clients gradually become more comfortable about revealing feelings, beliefs, and attitudes. The trick is to do so without eliciting judgmental statements by other members. On occasion, there is likely to be confrontation among members of the group. This is normal and to be expected. Group members should not feel pressure to self-disclose before they are ready. A good guideline is that no one has to talk unless they want to, and no question *must* be answered. Still, members must feel that their individual needs are being considered. Finally, members must be reassured of the confidentiality of the group's discussions (Luterman, 1991).

Structuring Group Activities

Ideally, group meetings should be held in a large room with comfortable seating. A degree of privacy is preferred (Levy, 1983), and if relaxation and imagery activities are to be conducted, the area must be quiet. It is also useful if the room is large enough for public speaking and able to be divided into areas for small-group discussion or role-playing. Some nearby access to outside speaking situations is helpful so that group members can leave the building, conduct brief speaking assignments, and return to evaluate the experience. Of course, arranging the participants in a circle is useful in enhancing conversation as well as promoting eye contact and allowing the clinicians and clients to read each other's body language (Luterman, 1991).

Once the group's structural and procedural norms have been established, the group can conduct specific activities.

Relaxation-Imagery Exercises. Many of the activities that are done in group meetings for fluency disorders are useful for anyone, regardless of the quality of their speech. This is clearly the case with this category of techniques (Kirby, Delgadillo, Hillard & Manning, 1992). It is not necessary or even desirable to be extremely relaxed in order to produce fluent speech. However, being able to relax in the midst of life's many anxiety-producing stimuli is a valuable skill for anyone. The process can be done anytime during the meeting, but often it works well to begin the meeting with these activities. Assuming the meeting is taking place in a reasonably quiet room with comfortable seating, the lights are dimmed. Playing quiet relaxing music can be helpful. Each group member closes his eyes and gradually focuses his thoughts on the instructions being delivered by a member of the group. The instructions direct each participant to sequentially relax groups of his skeletal muscles, eventually focusing on the muscles of respiration, phonation, and articulation. The emphasis is on slowing and smoothing breathing as well as visualizing an open vocal tract with cool air smoothly flowing through and out of the oral cavity. Participants are asked to imagine themselves in a serene and natural setting. Once relaxed, they are led through images of success, which include speaking activities. They are asked to remember the positive feelings associated with each success.

The process usually lasts approximately ten minutes. Often, a relaxed state is created that carries over into the remainder of the group session. Initially, the responsibility of leading this portion of the session can be directed by a clinician. However, the instructions, as they should be delivered slowly and smoothly, provide an ideal speaking situation for clients who have limited experience speaking in front of a group.

Relaxation has been advocated as a way of promoting fluency for many years. In and of itself, relaxation is far from a solution to the problem of fluency disorders. Such techniques can, however, contribute to the learning that takes place during a comprehensive treatment program. The goal is not to promote fluency per se but to teach the client better ways of responding to stress-producing situations, whether giving a presentation to a large audience or having dental surgery. Some members of the group will respond more readily to this experience than others, and some will be better able than others to make use of the relaxation and imagery skills in everyday situations. It takes consistent practice for these skills to be available when needed.

Role-playing. The acting out of real-life situations is facilitated by group treatment sessions. This exercise is useful in helping the stutterer work through feared moments he has previously encountered. Such situations may include ordering food at a restaurant or drive-through window, taking an oral exam for certification, giving a formal oral presentation, exchanging marriage vows, or dealing with threatening or confrontational situations at home, work, or school. Role-playing activities by the group lend themselves to creativity and role-reversal. It provides an opportunity to become desensitized to past fluency failures and future anxiety-provoking situations. Observers can analyze the interpersonal aspects of the situation and offer constructive feedback and alternative ways of responding to the situation.

Public Speaking. Public speaking is a highly feared situation for nearly anyone, and the group session provides a forum for speaking before a group. Depending on the level of each member's experience and upcoming demands at work or school, public-speaking situations can be created during the session. Clients have the opportunity to experience the preparation of different types of presentations (informative, demonstration, storytelling, extemporaneous) and to practice responding to questions from the audience. Participants also have the opportunity to improve important speaking and organizational skills and to learn to sequence and present their ideas in front of a group. Public speaking can be done in the same room where the group session normally takes place or in a more formal setting such as a classroom or auditorium, sometimes making use of a microphone and amplification system. During the final stages of preparing for a presentation at work or school, the individual or the entire group can meet at the site. Of course, when it comes time for the actual presentation, the group members can share in the success of the event by actually being there or by viewing the presentation on videotape.

Demonstration of Client Skills and Progress. During the group meeting, each client has the opportunity to demonstrate techniques being worked on during the individual treatment sessions. For example, each group member can explain, demonstrate, and respond to questions about the use of specific techniques. Voluntary stuttering is a good example of such an activity. Other activities involve demonstrating examples of decreased avoidance behavior, providing examples of risk-taking activities, and describing humorous situations that occurred as a result of potential or real stuttering.

TREATMENT OF ATYPICAL FLUENCY CASES

As discussed in Chapter 4, the large majority of the people who seek assistance for fluency disorders have a long history of developmental change with etiology of unknown origin. While each client has his own story and his own intrinsic and surface characteristics, he is usually physically and psychologically normal. Although the most common client is the otherwise normal, healthy person, some clients are considerably less common (St. Louis, 1986b) and require modifications to the typical treatment procedures and additional clinical decisions.

Neurogenic Stuttering

Fluency-modification techniques appear to help facilitate fluency in those speakers exhibiting neurogenic stuttering. Having clients speak at a slow rate may be especially helpful in improving fluency. In addition, since word finding has been mentioned as a common problem in neurogenic fluency disorders and may contribute to fluency breaks (Brown & Cullinan, 1981; Meyers, Hall, & Aram, 1990), a slow rate of production may also assist the speaker by providing more time for retrieval. Other fluency-enhancing techniques such as the initiation of airflow, gradual onset of phonation, easy articulatory contacts, and desensitization may also be helpful (Market, Montague, Buffalo, & Drummond, 1990; Meyers, Hall, & Aram, 1990; Rousey, Arjunan, & Rousey,1986).

Several authors have reported an improvement of fluency in clients with neurogenic stuttering who have suffered further damage to their central nervous system (Helm, Yeo, Geschwind, Froedman, & Wenstein, 1986; Jones, 1966; Manders & Bastijns, 1988; Van Riper, 1982). The additional trauma apparently resulted in an improvement of function for fluency. These observations suggest that of all the forms of fluency disorders encountered, pharmacological treatment may be most beneficial for this group of clients (Helm-Estabrooks, 1986).

Psychogenic Stuttering

The treatment of choice is debatable for people with psychogenic stuttering, for it depends on the characteristics of the fluency and the speaker. Perhaps more than in any other form of fluency disorder, each case is highly unique. Fortunately, these cases comprise what is perhaps the smallest number of clients who present with a fluency disorder. There are few empirical studies of such clients, and there is a clear need to document the nature of their recovery. Roth, Aronson, and Davis (1989) recommend "traditional fluency treatment" in combination with counseling from a psychologist or psychiatrist. According to Roth et al., these patients are receptive to both stuttering- and fluency-modification procedures. In order to promote progress in treatment, these authors stress the importance of encouragement and optimism on the part of the clinician. For some clients, of course, the expense of this combination of treatments may be prohibitive. The very nature of a conversion disorder—responding to a problem by developing some dysfunctional behavior—suggests that these clients may not naturally choose the difficult road of treatment with all its challenges. There is little information on the course of treatment with this population, but it appears that for those clients who continue for a time in treatment, fluency can be enhanced and the handicap decreased as a result of stuttering and fluency modification in conjunction with cognitive-restructuring activities.

Cluttering

As with the diagnosis of cluttering, treatment for this disorder, especially when it presents in combination with stuttering, can be perplexing. Because the problem is broad based, involving many linguistic, motoric, emotional, and pragmatic features, treatment can also be complex. St. Louis and Myers (1995) suggest three principles of slowing rate, heightening self-monitoring, and developing the ability to encode language, including the pragmatics and turn-taking aspects of communication. These authors suggest that focusing on these principles often results in improvement in articulation and intelligibility as well as fluency. St. Louis and Myers (1995) provide a detailed list of treatment activities, particularly for children and adolescents.

One of the most difficult aspects of treatment is the aversive attitude frequently taken by these clients. As Daly (1986) points out, clients can be aggressive and extremely defensive, characteristics that make it difficult to develop a workable clinical relationship. On the other hand, intelligibility and fluency can often be dramatically improved as these speakers develop the ability to monitor their speech. These speakers need to concentrate almost totally on *how* they are speaking rather than on what they are saying. As the speaker is made aware of his irregular and rapid speech, he will typically be able, at least for brief periods, to make appropriate alterations in his production, often even without specific instruction. As the client is shown techniques for self-managing his speech and the effects on others, his fluency will improve, as will his expressive language and articulation. Unfortunately, without the development of self-cuing strategies, the improvement is often short-lived. Temporary success often occurs rapidly, but the speakers quickly lose their motivation for self-monitoring activities. In addition, the client often finds it difficult to tolerate speaking at what seems to him an exceedingly slow rate. The "driven" quality described in Chapter 4 becomes obvious after even a brief period of speaking at a slower rate.

The essence of treatment with these clients involves varying the rate of speech production and increasing their ability to monitor output. A variety of stuttering-modification and fluency-modification techniques have been found to have a positive effect. Van Riper (1992b) provided a summary of techniques that he found assisted clutterers in modifying their speech.

- Read in unison with the client, beginning with a fast rate and systematically changing speed while the client shadows the clinician's rate changes.

- Have the client write down the words he wants to say before he utters them.

- Have the client repeat phrases using different tempos, altering the stress placed on different words or syllables.

- Using recorded samples, have the client analyze the audio- or videotape and instruct you about his speech, explaining the repetitions, misarticulations, revisions, interjections, and so forth.

- Using modeling and signals, have the speaker increase his ability to pause for gradually increasing lengths of time. Use the natural pauses afforded by punctuation and clause boundaries. Do this in reading as well as paraphrasing of pictures of events. Role-playing of extratreatment events can also be useful here.

Other authors (Daly, 1986, 1988; Trotter & Silverman, 1973; Weiss, 1964) have suggested the use of masking devices (Dewar, Dewar, & Anthony, 1976) or delayed auditory feedback (Daly, 1992) in order to heighten the speaker's ability to monitor his speech proprioceptively. The slowed speech rate resulting from these devices also improves intelligibility and fluency. The use of a metronome (or tapping with a finger, pencil, etc.) may also facilitate concentration on how the client is speaking. Using a window-card so that one or a few words are visible to the client or reading backwards one word at a time may help to increase the speaker's ability to tolerate something other than his typical excessive rate. Fluency-modification programs, because of their tendency to incorporate rate variation and control as well as specific alterations of the vocal tract and articulators, are often especially useful with individuals who clutter.

As with the other "atypical" fluency disorders, treatment for cluttering is more appropriately done with a team approach, for these speakers are likely to have other educational, emotional, and learning difficulties. The prognosis for success is not particularly good but, as always it is better for children than adults (Daly, 1986, 1993; Luchsinger & Arnold, 1965; Myers & St. Louis, 1992; Silverman, 1995; Weiss, 1964).

CONCLUSION

For the clinician who understands the surface behaviors as well as the underlying cognitive and affective components of stuttering, treatment decisions become reasonably obvious. In contrast to the young person who stutters, the adolescent or adult client comes to treatment with a well-developed syndrome. The client's patterns of behavior and his thinking about the problem are tightly bound together with anxiety and fear. The speaker has made many subtle adjustments to his communication problem. Not only does the older client have to learn new ways of thinking and speaking, he may have to discard his old patterns and beliefs about himself and his speech.

The experienced clinician recognizes that, in many ways, it is the client who will lead the treatment process. What is possible during treatment is often determined by treatment variables such as the availability of services, the setting, and cost. Ideally, treatment will result in spontaneous fluency. Often for adult speakers, however, controlled or acceptable fluency is the outcome. More important, however, it is possible to reduce the severity of the handicap. That is, the person will become able to make choices that are not influenced by the possibility of stuttering. Treatment for adults often includes many features of both stuttering- and fluency-modification strategies. Fluency-modification techniques can help adult clients learn how to speak with greater fluency. However, those speakers who are able to achieve controlled or acceptable fluency also need to be able to repair their fluency breaks in an efficient and effortless manner. Thus, the clinician must decide how to sequence and blend the variety of strategies and techniques for each client.

Fluency treatment for adults often requires arduous work over many months or even years. The cognitive changes that occur can take some time to catch up to the behavioral changes taking place on the surface. Group meetings can serve as an essential part of treatment, providing information, support, and insight that are otherwise unavailable. The group activities provide the client with an opportunity to practice skills learned during individual meetings, try out new speaking roles, and test new perceptions with others who share the same problem. As a group leader, the clinician must develop the skill to carefully walk the line between giving the group direction and promoting flexibility of discussion.

RECOMMENDED READINGS

Culatta, R., & Goldberg, S. A. (1995). *Stuttering therapy: An integrated approach to theory and practice*. Boston: Allyn & Bacon (See especially the chapter, "A Synopsis of Approaches to the Treatment of Stuttering.").
Van Riper, C. (1973). *The treatment of stuttering* (2nd ed.). Englewood Cliffs, NJ: Prentice-Hall. See Part 2 of the book, "Our Therapeutic Approach."

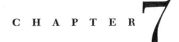

C H A P T E R 7

Counseling Strategies and Techniques

INTRODUCTION

Telling someone how to conduct counseling is like telling someone how to have a relationship. How you do it . . . "depends." It depends on the people who are involved and on the issue that brought the person to counseling to begin with. How to counsel also "depends" because counseling is client-centered and each client is unique. Of course, it is also hard to tell someone how to counsel because counseling need is a hands-on, dynamic experience rather than an academic exercise.

Responding to the question, "How do you do counseling?" reminds me of questions I am asked when giving presentations about treatment for fluency disorders. Someone in the audience will ask what to do with a particular client during treatment. For many years I tirelessly tried to answer each of these questions, but today I no longer do so. Now I am more likely to elicit a quizzical look from the audience by saying something like, "You know, I have no idea." Some expert—but beyond giving a technical answer that is based on some treatment protocol, I do not believe you can really *know* what to do in treatment with another person until you begin to establish a relationship with him. Establishing that relationship normally takes at least three or four sessions. Before I can make accurate and reasonable clinical decisions, I need to know how motivated the client is. I must know his story and begin to understand his situation in order to develop empathy for this person. I need to have a sense about his personality before I can probe and challenge him. Moreover, I need to get a feeling about how tough he will be when asked to apply his treatment techniques in the real world.

THE NECESSITY OF COUNSELING

Ackoff (1974) calls human problem solving "mess management." Clients as well as clinicians tend to be unsystematic and irrational in their decision making (Egan, 1990). The information on which we act is often incomplete, incorrect, or colored with emotion. The information we use to make our decisions tends to be distorted and far from objective. We must accept uncertainty and inconsistency. Clearly, this is also the case with our clinical decisions, based as they are on a combination of facts (or what seem, at least, to be facts) and the intuitive feelings achieved from the clinician's experience and insight. Although this collection of less-than-accurate information may be complex and even confusing at times, as Egan (1990) points out, it also reflects the richness of the human condition.

Should speech-language pathologists even be dealing with counseling issues? Should issues such as affect, emotions, and cognitive change be left to the professions of psychology, psychiatry, or counseling? If we find ourselves working with clients who have chronic life-adjustment problems, the answer is most likely yes. However, the vast majority of our clients are ordinary people experiencing a normal reaction to a communication disorder (Luterman, 1991). Serious communication disorders create genuine stress and anxiety. As Luterman indicates, such people are generally experiencing normal emotions in the face of an important problem. Clearly, then, speech-language pathologists should be doing counseling with their clients. Actually, we have no choice but to counsel them if our goal is to provide truly comprehensive treatment.

Many things are good for people. Exercise is one of them, having a network of good friends is another, and there is no question that counseling is beneficial for humans, especially those of us who have specific problems. This is true for communication disorders in general and fluency disorders in particular.

In the field of counseling, research has shown (Egan, 1990) that success rates typically have more to do with the therapist than the type of treatment. When reading through the current literature in counseling, the word that comes up more than any other is *relationship*. As Backus proposed in 1957, the learning and the substance of what goes on in the therapeutic relationship between the client and clinician are more essential than the materials. That relationship is also likely to be more crucial than the treatment strategies or techniques that are employed. In a review of research findings, Goleman (1985) discovered that the best predictor of success in the helping process—a better predictor than the therapy used, the attributes of the clinician, or the problems of the client—is the quality of the relationship between the client and the clinician. Patterson (1985) stated that counseling not only *involves* the relationship, it *is* the relationship.

As a participant in the counseling relationship, the clinician plays a pivotal role. In order to be an effective counselor, the clinician must be well trained and clever. However, the clinician must also be wise. As Egan (1990) states, we clinicians must understand the limitations of our profession, the shortcomings of the treatment strategies and techniques, and the strengths and weaknesses of both the clients and ourselves. We must recognize that the dogma of treatment approaches and book learning can filter, and on occasion bias, what we would otherwise understand about the person we are trying to help. Egan (1990) cautions that learning must be sifted through experience in order for the person to be wise.

Although as clinicians we learn about counseling strategies and techniques primarily in order to help our clients, it does not take long to realize that we can apply these same techniques to ourselves and the relationships in our own lives. For example, as a part of his rational emotive therapy (RET), Ellis (1977) provides a list of irrational ideas to which most of us adhere. Obviously, we would be healthier and happier if we could change our attitude about the following issues:

- It is a dire necessity for an adult human to be loved or approved of by virtually every "significant other" in his community.

- A person should be thoroughly competent, adequate, and successful in all possible respects if he is to consider himself worthwhile, and he is utterly worthless if he is incompetent in any way.

- Certain people can be labeled bad, wicked, or villainous, and they deserve severe blame or punishment for their sins.

- It is awful or catastrophic when things are not the way an individual would very much like them to be.

- Human unhappiness is externally caused, and individuals have little or no ability to control their sorrows and disturbances.

- If something is or may be dangerous or fearsome, one should be terribly concerned about it and should keep dwelling on the possibility of its occurrence.

- It is easier to avoid certain life difficulties and self-responsibilities than to face them.

- An individual should be dependent on others and needs someone stronger than himself on whom to rely.

- A person's past history is an all-important determinant of his present behavior, and because something once strongly affected his life, it should continue to do so.

- An individual should become quite upset over other people's problems and disturbances.

- There is invariably a correct, precise, and perfect solution to human problems, and it is catastrophic if this perfect solution is not found.

COUNSELING IN PSYCHOLOGY

Counseling is an everyday experience. Indeed, we counsel others in an informal manner as we help our friends and colleagues deal with life's problems. Egan (1990) suggests that the goal of professional counseling falls somewhere on a continuum between telling the client what to do and leaving him to his own devices. The ideal location on the continuum is a point where we are able to help our clients make their own decisions and act on them (Egan, 1990).

One helpful way to characterize professional counseling is to say that the primary focus is on the person and the secondary focus is on the problems. Along with the problems the individual may be facing are emotions associated with them. Another issue in counseling that applies to clients with communication disorders is the concept of missed opportunities. These are not so much specific problems per se, but situations of daily living that the client may suspect could be handled better. In many instances, counselors are asked to help with both issues: specific problems and missed opportunities.

Another useful way to consider the nature of counseling is to think in terms of "stuckness." People go to counseling because they are stuck (Ivey, 1983; cited in Egan, 1990, p. 270). Often, along with being stuck, clients feel helpless to do anything constructive about their situation. As Ivey (1983) submits, it is the responsibility of the counselor to get them unstuck. Often there is no distinct way to accomplish this. It takes experience and wisdom on the part of the clinician to assist the client to progress from the stuck and helpless feelings to better ways of dealing with the situation. However, as Ivey (1983) indicates, it is not an easy task to describe the "possible self" one can imagine and become.

At its most basic level counseling requires the clinician to respond with nonjudgmental respect for a client's unique differences and a willingness to listen instead of prescribe (Luterman, 1991). Furthermore, to be a counselor one must go beyond being a technician. The effective counselor is one who frequently does much more than the traditional requirements of the job.

One of the most misunderstood but at the same time more helpful insights concerning counseling is that the goal of counseling is not to make people feel better. Rather, the primary purpose is to enable the client to separate his feelings from his nonproductive behavior (Luterman, 1991). Moreover, although the problem or the pain may not go away (as with the loss of a loved one or the realization of a son or daughter's handicap), with successful counseling the client should be better able to manage the situation (Egan, 1990). As Egan states: "Helpers are effective to the degree that their clients, through client-helper interactions, are in a better position to manage their problem situations and/or develop the unused resources and opportunities of their lives more effectively" (1990, p. 5). Experiencing emotional pain in the face of great difficulty is normal. As Peck (1978) states in the first sentence of his book, *The Road Less Traveled,* "Life is difficult" (p. 15). It is normal and acceptable for people to feel sad when undesirable or bad things happen to them. The goal of counseling is to help the client disengage the feelings from behavior that is self-defeating.

On the other hand, it is not the task of the clinician to "rescue" clients (Luterman, 1991). In other words, the purpose of counseling is not necessarily to "solve" anything. In the case of fluency disorders, we are not necessarily solving or curing stuttering. Although it is possible, especially with young children, to essentially do away with most or all the behaviors associated with stuttering, it is not possible to "cure" attitudes or ways of thinking about a problem. Accordingly, counseling is not something that clinicians *do* to clients. Rather, it is a collaborative process between the people involved. As Egan (1990) suggests, in many ways counselors stimulate clients to provide services to themselves. We help them to have "more degrees of freedom" for making choices in their lives (Egan, 1990, p. 6).

Of course, it is true that as a result of counseling, clients sometimes feel better. However, it is even better if what the client is feeling good about are his accomplishments outside the counseling setting. Feeling good about a counseling session is of some benefit and such feelings may be thought of as the "perceived" gain (Egan, 1990). It is also possible, of course, that the counseling sessions prove painful. Sessions can be difficult simply because changing and growing are often painful.

However, in order to be effective, the counselor must help the client translate his choices into *action*. Thinking—even clear, creative, healthy thinking—will not change anything. It is the taking of action by the client that will result in more effective living. As Egan (1990) indicates throughout his book, *The Skilled Helper*, counseling is not about talking, it is about acting. If people want to manage their lives in a better way, they usually have to act differently.

Contemplating the situation is fine, but too much thinking can paralyze a person. When counselors fail, Egan suggests, they most often do so by not helping their clients to act, for counseling can too easily become a process of too much talking and too little action. We all know people who frequently talk about losing weight, running a marathon, taking a trip, or writing a grant and yet never get around to actually doing any of those things. Wonderful things often take place during the treatment or counseling session, but this is of little consequence if no action takes place in extratreatment situations.

The counselor provides the security and insight necessary that allows the client to explore new possibilities, go into action, and take risks. Support by the counselor makes it possible for the client to move into a future of his own creation. As Egan eloquently states, at the conclusion of successful counseling the clinician may be able to say about the client:

> Because I trusted him, he trusts himself more; because I cared for him, he is now more capable of caring for himself; because I invited him to challenge himself and because I took the risk of challenging him, he is now better able to challenge himself. Because of the way I related to him, he now relates better both to himself and to others. Because I respected his inner resources, he is now more likely to tap these resources. (Egan, 1990, p. 59).

Trust is understandably an essential part of a successful and therapeutic relationship and may be particularly important when working with adolescents (Daly, Simon, & Burnett-Stolnack, 1995).

COUNSELING IN COMMUNICATION DISORDERS

Many of the counseling principles discussed here obviously apply to clients with communication disorders. In the case of fluency disorders, the "problem" is usually apparent. What may not be so obvious, however, is the client's response to his situation.

In the field of communication disorders, there is cause for concern that few of our students receive adequate preparation for counseling our clients. McCarthy, Culpepper, and Lucks (1986) found that only one-third of the programs in communication disorders require a course in counseling. These authors noted that only 12 percent of clinicians who responded to their survey felt that they were adequately prepared to counsel their clients. According to Luterman (1991), far too many clinicians, although knowledgeable about the field, are clinically and interpersonally inept.

It is understandable that students are apt to feel uncomfortable taking on the role of a counselor. After all, most students are likely to be in their early twenties and should feel cautions, or at the very least sensitive, about counseling adults and parents who have considerably more life experience than the student has had the opportunity to obtain. Although the new clinician can appreciate that she is not an expert in all areas, she is in the process of becoming an expert in communication disorders. Gregory states it nicely:

> Because we are the specialists in communication disorders, no one else can counsel in this area as well as we. The first requisite of counseling is to understand the nature of the problem, and no other professional group knows as much about stuttering as the speech-language pathologist. (1995, p. 198)

To many clinicians, counseling means giving information and advice. However, as Luterman cautions, counseling by informing or persuading is a seductive model. It presents the view that "I as a professional have all of this information and experience. You as clients are ignorant of so many things that you need to know; therefore, I can make a better decision for you than you can for yourself" (1991, p. 3). Not only is this information-giving approach likely to result in the clinician "playing the role" of a counselor, but over time, it results in the job becoming a bore for the clinician and contributes to burnout.

Luterman (1991) suggests that a better approach is learning how to relate to our clients. By listening and valuing the client's story, we allow more affect to enter into the relationship. If the client is viewed as possessing the inherent wisdom to ultimately make good decisions for himself, we are less likely to take a role of lecturer, providing information that we assume will be helpful to this person. By listening and valuing, however, the counselor is more apt to assign the responsibility for change and action to the client. This strategy also increases the client's control, as well as his options.

EMOTIONS ENCOUNTERED DURING TREATMENT

Emotions are brought to the treatment session, not only, of course, by the client, but also by parents, spouses, and friends. Because clinicians working with fluency clients tend to believe their clients are so fragile that any mistake might do damage or at least result in increased stuttering (Cooper and Cooper, 1985b; 1992), clinicians tend to be careful about exposing their own feelings.

According to Luterman (1991), an underlying principle for counseling is that emotions are neither good or bad; they just are. Emotions (generally of the client but, on occasion, also those of the clinician) need to be acknowledged and accepted rather than judged. This, of course, is not necessarily an easy thing to do. There is often deep pain in those involved in a communication disorder (Luterman, 1991). In many cases, that pain is not going to go away. It is appropriate to acknowledge it for what it is—a normal reaction to an unwanted situation. In any case, as Luterman points out, it is always a mistake in any relationship to tell people that they should not feel a particular way. No matter how you do it, it is likely to make them feel guilty about their feelings.

There are several sources of emotions during treatment. The emotions of everyone who may be involved in the treatment process, including the client, the clinician, parents, spouses, siblings, and friends, all come into play. Luterman (1991) describes several of these emotions.

1. Grief: grief may be more likely to be associated with a communication problem if there is a relatively sudden onset such as with a stroke or traumatic brain injury. However, grief also exists for other problems, including fluency disorders. Clients and parents may move through the stages of grief—denial, anger, bargaining, depression, and acceptance. However, as Luterman (1991) suggests, the process is likely to be cyclical without set boundaries separating the stages. Participants will find themselves back in stages of grief that they have visited before. Luterman (1991) cites a wonderful story by the parents of a handicapped child who describe how they accepted the realization that they will spend a lifetime dealing with the fact that their child, although lovely and special, is not the child they expected. By recognizing and confronting grief and loss, one is able to slowly appreciate the goodness that is nonetheless available. Similarly, although it can be helpful to accept

the grief associated with having a fluency disorder, the client can, nonetheless, continue to strive to self-manage his situation.

2. Inadequacy: there is great frustration in being unable to "fix" a problem. Clinicians as well as parents feel a great need to help the person with an obvious problem. However, Luterman (1991) calls attention to what he terms the Annie Sullivan syndrome (referring to the teacher, counselor, and caretaker of Helen Keller). There is a danger in *rescuing* the client. There is a profound difference in taking charge of the situation (and the client) rather than empowering the client or the parents to manage it themselves. Luterman makes a convincing case for keeping ourselves from rescuing the client and thus making him codependent on a clinician. As in parenting, the ultimate goal in treatment is for the client to become independent. The clinician needs to be aware of her own need to be needed, and the client must be aware that his situation is his responsibility to handle.

3. Anger: anger has many sources, one of which is a violation of expectations. Clients, parents, and spouses have many expectations about themselves and each other. Clinicians and clients also have expectations of each other. When these expectations and hopes are not realized, anger is a common result. Communication problems typically restrict many options for the client and his family, which can be extremely frustrating for all involved. Moreover, as we see every day, when people are frustrated sufficiently often, anger will surface. Another source of anger is loss of control. As Luterman (1991) compassionately illustrates on several occasions throughout his book, having a loved one, especially a child or a spouse, hurting in some way makes one angry. Ask yourself how you feel when your choices or options are taken away. What is your response when you feel that you no longer have complete control over your life? Anger is not the only response, but it is certainly a basic one. The real danger is that such anger eventually can be displaced to others or turned inward to become depression.

One way not to be angry is not to care, to become numb. Of course, however, it is generally better to recognize anger. For example, professionals have the right to be angry at clients. If the client means enough to the clinician, the behavior that provokes anger, such as not completing his part of the clinical contract, should be acknowledged. In some cases, anger can be healthy, for as Luterman (1991) points out, there is a great deal of caring and energy therein. As Luterman suggests, the energy contained in anger can become the fuel for change.

4. Guilt: along with anger, guilt is another common emotion experienced by families of clients. This is most often the case with mothers where their children are concerned. Luterman (1991) makes the interesting observation that guilt is often a statement concerning power. It says, "I have had some power to influence or cause this bad result." Feeling guilty about something (or worrying) implies that the person can control the situation. It is a little like worrying about the weather or your safety before leaving for a trip. Obviously, it is possible to do appropriate and judicious planning for the weather or a trip, but worrying will not control the situation or save you from harm.

Luterman points out that guilty parents may overprotect their children. Such people can be the ideal parent for the clinician or teacher to work with. Although they are usually able to work well with younger children, difficulties typically arise when the child is a teenager and the parents face the prospect of letting go. On the other hand, guilt can fuel a commitment to rectify the problem and to undertake creative and demanding solutions.

5. Vulnerability: we are all vulnerable. Luterman states, "If we live long enough something bad will happen to us, and if we don't live long enough then something bad has already happened" (1991, p. 62). Speakers who stutter can be especially vulnerable in social settings. The ability to separate the problem (stuttering) from the client's reaction to the problem (feelings of vulnerability) is one measure of progress. Fortunately, vulnerability is usually easier to deal with than guilt and can actually be a positive force. Once our vulnerable and finite nature is acknowledged, and even accepted, we are free to take action to do what we can to improve our situation.

6. Feelings of Confusion: communication disorders can be, not only anxiety producing, but confusing, especially for parents. It is difficult to know what to do and whom to turn to for assistance. By giving information-based counseling, the clinician can add to feelings of confusion by providing information before the client is ready to receive it. On the other hand, such information can function to establish the credibility of the clinician at the outset of treatment. In any case, confusion on the part of the client can become a motivating force for learning.

In summary, the clinician's task is to acknowledge and accept all these emotions. They are, for better or worse, part of the syndrome and a component of the treatment process. While we will not always be able to make our clients feel better, we can help them by preventing the many emotional components of the problem from developing into inappropriate behaviors and secondary, negative feelings such as feeling guilty about feeling guilty, or being depressed as a result of anger.

COUNSELING STRATEGIES

Egan cautions that we should "beware the person of one book" (1990, p. 26). The message of a single book or single author can too easily become a calling. It is true that the discovery of *the method* can be empowering and give a sense of direction to the clinician and, therefore, the client. However, as Egan points out, such devotion to a single treatment path can also lead to a closing down of new ideas and new growth. The basis for choosing a strategy or technique for a professional should not be the method, but the nature and needs of the client.

Several years ago, at a professional meeting of a state association of speech-language pathologists, I was a member of a panel that was asked, along with the audience, to view a series of videotapes of children and adults with fluency disorders. The panel's task was to react to these hypothetical clients and discuss the strategies and techniques we speculated might be appropriate to use with them. As we took our turns offering suggestions about each tape segment, it became apparent that one member of the panel was giving the same response each time. Regardless of the client's age, severity, or nature of the fluency breaks, this clinician would take the microphone and say something like: "I believe strongly in the _____ method and feel that this approach would be ideal for this client. I have seen this method work for many clients and would use this approach with this person."

Regardless of the demonstrated efficacy of this particular method we were all witnessing a clear example of a "one book" approach to helping clients. Just as in any treatment, the choice of a counseling strategy *must* be driven by the needs of the client rather than the dogma from a book. As discussed in Chapter 1, if you want to be a technician, you may make your clinical decisions according to the treatment manual. If you want to be a professional, however, you must make your decisions primarily according to the needs of the client.

According to Luterman (1991), there is no experimental evidence supporting the superiority of any one counseling strategy. An approach is often selected because it coincides with the personality of the clinician and her view of reality. Webster (1966) suggested that the risk of hurting a client may be heightened by using a prescriptive approach with a nonaccepting and noncompassionate clinician. If in doubt about what strategy to employ, she recommended a less direct approach since she believes it is virtually impossible for the clinician to damage a client by listening and trying to understand what his world looks like. On the other hand, Luterman (1991) indicates that the safest approach is not a nondirective approach because this can generate client anger when it violates expectations of what the clinician should provide. He suggests that the safest choice is a cognitive approach that advises clients to restructure the view of their situation. People can survive bad advice, he suggests, for we have been doing it for most of our lives.

Luterman (1991) describes four general approaches to counseling: behavioral, humanistic, existential, and cognitive.

Behavioral Counseling

Behavioral counseling can be an attractive strategy, especially for new clinicians. It provides a distinctive structure whereby the clinician can break down the behavior to be changed into a series of subtasks, each with successive approximations toward the desired goal. This approach is relatively easy to teach because of the concrete nature of the techniques and the specific, overt criteria for moving on to a new level.

Humanistic Counseling

This approach was developed by Carl Rogers (1951) and Abraham Maslow (1968). The underlying concept of this strategy is that humans have an innate drive toward self-actualization (e.g., the true Buddha is within oneself). The basic elements of this approach include the concepts of congruence (bringing into parallel the parts of the self, particularity the intellectual and emotional components), empathy, self-actualization, and unconditional positive regard for the client. Without labeling him the clinician attempts to release the client's self-actualizing drive so that he can take appropriate actions to solve his problems. Luterman (1991) points out that, because of the abstract nature of the basic concepts involved, this approach can be difficult both to teach and to learn. Furthermore, the responsibility for change rests almost completely on the client and, for some clients, it is difficult to accept that the self-actualizing drive will take effect. According to Luterman, this approach does not work well with severely involved adults and children or those with limited abilities.

Existential Counseling

This approach comes from the French intellectual movement of the mid-1800s and the work of the Danish philosopher Søren Kierkegaard. This view holds that many human problems are a result of anxiety due to the facts of our existence. That is, we must die, we have freedom to make choices, we are alone, and life is meaningless. This view is different from traditional psychoanalytic theory, where the source of anxiety results from the conflict between the id (the pleasure drive) and the superego (social restrictions). In existential theory, there is no clinical value in understanding the client's past history or behavior.

For individuals whose response to life is to avoid the basic facts of human existence, there are some interesting results.

Death: existentialists hold that anxiety resulting from our eventual death can result in the avoidance or postponement of activities or decisions. Furthermore, it can result in a decreased ability to appreciate our everyday existence. By not recognizing the boundaries of our existence, we are likely to miss the beauty of the commonplace. The greater this death anxiety the more one is likely to experience a restricted and unfulfilled life. The recognition that nothing is permanent enables us to value what we have been given while we can.

Responsibility: each of us is responsible for our own actions. Whether we admit it or not, in many respects at least, we are in charge. Because of this, the clinician should not feel sorry for the client with a problem. The client has a choice about what to do about his situation and about what to tell himself about his circumstances. If he chooses, his problems can be approached as challenges, as opportunities to grow. Virtually every writer in counseling agrees that the starting point of therapeutic change is the *assumption of responsibility* by the client and a decision to change (DiClemente, 1993). However, acknowledging this responsibility frequently results in anxiety. As Luterman (1991) points out, the assumption of responsibility by the client implies that we ought not to play the role of the rescuer. Rather, the clinician ought to empower clients to assume the major responsibility for their situations. To the degree that we rescue clients they will continue to feel powerless.

Loneliness: as Luterman states, "We are alone and that crushing fact is central to existential thought" (1991, p. 19). We are all lonely at times, but clients with communication disorders are apt to be uncommonly so. By confronting our loneliness, we are able to generate an unconditional regard for humanity in general.

Meaninglessness: as if loneliness were not difficult enough to face, existentialists propose that there is no extrinsic meaning to the world, which cannot be judged good or bad. The world just is. Nevertheless, as Luterman (1991) points out, it is possible to find meaning in the solution of a problem, a strategy that often results in success for families or individuals.

Existentialist philosophy suggests that it is the counselor's mission to help the client face these facts of existence and find more appropriate and non-pathological ways of managing his life situation.

Cognitive Counseling

This view holds that any human problem is, in many important ways, is a disorder of thinking. The clinician helps the client to identify specific misconceptions and unrealistic expectations that underlie his behavior. This strategy results in a confrontational approach whereby the client is challenged to examine the underlying "irrational" assumptions that are reflected in his language. Ellis's (1977) list of irrational thought processes presented at the outset of this chapter and his rational emotive therapy (RET) comprise a good example of this approach in counseling psychology. In the area of fluency disorders, there are a number of authors who report using this general strategy with clients (Bryngelson, Chapman & Hansen, 1944; Emerick, 1988; Fransella, 1972; Hayhow & Levy, 1989; Johnson, 1946; Manning, 1991; Maxwell, 1982; Van Riper, 1947, 1982; Williams, 1979).

COUNSELING TECHNIQUES

According to Luterman (1991), good counseling technique flows from personality. He suggests that specific techniques should not be easily apparent to the person being counseled or to an observer. "If clients know they are being counseled, the counselor is probably doing it poorly" (Luterman, 1991, p. 87). Ideally, the techniques become congruent with the personality of the clinician and blend into the treatment process. If the clinician acts mechanically the technique is likely to fail because it will be discontinuous with the authenticity of the relationship.

Moreover, although specific counseling techniques are helpful, in and of themselves, they are not counseling. For example, Rogers (1980) spoke against the appalling consequences of overemphasizing microskills during counseling. Rather, to be effective, the clinician must approach counseling as a *fully human endeavor.* The clinician's counseling skills must become extensions of the helper's humanity, not just bits of technology.

A good example of this idea is the use of silence during treatment. Less-experienced clinicians are often uncomfortable with silence. Silence can be embarrassing for the client as well as the clinician, and its intensity will eventually force the inexperienced clinician to act. Luterman (1991) suggests that silence forces inexperienced clinicians to become role bound. The clients, meanwhile, sit back and watch. Actually, silence can be a powerful technique to facilitate change, for where there is silence, there is often growth. Indeed, silence can be a powerful motivator for client action.

Silence is not a void, but a part of the process. As in Oriental ink drawings, the open spaces are an intentional and important part of the overall composition. The deepest feelings in a relationship can take place in silence, for there is companionship in thoughtful silence. Observe couples who are congruent. There is much communication during the silence. This is observable also in the process of a dynamic clinical relationship. As a clinician with whom I worked years ago used to say, "I knew we were friends when we could share the silence."

Nonverbal Behaviors of the Clinician and Client

Most clinicians today are aware that the use and appropriateness of many nonverbal behaviors are culture specific. The array of just what is and is not considered appropriate across the categories of age, gender, race, and nationality makes for fascinating study and interesting accounts. It can also make a clinician inhibited, for even the most cursory study of cultural traditions makes one aware of the serious consequences of misreading cultural or ethnic responses. It is difficult, if not impossible, for the clinician to fully understand all the possible microcultures present in a pluralistic society. We must, of course, continue to learn as much as we can about the populations we are likely to encounter in our clinical practice. As Culatta and Goldberg state:

> Speech-language pathologists cannot be expected to be experts in anthropology. Nor can we be expected to be intimately aware of all the microcultural variables of each cultural subgroup in our country. Sensitivity toward the existence of differences within a pluralistic society, however, is critical. (1995, pp. 116–117)

With this in mind, we provide the following recommendations for facilitating interpersonal communication. With an awareness of these behaviors, the clinician should be able to monitor her nonverbal reactions to client's comments in terms of such responses as defensiveness, anger, surprise, and encouragement. Egan (1990) suggests the following acronym to recall the relevant behaviors: SOLER.

S   Face the client *Squarely*, with a straightforward posture.

O   Adopt an *Open* posture; do not cross your arms or legs, as the open posture indicates confidence and involvement.

L   At times, *Lean* toward the client; leaning forward or backward indicates the degree of involvement and the equilibrium during a discussion.

E   Maintain good (appropriate) *Eye* contact.

R   Be relatively *Relaxed* or natural.

Another aspect of nonverbal behavior involves calibrating yourself to the client. A good way to think of this process is that the clinician should be doing something well beyond what a tape recorder could do. Rather than merely recording the client's words, you are observing and interpreting cues, such as his posture, facial expressions, movement, tone of voice, and general grooming. As Egan (1990) suggests, a person's nonverbal behavior has a way of *leaking* messages to others. In addition, Egan suggests that nonverbal behaviors can serve to punctuate verbal statements, to confirm or enhance, to reveal inconsistencies, and to send controlling or regulating messages to others.

VERBAL BEHAVIORS

The verbal behaviors of the clinician combine with nonverbal actions of the client and the clinician to indicate the status of the therapeutic relationship. The clinician has several options for verbally responding to the client's questions and circumstances. Luterman (1991) provides some general categories of verbal responses from which the clinician can choose.

Content Response

The content response is the most commonly used. Such responses tend to keep the relationship at an expected and predictable level. Content responses are most likely used at outset of treatment, especially if the participants anticipate that the treatment will be short term. The client may ask, "What is the likelihood of relapse following intensive treatment for fluency disorders?" to which the clinician will provide an answer.

Counterquestion Response

Luterman (1991) points out that most people do not really want advice. What they seek is confirmation for a decision they have already made. Although their statement may take the form of a question, what they are asking for is not an answer, but a confirmation of their decision. Luterman points out that people do not learn from (or even listen to) advice. Furthermore, if the advice works, the client will come back for more, while if it does not, he may be angry. Luterman suggests that the most productive response one can give to a confirmation question is a counterquestion. The client may ask, "Am I making progress in therapy?" and the clinician may respond, "What behaviors and attitudes have you changed?"

Early in the therapeutic relationship, before trust has evolved, there are apt to be many questions (Luterman, 1991). However, with the development of a secure relationship, there tend to be fewer questions and more observations and statements. Luterman suggests that the counterquestion can be a powerful tool for moving a relationship beyond the initial stages.

Affect Response

The affect response by the clinician is also helpful for building the counseling relationship. Rogers (1951) called this empathetic listening. Examples of this type of response would be comments by the clinician such as, "You must be very frustrated by this situation," or, "You must feel extremely helpless when that occurs."

Reframing Response

This response takes the form of restating the client's question in a different context. "Why should I have a stuttering problem?"—"Why shouldn't you be someone who stutters?" This response involves reconstructing the situation (problem) as a chance to learn and grow. Luterman (1991) suggests that this is a powerful tool for anyone in an undesirable situation.

Sharing Self Response

The sharing self response is quite natural for some clinicians but less likely to be a reply of the professional who has a need to be in control at all times. By sharing our own doubts and uncertainties, we become more genuine. The clinician is free to honestly answer a question by saying something like, "At the moment I don't have any idea what would be best for you [or your child]." The clinician may acknowledge that the process of treatment is difficult or that she is uncertain about the next therapeutic step. Luterman (1991) indicates that it is permissible to ask the client if he has any ideas about what to do next (a form of assigning responsibility and independence and increasing the internal control of the client). According to Luterman (1991) it is not advisable for the clinician to do this too early in treatment, for she may lose credibility if she has not yet proved herself. Once the client has achieved a higher degree of self-esteem, such sharing responses can emerge, however.

Affirmation Responses

In this response, the clinician affirms the client and provides a sounding board for the client to explain and ventilate the emotions associated with his situation. The clinician listens to the speaker and nonverbally indicates that the client is free to express himself. As Luterman indicates, "It often shows a fine command of language to say nothing" (1991, p. 94). Of course, in order to know which of the possible responses may be best, the clinician must actively monitor both the client's verbal and nonverbal messages.

ACTIVE-LISTENING TECHNIQUES

Active-listening techniques are essential for facilitating the development of any relationship. In a clinical relationship, active listening is vital if the clinician is to effectively probe and challenge the client. Listening actively implies something beyond understanding the client's verbal and nonverbal messages. It involves "being with" the client, both physically and psychologically, in order to communicate empathy (Egan, 1990).

In the active-listening process, the clinician uses both verbal and nonverbal cues to recognize the client's core messages and cognitive patterns. The clinician continually asks the question, "What is it that the client wants me to understand?" The task takes persistence and concentration. Furthermore, the clinician must be aware of possible cultural biases. As Egan (1990) suggests, if the clinician's cultural filters are strong, there is a greater likelihood of bias and distorted understanding. He also cautions that (as discussed earlier) book learning can distort perception. It is important to keep academic theories in the background and the client in the foreground. In addition, it is helpful for the clinician to keep from rehearsing a possible response to the client before he has completed what he has to say. Rehearsal puts a stop to active listening by the clinician. Finally, interrupting the client can be permissible if it is done appropriately, especially for clarification. However, it must not be done simply because the clinician has something to say.

Expressing Empathy

The clinician who is able to express empathy has a way to get inside another's world. As Egan (1990) explains, "being with" the client is temporarily living another's life, as a means to viewing the person without labels, interpretation, or categories. Rogers suggested that empathy is, in and of itself, a healing agent. "It is one of the most potent aspects of therapy, because it releases, it confirms, it brings even the most frightened client into the human race. If a person is understood, he or she belongs" (1986, p. 129).

Egan (1990) indicates that while listening to the client helps the clinician get in touch with the client's world, empathy helps the clinician to understand that world. He noted that clients rate understanding as the thing they find most helpful during counseling. Unfortunately, the clinician's ability to indicate empathy is not a skill that comes naturally. Of course, the clinician must first *be* empathetic before empathy can be expressed (often without words but rather with a glance or touch). The expression of empathy involves the clinician's shared understanding of the client's experiences, behaviors, and feelings. It is important to distinguish empathy from sympathy. Sympathy denotes agreement, whereas empathy denotes *understanding* and *acceptance* of the person.

The clinician's perception of the client must be accurate. Furthermore, in order to be helpful, the clinician's understanding of the client must be presented to the client, and the clinician must be assertive enough to act when the time is right. Egan (1990) suggests that once the clinician has formulated an accurate understanding of the client's situation the clinician can try the formula, "You feel _____ because _____." Egan indicates that the client will help the clinician stay on track by responding with silence, correcting her, or restating her understanding. If, on the other hand, the clinician is accurate in her perception, the client will often respond by moving on. Other helpful suggestions for responding with empathy include allowing yourself time to reflect on what the client said, using short responses (i.e., do not give speeches), and being yourself in your choice of words and style.

Probing the Client

The purpose of probing is to highlight the client's blind spots about his situation. Egan (1990) describes probes as verbal tactics that help the client talk about himself and define his problem in terms of specific *experiences*, *behaviors*, and *feelings*. The goal of probing is not to identify a single, momentous piece of information but rather to increase understanding. This is usually accomplished by asking the client to become more specific. With accurate probing there should be an increase in the quality of the information the client can use in making better decisions. The speech-language pathologist working with a client who stutters is not likely to probe as often or as deeply as the psychologist who is working with a client with a personality disorder. Nonetheless, on many occasions throughout treatment, clinicians need to obtain more specific information concerning a client's behavior, motivation, and cognitive processes.

Egan (1990) provides some guidelines for probing:

- Do not assault your clients with too many questions, don't grill them.

- Ask questions that serve a specific purpose. Use questions that challenge the client to think, questions that have teeth but not fangs.

- Ask open-ended questions that get clients to discuss specific experiences, behaviors, and feelings.

- Keep the focus on the client, keep placing the ball in his court.
- Keep in mind the value of using nonverbal communication to prompt the client.
- Consider the possibility that if you ask two questions in a row, it may well be that they are poor questions.
- Think of verbal probes as the spice of the communication process. They should remain condiments.

Challenging the Client

Closely related to probing techniques is the skill of challenging the client. This is similar to challenging and pushing the client, as described in Chapter 1. As the clinician determines the client's strength and resilience, it is often necessary to push him into attitudes and behaviors that he is likely to resist. It is possible, of course, to challenge someone and still be "for" that person. Challenging another person signifies that you take him seriously enough to respond when his choices are not in his best interest. It also indicates the clinician's belief in the client's potential. As Fisher and Ury (1981) suggested, it is best to be soft on the person and hard on the problem.

USING HUMOR

As discussed in Chapter 1, humor can play an important part in the clinical relationship. Humor allows the clinician to challenge the client and discuss things that would otherwise be risky. Humor involves aspects of distancing oneself from a problem, conceptually shifting one's view of the situation, and mastering events and situations that were previously avoided or anxiety producing. As Rusk (1989, cited in Egan, 1990) suggests, deliberate self-change requires a willingness to (a) stand back from yourself far enough to question your familiar beliefs and attitudes about yourself and others, and (b) persist at awkward and risky experiments designed to increase your self-respect and satisfy your needs. Not only can humor facilitate such self-change, but for the clinician, humor provides a window for viewing the cognitive changes associated with a problem.

CLIENT RESPONSIBILITIES

At the core of the helping process is the assumption that, within limits, people are capable of making choices and controlling their destinies. Egan (1990) argues that many people adopt a deterministic view of life without realizing it. Moreover, while it is true that many limits are imposed on us by social, political, economic, and cultural forces, accepting responsibility for one's own life is at the heart of self-respect and happiness. Egan cites Farrelly and Brandsma (1974), who suggest a view of the client that is both encouraging, and, probably, accurate.

- clients can change if they choose to do so
- clients have more resources for managing problems in living than most clinicians assume
- the psychological fragility of clients is overrated both by themselves and others
- maladaptive attitudes and behaviors of clients can be significantly altered, no matter how severe or chronic
- effective challenge can provide in the client a self-annoyance that can lead to a decision to change

Often we need to hit an emotional bottom in order to move on with the coping process. As a result of growth, we begin to recognize that denial is not the best response to a situation. It really is possible to accept the associated pain and move along with it. The goal of counseling may not be a matter of going exactly where we think we should go or even reaching what we may think of as normalcy. *Rather, the goal is to live life to the fullest in the face of the situations with which we are presented.*

Metalinguistic Indicators of Change

The language a person uses to describe his situation provides important clues about who he is and where he is going. The way a person depicts his situation or problem can indicate signs of progress during treatment. Moreover, as described earlier, in the discussion of cognitive restructuring approaches to counseling and treatment, by changing the way we describe a problem, we can often change the problem itself. However, changes in the way the client talks about himself need to be made gently. Encouraging such changes is less appropriate early in treatment when his affect is high and it may be all the client can do to accurately tell his story and describe his situation. Furthermore, as Ellis (1977) indicates, trust in the clinician must be high or else linguistic alterations will be seen as interfering and annoying. Ellis provides some recommendations for changing the way we talk about ourselves and our situations. As Luterman (1991) suggests, these ideas can be of great help in both professional and personal interactions. The client's language will reflect his level of "stuckness" and degree to which he is able to assume responsibility for his choices and his world.

- *Should* and *ought* may be changed to *want to* or *not want to*, as in changing "I should use my new fluency modification techniques" to "I want to [or do not want to] use my new fluency modification techniques."

- *Have to* can be changed to *want to* or *choose to*, as in changing, "I have to stay home and not speak to people," to, "I want to stay home," or, "I choose to stay home and not risk a stuttering moment."

- *We, us, society* may be changed to *I*, as in changing "We are unhappy with this treatment program or technique" to, "I am unhappy with this approach [therefore, I can do something about it if I choose to]."

- *To be* verbs can be modified from, "I am a dumb person," to, "Although I did a dumb thing I am still a smart person."

- The word *but* can be changed to *and*, as in changing, "I want to speak in public but I am afraid," to, "I want to speak in public and I am afraid."

More accurate and appropriate ways of using language to describe a situation can force the person to take responsibility for his behavior and the associated self-talk concerning it.

Choosing a Future

According to Lindaman and Lippitt (1979), in order to shape a future, we need to hold in our minds an image of what it is that we truly want. Imagination is one way for the client to propel himself into the future. Egan (1990) points out that the use of imagery is slowly moving back into the mainstream of counseling after many decades of disfavor. He suggests that the use of conscious and creative imagery can help to overcome inertia. Egan asserts that inertia tends to permeate life and influence our decisions and is one of the principal mechanisms for keeping individuals, organizations, and institutions mired in the *psychopathology of the average* (Maslow, 1968).

Some procedures for realistically defining the future include having the client find new models for configuring their own lives. Egan (1990) recommends using as a model biographies of current or previous clients, keeping in mind issues of confidentiality. Clients can be asked to write about a desired future or construct their own epitaph. Based on his experience, Egan points out that many clients are much better writers than most people realize and can use this ability to define a new future.

Possible Negative Responses

Because change is difficult, clients will sometimes be resistant. As suggested in Chapter 1, as clinicians, we sometimes have to be demanding and push the client into areas of thinking and behavior he does not want to enter. It is possible, on occasion, that the clinician will encounter a variety of negative responses. Egan (1990) provides a description of three such characteristics: passivity, learned helplessness, and disabling self-talk.

Passivity. Egan (1990) indicates that few people bring more than about 10 percent of their human potential to the problems and challenges of living.

He suggests that, in the field of counseling, untapped human potential is probably a more frequent problem for most people than emotional disorders. Citing Schiff's (1975) description of passive behavior, Egan indicates that people tend to evade problems by doing nothing, overadapting and uncritically accepting goals proposed by others, engaging in random behavior, or becoming incapacitated by shutting down or blowing up.

Learned Helplessness. Many clients tend to believe that there is nothing they can do about their situation, resulting in depression. Clients who are minimally helpless tend to be minimally depressed. Obviously, clients will not be able to control everything, but each one must learn those things that they can self-manage and those they cannot.

Disabling Self-Talk. Clients may say they "can't do it," "can't help it," or "aren't able to cope." Clearly, such a pattern of thinking can also lead to a negative self-image and depression.

CLINICIAN CHARACTERISTICS

This chapter began with a discussion of the importance of the clinical relationship. The characteristics of the clinician have a primary impact on the nature of that relationship. We discussed many of the characteristics of the clinician in Chapter 1 and will include a few additional qualities here as they relate specifically to the counseling relationship. As Luterman (1991) comments, if the literature on the desirable personality characteristics of the ideal counselor were examined, the only ones who might conceivably have a chance to qualify would be some of the more outstanding saints. However, as Egan (1990) argues, it is not necessary for the effective clinician to be an entirely self-actualized person. It is critical, he states, for the clinician to be a person who has a deep interest in people and a sensitivity to others. The competent counselor needs to be a caring individual who does not impose his or her beliefs on others, who maintains a constant awareness of self, and who does not hide behind the role of professional. Luterman states:

> I think the key to counseling is the congruence of the counselor. As I become more congruent, technique slips away or, more accurately, becomes incorporated into everything I do. I think the most important thing a counselor brings to the helping relationship is self. The importance of the congruent professional far exceeds the value of any diagnostic test or specific techniques in counseling. (1991, p. 180)

In a similar manner, Egan indicates that, for a clinician to be an effective counselor, it is essential that she understand herself, including her own assumptions, beliefs, values, standards, skills, strengths, weaknesses, idiosyncrasies, style of doing things, foibles, and temptations. She needs to appreciate how her characteristics will be apt to influence her interactions with her clients. To begin the process of introspection, Egan suggests the following questions (1990, p. 25):

- How did you decide to be a helper?
- Why do you want to be a helper?
- With what emotions are you comfortable?
- What emotions—in yourself or others—give you trouble?
- What are your expectations of clients?
- How will you deal with your clients' feelings toward you?
- How will you handle your feelings toward your clients?
- To what degree can you be flexible, accepting, gentle?

One critical characteristic for an effective clinician and counselor is her overall competence. Whatever true competence may be for each professional, it is likely to be a lifelong pursuit. Particularly in the areas of human behavioral science, competence means more than simply understanding models, strategies, and techniques. It means being able to "deliver the goods" to the people you are trying to help. All effective counselors must continue to learn—it is basic for counseling and for life. Beyond learning, the effective counselor must model the things she challenges her clients to do. More than learning and thinking must be modeled—action must be modeled as well. As Egan (1990) suggests, if the clinician wants her clients to act, she must be active in her own life in regard to her own problems. Berenson and Mitchell (1974) forcefully suggest that only those counselors who are committed to living fully themselves deserve to help others.

Being competent does not mean having solutions to all the problems you will face. Difficult cases will, as Luterman (1991) suggests, cause the icy finger of possible failure to threaten and test our confidence. Nonetheless, if the clinician is learning, if she is a truly responsible professional, she should be operating on the *fringes of incompetence*. Effective counselors, clinicians, and people in general should take risks and occasionally make mistakes or they will not grow.

At the end of his book, Egan has a wonderful paragraph discussing the need for the counselor to go beyond the technology of helping and move toward becoming authentic. He indicates that our clinical and other life experiences can be either a teacher or a tyrant. Going through these experiences provides us with the opportunity to recognize and accept the shadow side of ourselves, our clients, and the world. To do so without becoming a victim is crucial but not the reward of the experience. The events of each life need to be wrestled with, reflected on, and learned from. Only then can these events become our teacher and friend. Wrestling with our self, our colleagues, our friends, our demons, and our God will provide us both pain and comfort. It is that struggle that will help the skilled helper become the wise helper (Egan, 1990, p. 409).

CONCLUSIONS

Even though clients with fluency disorders do not tend to have chronic life-adjustment problems, they experience real and normal reactions to a serious communication disorder. To influence how clients respond to this fact is the goal of counseling. If clinicians are to provide a comprehensive response to their clients, they have no choice but to provide some form of counseling. The need for counseling may be most obvious for the parents of a child who stutters, but clinicians also serve a valuable counseling role for adults.

At the center of the counseling process is the relationship of the client and the clinician. The clinician can enhance this relationship, not by playing the role of a counselor, but by providing a nonjudgmental response and actively listening to the client's story. The degree of directiveness will be determined by the needs of the client, and an ideal response is likely to fall somewhere between telling the client what to do and letting him make his own decisions. The goal of counseling is not to make clients feel better or solve their problems. Clients will feel genuinely better as a result of the *actions* they take following treatment. The emphasis is on clients taking action to design a new future for themselves. The goal is to deal more effectively with the situations with which they are presented. To the degree that the clinician can model this response to problems the client is more likely to modify his own behavior. The client's manner of changing and adjusting to his communication disorder will determine the long-term success of treatment and the possibility of relapse.

RECOMMENDED READINGS

Albach, J., & Benson, V. (Eds.). (1994). *To say what is ours. The best of 13 years of letting GO* (3rd ed.). San Francisco, CA: National Stuttering Project.

Egan, G. (1990). *The skilled helper, A systematic approach to effective helping* (4th ed.). Pacific Grove, CA: Brooks/Cole Publishing Co.

Luterman, D. M. (1991). *Counseling the communicatively disordered and their families* (2nd ed.). Austin, chs. 1 ("Counseling by the Speech Pathologist and Audiologist," pp. 1–8), 4 ("The Emotions of Communication Disorders," pp. 49–76), 8 ("Working with Families," pp. 135–166), and 9 ("Counseling and the Field of Communication Disorders," pp. 167–180).

Webster, E. (1966). Parent counseling by speech pathologists and audiologists. *Journal of Speech and Hearing Disorders, 31,* 331–345.

Indicators of Progress during Treatment

INTRODUCTION

Peck, in a discussion of the psychotherapeutic process, indicates, "The majority of patients, even in the hands of the most skilled and loving therapists, will terminate their therapy at some point far short of completely fulfilling their potential" (1978, p. 180). This is also the nature of intervention for fluency disorders. Not all clients make as much progress as we would like, but almost any client who is ready and motivated enough to face his communication problem head-on is likely to make some progress during treatment. As the client meets with a competent clinician, he will begin to learn something about himself and his communication problem. As he is guided through the features of his stuttering, he is likely to become desensitized to the problem. He will develop a more accurate and broader view of his communication disorder, and he will gradually begin making better decisions that are less influenced by the fact that he happens to be a person who stutters. Gradually, as these and other changes occur, he will become less handicapped.

Therapeutic progress is much more than the changes that take place during the time the client is immersed in formal treatment. An important aspect of the client's long-term progress is the continuum of *formal versus informal treatment*. Formal treatment may be thought of as that time when the client is receiving and paying for the services of a professional clinician. Informal treatment may be regarded as the much longer time following formal treatment, when the client is on his own. During informal treatment, there is minimal or no contact with the professional clinician. In many important ways, this latter stage of treatment is the most critical part of the overall treatment process. It is the client who is doing the changing, and the process of change cannot cease at the conclusion of formal treatment. The months and years that follow formal treatment will provide the true measure of treatment efficacy. Can the client, once he is on his own, make consistent use of the strategies and techniques acquired during formal treatment? Will he take the time to expand his ability to monitor and modify his fluency? Will he gather the energy to cultivate the cognitive and affective changes that are necessary to reduce the handicap of the syndrome, or will relapse, to a greater or lesser degree, dictate additional periods of formal intervention?

This chapter will discuss ways of considering the major variables that appear to influence progress during formal treatment. Progress will be discussed in terms of the most obvious surface feature of the syndrome, the frequency and nature of stuttering. However, other directions of change during treatment will be suggested, changes that are more likely to indicate the successful long-term modification of the syndrome. The variables discussed in this chapter will set the stage for the final chapter, where success following formal treatment is considered.

DEFINING PROGRESS

Identifying progress during treatment is more intricate than it may first appear. It is a more complex issue than assessing the nature of the syndrome at the outset of treatment. Certainly, clinicians will interpret progress differently, depending on the overall treatment strategy and associated techniques that are used. An indicator of progress for a client taking part in a treatment program emphasizing fluency enhancement will not necessarily be thought of as progress for another client who is taking part in a program where stuttering modification is the major focus. Determining progress during treatment is an intricate issue, as suggested by the fact that treatment efficacy is only recently being addressed in an orderly manner. (For a review on treatment efficacy research in stuttering see volume 18, numbers 2 and 3, of the *Journal of Fluency Disorders*, 1993). In discussing this issue with children, Conture and Guitar (1993) suggested that treatment can be considered successful if the child begins to communicate easily whenever and to whomever he or she chooses. This also seems to be a reasonable approach to take with adults.

The Variability of Progress

Just as fluency itself can be highly variable, progress during treatment is variable. In addition, fluctuations in some features of the syndrome are better indicators than others. Changes in some features (the percent of words stuttered) may indicate short-term progress, while changes in other features (decreased avoidance of words) provide a better indication of long-term treatment effects. Furthermore, the rate at which these features will change is influenced, not only by the particular treatment strategy, but by the treatment setting and the clinician.

As discussed in Chapter 1, the clinician plays a crucial role in motivating and guiding the client. It is likely, however, that the most influential variable is the client himself, for personal change and growth are highly individualized. Not all clients will make the same degree of progress during formal treatment. There are, of course, clinicians who describe impressive levels of success for their treatment program, but a closer examination of these reports often indicates that the selection process for inclusion in the program was highly restrictive (e.g., only clients who are highly motivated, could afford the time and cost, or were responsive to the diagnostic tasks were included in treatment). In other instances, the criteria for success are overly simplistic, for example, the percentage of syllables stuttered within the clinic environment.

Regardless of the particular treatment strategy, clinicians who have written about treatment efficacy for adult clients seem to accept what could be called the *one-third rule*. That is, regardless of the overall treatment strategy, and everything else being equal in terms of client motivation and intelligence, clinician experience, and the timing of intervention, one-third of clients will make good progress; one-third, moderate progress; and one-third, often because they prematurely drop out of treatment, little or no progress.

Of those speakers who make good progress, there will be some that do extremely well and conclude formal treatment exhibiting little or no stuttering behavior. Perhaps even more telling, if these speakers should experience a break in their fluency, they are not likely to panic. They are able to analyze what it is they are doing and modify their breaks into smooth and comfortable forms of stuttering. They are assertive, choosing to enter into new and demanding speaking situations. When these clients are faced with a difficult communication situation, they are able to adjust to a smooth speech mode and achieve fluency-shaping targets that enable them to move through feared words and sounds. Finally, after formal treatment concludes, they are able to maintain these behaviors and attitudes about their fluency disorder.

Other clients, while not showing such marked change, will make good progress. They will regress somewhat from their levels of fluency during formal treatment. They will continue to stutter but with less frequency and struggle than they did prior to treatment, and they will slowly become less afraid of the stuttering experience. The fact that they are people who stutter incrementally plays a much smaller part in their lives. To be sure, they stutter on some occasions, but they also maintain their ability to make significant changes in the form of their stuttering. They gradually learn to avoid less and are progressively less likely to be at the mercy of a possible stuttering event.

Of course, there is the final 33 percent of all clients—those who make little or no progress. Often these are individuals who attend treatment for a relatively short time. As they realize the effort and time it will take to change all the features of their syndrome, their motivation begins to fade. Attendance becomes inconsistent and ceases. If change has occurred, it is enough for now, and the cost of additional change is not deemed worth the effort. Perhaps we should decline to see such clients until they demonstrate acceptable levels of motivation at the outset, or maybe a little knowledge and some new insights will set the stage for later progress and we should attempt to do what we can when we have the opportunity.

In a review of thirteen clinicians and their associates Martin (1981) came to a similar conclusion about progress. He determined that one-third of the clients achieved and maintained satisfactory fluency, one-third achieved fluency during therapy but regressed over time, and one-third either failed to complete treatment programs or were unavailable for follow-up assessment. He stressed that a major problem preventing a complete interpretation of the data was the fact that many clients left treatment prior to completion of the therapy program. Prins (1970) found similar results, noting that 67 percent of ninety-four male clients taking part in an intensive residential program completed questionnaires indicating "much or complete" improvement. Interestingly, 65 percent of the subjects indicated that little or no posttreatment regression had occurred in terms of *morale*. In addition, Prins noted that, once they occurred, interpersonal changes were more durable than the level of fluency or decreased avoidance of words.

Chronic Perseverative Stuttering

There is one other distinct category of clients that can be included in a discussion of therapeutic progress. These people would most likely fall into the second or third of the three groups discussed in the previous section. Cooper (1986a, 1987) argues that there is a significant group of stuttering individuals for whom fluent speech is an unrealistic goal. Any clinician who has worked for several years in the area of fluency disorders will recognize this pattern of behavior. Cooper describes this group as Chronic Perseverative Stutterers (CPSs). These speakers are adolescents or adults who have stuttered for several years (at least ten) and for whom stuttering will always be a problem. Cooper indicates that these clients typically respond to treatment with increased fluency, only to experience profound levels of relapse shortly after completing formal treatment. Their predominant self-perception is that of a stutterer. They demonstrate some degree of obsessive striving for normal speech as well as a deep fear of fluency loss, even though such loss may occur infrequently.

Cooper suggests that if clinicians are unwilling to recognize that fluent speech is *not* a possibility for these CPS speakers, they are likely to create and perpetuate unwarranted feelings of guilt on behalf of their clients. He argues that an acknowledgment of this syndrome by clinicians results in a profound relief for clients who see themselves as Chronic Perseverative Stutterers. Whether this view would predispose a client to failure is debatable. Accepting the fact that some people who stutter will always have a chronic problem is simply being realistic. It is, however, important to point out that, although these speakers will always have a degree of obvious stuttering present in their speech, they may be able to alter their stuttering to the degree that they can communicate more effectively.

Paper-and-Pencil Measures

Determining progress during and following treatment is most often accomplished by client observation in a variety of settings and by administering paper-and-pencil measures of change. Many of these measures are similar to those used at the outset of treatment during the diagnostic session (see Appendix A). Baseline measures obtained with these procedures can, of course, be used to indicate change during treatment. Just as the diagnostic process is a multidimensional one, so is the estimation of progress during the treatment process. The procedure for determining progress should be appropriate for the age of the client and the attitude, cognitive, or behavioral aspects of the syndrome one wishes to assess. In some instances, other characteristics such as the time it takes to administer the measure or the availability of the measure becomes important.

   As the period of formal treatment comes to a conclusion, it becomes increasingly important to determine the client's performance and response in extratreatment speaking situations. Some assessment measures, although useful for obtaining initial diagnostic information, are specifically devised to determine progress during and following treatment. That is, they are designed to assess both intrinsic and surface features in a variety of extratreatment settings. As with diagnostic procedures, there are a wide variety of protocols for determining progress and selecting criteria for termination (from formal treatment) criteria. The protocols vary in length and the nature of the quantitative or qualitative data obtained, as well as in reliability and validity. Examples of paper-and-pencil procedures that were designed specifically for assisting the clinician to make decisions concerning termination from formal treatment are the Locus of Control of Behavior Scale (Craig, Franklin, & Andrews, 1984) and the self-efficacy scaling techniques for adults (Ornstein & Manning, 1985) and adolescents (Manning, 1994).

Locus of Control of Behavior (LCB). This seventeen-item Likert-type scale was developed by Craig, Franklin, and Andrews to "measure the extent to which subjects perceive responsibility for their personal problem behavior" (1984, p. 174). This scaling procedure is designed to indicate the ability of a person for taking responsibility for maintaining new or desired behaviors. Subjects are asked to indicate their agreement or disagreement to each of the seventeen statements about personal beliefs using a six-point scale. The scale was designed for use with adults. It has good internal reliability and scores are not influenced by age, gender, or social desirability of responses. The scores of the seventeen statements are summed to yield a total LCB score (items 1, 5, 7, 8, 13, and 16 are scored in reverse order). Higher scores on this scale indicate a perception of external control (externality), while lower scores indicate the perception of greater internal control (internality). Since all forms of intervention for stuttering in one way or another ask the client to gradually assume responsibility for changing his speech, the locus of control concept is intuitively appealing. As Boberg, Howie, and Woods (1979) have suggested, individuals who continue to rely on the clinician and the clinical environment for reinforcement and who fail to take the necessary responsibility for their fluency are more likely to relapse once formal treatment is completed.

Craig, Franklin, and Andrews (1984) administered the LCB scale to a group of forty-five adult stutterers who had received treatment in the fluency modification program at the Prince Henry Hospital in Australia. Stuttering subjects averaged scores of 32.0, while a nonstuttering control group averaged 27.0, a difference that was found to be statistically significant. Following treatment, thirty-two of the subjects maintained fluency levels ten months posttreatment, and thirteen subjects showed relapse (more than 2% syllables stuttered). Twenty-eight of the thirty-two subjects who maintained fluency also showed increased internality on the LCB scale during treatment. Of the thirteen subjects who relapsed, eleven either had no change or became more external during the three-week program. These results were replicated by Craig and Andrews (1985).

Madison, Budd, and Itzkowitz (1986) studied locus of control (LOC) with seven- to sixteen-year-old children and found that those subjects who had a more internal locus of control *prior* to treatment tended to achieve more fluent speech during treatment. They did not, however, find a significant relationship between pretreatment LOC values and fluency levels at two follow-up measures taken two and six months posttreatment.

The results were less encouraging for the ability of the LCB to predict long-term change in a more recent study by deNil and Kroll (1995). These authors studied twenty-one adult subjects who had been enrolled in a three-week intensive behavioral treatment fluency-shaping program (the Precision Fluency Shaping Program [PFSP] of Webster, 1975). Thirteen subjects were contacted two years following treatment. While the follow-up measures indicated that the fluency gains achieved during treatment were maintained by most clients, no predictive relationship was found between LCB scores and the client's percent words stuttered. There was a significant decrease in LCB scores from pre- to posttreatment, indicating increased internality. The use of a stepwise regression analysis procedure indicated that LCB scores were found to be predictive of the speakers' self-evaluation of fluency level. However, the results did not support previously reported findings that the amount of change in locus of control toward more internality during treatment predicted success two years after treatment.

DeNil and Kroll's (1995) findings supported the findings of Andrews and Craig (1988) that total LCB scores *alone* were of limited help in predicting treatment outcome. Moreover, as pointed out by deNil and Kroll as well as Ladouceur, Caron, and Caron (1989), the predictive value of locus of control is likely to be significantly affected by the nature of the treatment program. If for the client to assume control of his speech is a major focus of treatment (regardless of the individual's fluency level), LCB measures are more likely to change in their direction of internality. In addition, an intensive three-week period of treatment may not allow adequate time for the internalization of control.

Self-Efficacy Scaling. Based on the work of Bandura (1977) with perceptual self-efficacy scaling, the Self-Efficacy Scale for Adult Stutterers (SESAS) (Ornstein & Manning, 1985) is designed to measure the confidence that an adult who stutterers can both approach and maintain a level of fluency in fifty specific, extratreatment speaking situations. During the first section of the scale (SESAS approach), clients respond by indicating the likelihood that they could enter into each of the speaking situations by using a decile scale from 10 to 100. The fifty speaking situations are ordered in a hierarchy, from easy to difficult. Subject responses are averaged over the fifty situations to obtain the SESAS approach score.

The same fifty speaking situations are presented again for the second section of the scale (SESAS performance). For this section, clients are asked to indicate confidence that they could maintain a client-selected "level of fluency" based on their treatment program and current progress. Again, subject responses are averaged over the fifty speaking situations to obtain the SESAS performance score.

Ornstein and Manning (1985) administered the SESAS to twenty adults who stuttered and a matched group of control subjects. The authors found the SESAS total score to correlate with the Erickson Scale of Communication Attitudes (Erickson, 1969) at −.71 (sign in the expected direction) and with the Perceptions of Stuttering Inventory (Woolf, 1967) at −.52 (sign in the expected direction). In addition, test-retest reliability for the SESAS for ten of the experimental subjects averaged .95 and .84 for the SESAS approach and performance scales, respectively.

Ornstein and Manning found that the stuttering subjects scored significantly lower on both approach (66.2) and performance (55.8) portions of the SESAS than nonstuttering subjects. Interestingly, the fluent speakers had scores of 94.2 and 98.0 for the approach and performance scales, respectively, indicating that they were less confident about approaching situations than about speaking fluently once they were in a situation. The stuttering subjects, on the other hand, were more confident about approaching speaking situations than about maintaining fluency once they entered the situation. Subsequent investigation (Manning, Perkins, Winn, & Coles, 1984) indicated that with treatment, adult stutterers demonstrated increasingly higher scores. In addition, stuttering subjects began to normalize their approach and performance scores in the sense that performance scores were slightly greater than approach scores.

Blood (1995) noted an obvious improvement in SESAS scores during and following a successful cognitive-behavioral treatment program for three high school clients. Treatment consisted of twenty-five hours of intensive work on changing speech (a modified version of the Shames and Florance, 1980, fluency-shaping program), fifty hours of relapse prevention, and two (six-month and twelve-month) follow-up phases. All three clients showed gradual improvements in overall (approach and performance) scores which averaged 56.3 percent performance (baseline), 77.6 percent (post–speech change), 87.3 percent (post–relapse management), 89.7 percent (six-month follow-up), and 86.7 percent (twelve-month follow-up).

Hillis (1993) pointed out that the pragmatic nature of the SESAS approach may be interpreted as an indication of the scale's content validity. In addition, the construct validity of the SESAS approach is supported by a 28-point difference (effect size = 3.50 nonstuttering standard deviations; $p<.05$) found on the 100-point SESAS approach between twenty subjects who stuttered and the twenty who did not. The construct validity of the SESAS performance scale is supported by a 42-point difference between means (effect size = 11 nonstuttering standard deviations, $p<.05$) on the 100-point scale between twenty subjects who stuttered and the twenty who did not.

In order to decrease the uncontrolled variance resulting from the different levels of fluency selected by clients, Hillis (1993) modified the instructions for the performance section of the SESAS. Rather than using the original (Ornstein & Manning, 1985) instructions of having the client determine a "level of fluency" based on his stage of treatment when scoring this section, Hillis asked the client to define fluent speech as "speech [that] would be so fluent in a given situation that, in the client's opinion, a listener would not recognize that the client had a history of stuttering" (1993, p. 28).

Hillis (1993) also provided data on a variety of measures including the SESAS for an adult female stuttering client. Despite two relapses when the client's pauses per minute and stuttered syllables per minute increased (to less than pretreatment levels), there was continued progress in that the client was judged to be speaking in a natural and fluent manner by herself, the clinician, and an independent observer. Because this was not the case in speaking situations outside the clinic, this fluency was termed "clinical fluency." At the end of treatment the client was maintaining a high level of fluency, both inside and in selected extratreatment situations. Nevertheless, Hillis points out that the SESAS approach score remained less than 70 and SESAS performance score less than 80 at the end of treatment—something less than normalized scores. Hillis notes that even successfully treated clients rarely score much above 80 on the modified SESAS performance scale. It is more common, however, for clients to fall within the range of normal speakers reported by Ornstein and Manning (1985) of 74–100, still well less than the −1 standard deviation (8.0) of 86.2. Thus, it is likely that clients can demonstrate high levels of fluent behavior, but nevertheless be lagging behind in terms of cognitive change (SESAS approach) and speech performance in extratreatment performance (SESAS performance).

Paper-and-pencil measures provide helpful information for the clinician's decision making during treatment, but these measures are not without their problems. Some can be tedious to complete, and there tend to be sequencing effects associated with multiple administrations of the measures. Clients tire of completing the forms, may fail to take the task seriously, and become test-wise about the intent of the measure, filling it out the way they believe they "should" respond rather than indicating what they truly think or feel.

Asking the Client

Although paper-and-pencil measures provide practical ways of estimating change and progress, it is also important to keep in mind that when the clinician wants an indication of progress, there is also the possibility of asking the client. Asking a question as simple as, "How's your speech and what are you doing about it?" can yield a wealth of information to which the clinician can respond in the treatment setting.

One of the events that motivated the writing of this book was a presentation I attended at the annual meeting of the American Speech-Language-Hearing Association a few years ago. The six presenters who took the stage were provided as experts in the area of fluency disorders. They were charged with discussing selection criteria for matching clients to particular treatment approaches. After listening throughout the one and one-half hour session, I left with a sense of frustration. I suspected that, with the possible exception of one presenter, these speakers had managed to alienate a large portion of the approximately one hundred clinicians in attendance concerning the treatment of fluency disorders. What was imparted was a frustration with the data concerning the efficacy of different treatment strategies. The emphasis was data—the lack of data, inaccurate data, conflicting data. There was no recognition of the success that can and does take place during treatment. There was certainly little appreciation, either for the people doing the stuttering or the clinicians administering the treatment. The presenters were not giving clinicians credit for being able to identify progress. Even more so, there was no appreciation for the integrity of clinicians' decision-making abilities. Moreover, they certainly were not imparting much enthusiasm. It was a fine example of experimenters not being able to see the people for the data.

One of the presenters, in response to the frustration of the conflicting efficacy data, made the suggestion that the most useful data is right in front of us during treatment. "If you want data," he suggested, "try asking the client. He might have some good information for you about what is helpful and what is not."

Obviously, a professional clinician relies on a variety of data obtained during treatment as well as findings gleaned from descriptive and experimental research. Sometimes the patterns in the data are clear, but sometimes they are not, and often the numbers conflict. In experimental investigations, individual performance is often obscured by group statistics and methods of data reduction. Furthermore, the experimental or treatment group of subjects is typically composed of a group of individuals who are far from homogeneous. Each subject exhibits a unique response to the treatment strategies and the clinician. We rarely have all the data we would like for making clinical decisions, but we do have clinical experience, and we can try different approaches depending on the needs and response of the client.

The Multidimensional Nature of Therapeutic Change

Van Riper (1973, pp. 178–199) provided a comprehensive overview of ways to consider progress during treatment. His fundamental point is that any view of progress should be comprehensive and ought to make use of a multifactor approach. That is, several surface behaviors as well as many of the intrinsic features of the problem must be taken into account. Otherwise, success will be either overstated or unrecognized. As Sheehan suggested, the more trivial the criteria for improvement the greater the likelihood of success (1980).

As in the original assessment process, there are at least two major levels of change—change in the surface behaviors and change in the intrinsic features of the problem. The changes in the surface behavior of the client often occur relatively early in the formal treatment process. In some cases, these changes even begin to occur prior to treatment. Changes in the intrinsic features, such as attitude and cognitive aspects, lag behind (Emerick, 1988; Manning, 1991). The intrinsic changes that are reflected in the quality of the client's self-management and decision making are critical for long-term success. There are reports suggesting what seems intuitively correct, that the improvement of the surface behaviors will be more likely to be permanent if changes in the intrinsic features of the problem also occur (Emerick, 1988; Guitar, 1976; Guitar & Bass, 1978; Maxwell, 1982).

It has been shown by several investigators that change, at least in some of the surface behaviors of stuttering, can begin prior to the formal initiation of treatment (Andrews & Harvey, 1981; Bordeau & Jeffrey, 1973; Gregory, 1972; Ingham, Andrews, & Winkler, 1972; Ost, Gotestam, & Melin, 1976; Peins, McGough & Lee, 1972; Webster, 1979). For example, Andrews and Harvey (1981) measured 132 adult stutterers approximately eight months prior to the initiation of treatment and again immediately before treatment. The subjects showed significant improvements in the percentage of syllables stuttered (18.2% to 14.4%) and the rate of speech in syllables per minute (91.5 and 129.8). These changes became evident after the first three months on the waiting list. Changes in attitude, however, were much smaller. There was no significant change in the subjects' speech communication attitude, as measured by the S24 scale (Andrews & Cutler, 1974). Furthermore, no significant change was found in two of the three measures (perceived avoidance and severity of stuttering) indicated by the Stutterers Self Rating of Reactions to Speaking Situations (Johnson, Darley, & Spriesterbach, 1963). If, as suggested in Chapter 4, clients are apt to seek treatment when their problem is most severe, this regression toward the mean is not surprising. Furthermore, the very act of finding professional help and asking for assistance is an indication of change. The client's recognition that it is now time to work on the problem is a significant initial step in the direction of change. Seeking help indicates a degree of assertiveness that was not present before. Whatever the reasons, the problem has become important enough to take action. Even though formal intervention has not yet taken place, being included on a waiting list is a tangible step in a new direction and can provide a measure of support for the speaker.

The majority of investigations on treatment efficacy utilize reduction in frequency of stuttering as the dependent variable, for example, percentage of stuttered syllables or words (Andrews, Craig, & Feyer, 1983; Ingham, 1980; Ryan, 1980; Shames & Florance, 1980). That is, the frequency of this surface feature of the problem is the primary criterion for improvement—and to some degree this makes sense. A decrease in the frequency of stuttering obviously indicates change, and sometimes such change indicates progress. There are, however, others who argue that the intrinsic aspects of the problem, the attitude and cognitive features, are at least as important (and possibly more so) for determining long-term progress (Cooper & Cooper, 1985b; Rubin, 1986; Sheehan, 1970; Van Riper, 1973). In addition, studies on the quality of fluent speech (also referred to as *speech naturalness*) following both stuttering-modification as well as fluency-modification strategies indicate that the absence of stuttering, in and of itself, is not necessarily an indicator of successful treatment (Onslow & Ingham, 1987).

Many features associated with the stuttering syndrome will begin to change as a function of treatment. The time and the rate of change will depend on many variables such as the overall treatment strategy, specific treatment techniques, the nature of the fluency disorder, the age of the speaker, the severity of the problem, the needs of the client, and the intensity and the duration of treatment. As several authors have noted, to the degree that the fluency disorder is further complicated by problems such as excessive anxiety, psychological or social issues, or articulation or language disabilities, individually tailored therapy techniques become mandatory (Gregory, 1984; Riley & Riley, 1983, 1984; St. Louis, 1986b; Van Riper, 1973).

VARIABLES INFLUENCING PROGRESS

The treatment administered to a client is influenced, in large part, by the theoretical background received by the clinician during his academic and clinical training. The treatment strategy and techniques of choice are also influenced, or at least ought to be, by information gathered by the clinician during the reading of articles in professional journals and attendance at professional meetings. As pointed out in Chapter 6, the strategy is also likely to be influenced by the professional environment where the clinician is employed. In any case, there are several important variables that will influence the quality and quantity of progress during treatment.

The Treatment Strategy

The clinician's interpretation of progress will certainly be determined by the specific goals associated with a treatment strategy. As suggested in Chapter 6, clinicians who are using programs that emphasize stuttering modification will look for different signs of progress than those employing a program of fluency modification or enhancement. If a fluency-modification approach is used, a reduction of stuttering moments is considered one basic indicator of progress. However, if the modification of stuttered moments is a goal of treatment, a decrease in stuttered moments is not nearly as desirable and may, in fact, prevent the speaker from having the opportunity to identify and modify stuttered events. Furthermore, if a decrease in avoidance behavior is a primary goal of treatment, an *increase* in stuttered moments may be highly desirable and may result from an increase in speaker assertiveness and decreased avoidance of speaking situations or words.

The Nature of the Fluency Disorder

Many researchers, and probably the majority of clinicians, look to the frequency of stuttering as a primary, and sometimes the only, measure of change or progress. For some clients this measure may be a more valid indicator than for others. That is, for clients who clutter or exhibit a combination of stuttering and cluttering characteristics, the frequency of fluency breaks may provide a reasonably clear indication of progress. For these speakers, the surface behavior may be less obscured or influenced by the intrinsic features of the communication disorder. Measures such as the percentage of syllables or words that are stuttered are more likely to provide a direct indication about the severity of the problem. These speakers are either less interested in using, or less able to employ, techniques such as avoidance and postponement to conceal the problem. The decision-making aspects of the syndrome, while they are present, are not as likely to be a major component as they are with the more typical stuttering speaker.

The frequency of stuttering may also provide a more direct, and therefore, more valid indication of change for other subgroups of stutterers who are also less adept at concealing fluency breaks. Younger children, especially those who are in the early stages of developmental stuttering, usually have not yet developed sophisticated methods of hiding or avoiding their stuttering. The percentage of stuttered moments may also provide a relatively unencumbered picture of the stuttering syndrome for stutterers with psychogenic and neurogenic etiology. Moreover, there is also some indication that the surface behavior in the form of stuttering frequency may more clearly reflect progress for the retarded individual who stutters. Despite the fact that mentally retarded speakers who stutter typically demonstrate high levels of stuttering frequency (Cooper, 1986b), these speakers often appear generally unconcerned about fluency (Bonfanti & Culatta, 1977; Cabanas, 1954). Compared to nonretarded stutter they tend to show fewer avoidance and postponement behaviors, as well as relatively less anxiety, associated with stuttering moments. In this sense, the intrinsic features of such speakers resemble cluttering more than stuttering. However, for the typical developmental stutterer, the frequency of stuttering is only one of many features of the syndrome, and by itself it fails to provide a complete picture of the speaker's status.

The Age of the Client

The major focus for much of this chapter has been on the young adult who stutterers. Of course, there are similar indicators of progress among all people who stutter. However, there are at least three age groups that are distinct enough in their response to treatment that they should be considered further: young children, adolescents, and older speakers.

As discussed in Chapter 5, young children often have good success during both direct and indirect intervention for fluency disorders. They are relatively easy to work with, and the behavioral, attitudinal, and cognitive aspects of the syndrome tend to be responsive to change. Success with these speakers can be measured in increased spontaneity and enjoyment of speech production, increased rate of speech, and, of course, decreases in tension and fragmentation.

For the next age group, adolescents, it is quite another matter. Van Riper (1982) stated that adolescents are some of the clinician's most difficult cases. Motivation for change is relatively rare in adolescents. More recently, Daly, Simon, and Burnett-Stolnack (1995) explained that it is often extremely difficult to get adolescents to even take part in treatment. "Many adolescents drop out of therapy, miss sessions, or attend begrudgingly. [They may] downplay the effects of their stuttering on their communication and social interactions. . . . Student rationalizations for poor attendance or for not practicing are common" (1995, p. 163).

As Daly describes, adolescents are apt to be highly sensitive and easily give up during the treatment. Many teenage clients find great difficulty confronting their problem and strongly resist being singled out for anything that carries the potential social stigma of treatment. The importance of peer affiliation is a much more powerful force than the problems originating from their disorder. To complicate matters even further, adolescents often challenge the clinician's qualifications, clinical experience, and overall expertise (Daly, Simon, & Burnett-Stolnack, 1995).

In my own case, as a moderately severe high school stutterer, I firmly resisted the inconvenience and effort I knew would be necessary to work on my speech. After being referred by more than one classroom teacher for treatment, I promptly walked into the office of the two (male) clinicians and fluently announced that I had had enough therapy and wanted no part of it at this time. Daly, Simon, & Burnett-Stolnack (1995), quoted just above, described me exactly.

For this population of clients, progress may be measured by the consistency of attendance at treatment sessions, the level of interaction with the clinician, interest shown in the topics and techniques, requests for pamphlets on stuttering, or participation in group treatment. Assuming that adolescents are willing to take part, another major indicator of progress, given the high degree of peer pressure to conform and not stand out, is a decrease in avoidance behavior.

Progress can also be noted if the client is able to keep the presence of stuttering in his speech from becoming increasingly more handicapping in his educational and social lives. Even if the clinician is unable to achieve great change in the way of modification, she can begin to demystify the problem, explain the cause-and-effect relationships of the syndrome, and let the client and his parents know that, when they are ready, help is available from professionals who specialize in the area of fluency disorders. Thus, it may be possible to sow some grains of knowledge and understanding that another clinician can someday harvest.

The third group of speakers are older stutterers who have been coping with their lack of fluency for decades. Clients over the age of fifty are rarely seen in treatment and rarely included in research reports (Manning & Shirkey, 1981). This is unfortunate, for to fully understand a fluency disorder, it would appear to be essential to follow the development of the syndrome throughout the life cycle. Models of stuttering cannot be completed until the developmental changes that take place during the middle and late adult years are understood. A review of the literature, however, indicates that this subgroup of stuttering adults has received almost no investigation. Assuming a prevalence of at least .7 percent and the most recent census data (World Almanac Book of Facts, 1995), there should be nearly 1 million stutterers over the age of fifty in the United States alone.

It is known that few people over the age of fifty are seen for treatment (Manning, Dailey, & Wallace, 1984; Manning & Monte, 1981). The physiological, including articulatory and phonatory, abilities and psychological changes, including heightened introspection and personal growth, that occur during middle and late adulthood suggest the possibility of increased fluency (Manning & Shirkey, 1981). Travis told his students that death and old age were sure cures for stuttering, and that he never knew of an old man who stuttered (1978).

Anecdotal reports have indicated that stuttering is less of a problem for older individuals. The few data available indicate some support for this argument. Manning, Dailey, and Wallace (1984) obtained attitude and personality information from twenty-nine adults ages fifty-two to eighty-two years old who were members of two national self-help groups, the National Stuttering Project and the National Council of Stutterers. Scores on six paper-and-pencil assessment measures indicated that the older stuttering individuals scored minimally better than the typical scores for young adults who were about to enter treatment. Scores on the Perceptions of Stuttering Inventory (PSI) (Woolf, 1967) averaged 20.3 (standard deviation of 12.0) for the older subjects, in contrast to pretreatment scores for young adult stutterers of 21.1 (Manning & Cooper, 1969) and 27.2 (Ornstein & Manning, 1985). Responses to the S24 Scale (Andrews & Cutler, 1974; Erickson, 1969) for the older speakers averaged 16.0, in contrast to mean pretreatment scores of 19.4 (Howie, 1981), 20.0 (Guitar & Bass, 1978), and 15.6 (Ornstein & Manning, 1985). Scores on the Self-Efficacy Scale for Adult Stutterers (SESAS) (Ornstein & Manning, 1985) averaged 70.5 percent for approach items and 60.5 percent on the performance items, in contrast to 66.2 percent and 55.8 percent for young adult stutterers (Ornstein & Manning, 1985). In addition, the older stutterers ranked the approach tasks significantly higher than the performance tasks, just as the younger stutterers had done ($p < .05$) (Ornstein & Manning, 1985). Finally, responses to a twenty-five-item bipolar-adjective scale (Woods & Williams, 1976) indicated no significant differences between the twenty-nine stuttering and thirteen nonstuttering older subjects.

When asked to indicate whether the handicap associated with stuttering had lessened over the years, the large majority of the subjects agreed that this had been the case. Using a seven-point, equally appearing interval scale to rank their perceived severity as young adults and at the present time, subjects scored their current severity as significantly less ($p < 0.005$). Furthermore, in response to open-ended queries concerning past and current perceived severity, subjects responded with statements such as, "Stuttering is less of a problem now [since] there is not so much competition"; "I accept myself more now than when I was younger, I've become more insightful about personal problems as I grow older"; and "Stuttering has less of an all-consuming hold on me than when I was younger." Because of the way the subjects were selected, this group of older stutterers best represents those older stutterers who are actively involved in self-help groups. Nevertheless, the availability of data suggests that, although older speakers who stutter may be considered to be equally severely compromised as their younger counterparts, they consider themselves less handicapped by the problem.

The Intensity of Treatment

Intensive treatment is often desirable for many behavioral problems. When people are ready to change, the clinician must be ready to respond, and she must strike when the fire is hot. Often, if the client becomes totally immersed in the treatment process, he is more likely to experience rapid changes in the behaviors and attitudes that have persisted for many years (Gregory, 1983; Ingham, 1984; Shames & Florance, 1980; Webster, 1975, 1986). Azrin, Nunn, and Frantz (1979) and Webster (1975) have advocated short-term, intensive approaches, on grounds that it takes a big push to get off dead center and to begin moving in a new direction.

Intensive treatment often presents logistical problems. Many people are not able to leave their work for weeks at a time or cannot commute to and from the treatment site. Potential clients can't always afford the cost of intensive treatment. Moreover, while intensive programs can result in rapid behavioral change, treatment is sometimes followed by dramatic relapses (Kuhr & Rustin, 1985; Prins, 1970). An intensive program, especially if it involves having the client live apart from his typical environment, may yield rapid change in behavioral as well as cognitive aspects of the syndrome. However, for some people, the transition back to the typical world can be traumatic, especially if it is not well thought out and approached in a systematic manner. The old discriminative stimuli and expectancies, on the part of the speaker as well as the listener, are still operating. Relapse is often the case, even for those who practice diligently. Perhaps the suggestion by Cooper (1979a) provides the ideal situation. He advises intensive treatment to modify the surface behaviors, followed by less intensive treatment to allow for change in the intrinsic features of the syndrome and to also allow for maintenance activities.

In any case, if the time is right and the client is ready, significant progress can take place. Moreover, when the changes occur, the clinician must recognize the nature of the breakthroughs. She must recognize the victories when they occur, even though often they are small ones. If the clinician is unable to identify success—the small victories that signal progress—they will go unrecognized and unrewarded. The following section describes the nature of such victories by describing seven directions of progress.

DIRECTIONS FOR PROGRESS

Increasing the Client's Self-Monitoring Ability

A basic indicator of progress is the speaker's ability to tune into what he is doing when he stutters and what he is capable of doing in order to enable himself to speak fluently. Even if he is not yet able to *modify* his production, he may be able to accurately *monitor* what he is doing to make speaking so difficult. Accurate self-monitoring of any behavior or thought process is a preparatory step toward taking responsibility and transforming the event.

A good place to begin monitoring is to identify listener reactions. What are the subtle and not so subtle responses to stuttering in terms of body language and verbal responses? Role-playing, as described in Chapter 6, can be particularly helpful as both client and clinician portray responses observed in extra-treatment situations. Another target of monitoring activities can be the attitudes and behaviors of other clients. This can be done in person or using audio- and videotape segments of treatment sessions. Early in treatment, clients tend to have more success confronting and analyzing stuttering behaviors in others than in themselves. The clinician can provide realistic examples of stuttering behaviors for the client to identify. These can take the form of generic stuttering or replicate behaviors unique to the client. Of course, there will be many subtle aspects of the speaker's stuttering that may take some time and effort for the clinician to distinguish. Real-time analysis, whereby the client identifies stuttering events as they are happening, is usually too demanding at the outset of treatment. This is especially true if the client indicates high levels of fear and avoidance. Audio- or videotapes of the speaker are often essential prior to on-line analysis. Progress can also be noted in the ability of the client to identify progressively more subtle moments of stuttering. Moments of stuttering can be broken down into their component parts. That is, the speaker may have repeated the initial syllable of the word but also constricted the vocal tract at the level of the glottis, shifted his eyes to the side, and inserted the starter sound "ah" in order to postpone an upcoming feared word. It is essential that both the clinician and client be able to accurately identify the most subtle features of the client's fluency breaks before they can begin to systematically modify these aspects of the syndrome.

Eventually, the client will be able to monitor his own speech production via both auditory and, perhaps more important, proprioceptive feedback. Auditory feedback provides some indication of the nature and quality of fluent speech, but proprioceptive feedback provides a more direct indication of the status of the vocal tract and both the accuracy and ease of articulatory movement. Proprioceptive feedback provides a better way to monitor the quality of fluency—the degree to which the speech is produced in an open, flowing, and effortless manner. It is a major step in treatment as the client becomes able—using, for example, delayed auditory feedback and articulatory and proprioceptive training—to heighten his ability to monitor proprioceptively.

The value of accurate self-monitoring is illustrated by two investigations that considered the effectiveness of treatment. Martin and Haroldson (1982) studied twenty adult stutterers who were administered time-outs contingent on their stuttering moments during a behavioral-modification treatment program. All subjects showed significant reductions during treatment, but those stutterers who experienced *self-administered* time-outs showed significantly less extinction and significantly greater generalization than those who experienced only experimenter time-outs. Ingham (1982) investigated two adult stutterers who had failed to make progress in previous treatment. The subjects took part in a treatment program stressing the self-evaluation of performance. The subjects evaluated their own videorecordings for percent stuttering and words spoken per minute. If they achieved prescribed targets for these behaviors, they were able to decrease making the recordings and evaluations. Both overt and covert assessments of their speaking behavior indicated that self-evaluation training was associated with substantially reduced stuttering for up to six months posttreatment.

Self-monitoring will continue to be a critical element of long-term success. Van Riper reported that his own stuttering increased in frequency (although not, he felt in severity) after an initial heart attack at age sixty-five. He described "little sluggish prolongations" (1978) that mostly disappeared after his recovery. Following his retirement he again noticed an increase in the frequency and, occasionally, the severity of his stuttering. He found he was experiencing more frequent and longer tremors as well as some laryngeal blocks. Because these fluency breaks were surprising, he speculated that these changes were probably due to his lack of monitoring of his speech. He speculated that the hard work of closely monitoring his speech and "stuttering fluently" was no longer worth the effort.

During the initial stages of treatment, the client's monitoring is focused on the overt stuttering behavior. Although the focus early in treatment is on monitoring rather than the modification of stuttering events, as the speaker improves his ability to catch his behavior nearer to the initiation of the stuttering event, some instinctive and positive changes in the stuttering often take place. That is, the speaker will not only recognize what he is doing to make speaking difficult, he will begin to make some changes in his behavior. He may provide himself with some airflow; he may slightly decrease a constriction in his vocal tract that will assist him in smoothing his speech. These changes are small and transient victories to be sure, but the clinician should look for them and reward these subtle changes in the form of stuttering. As Conture (1990) indicates, the client's consistent identification at the beginning or the middle of stuttering events sometimes become associated with his ability to change his stuttering behavior.

As treatment progresses, such self-monitoring activities continue to be pivotal for long-term progress outside the treatment environment. In addition, self-evaluation also comes to mean the monitoring of the cognitive aspects of change, such as the self-talk the client provides to himself prior to and following successful, as well as less-than-successful, speaking situations.

Increasing the Client's Ability to Produce "Open Speech"

Victories can be observed during every treatment session by the clinician and the client if close attention is paid to the *form* of the fluency breaks. Early in treatment the fluency breaks are typically characterized by a greater degree of vocal tract constriction and effort. As the speaker begins to understand the nature of his speech production system and becomes able to modify moments of stuttering, progress can be observed in the form of greater airflow, increased smoothness, and blending of the sounds and words. Perhaps most importantly, he begins to produce speech with less vocal and articulatory effort. As he becomes able to monitor his production, especially via proprioceptive feedback,

he will be able to appreciate the difference between the tension and constriction of his old way of speaking and the new flowing and effortless production using an open vocal tract. The speaker as well as the listener can hear
the increased openness and ease of such speech movements. At each such
occurrence of enhanced airflow and smoothness of articulatory movement,
there is the opportunity for the clinician to reward the progress. The client's
speech may not be completely fluent, but the changes are obvious and satisfying. The result is a much easier form of stuttering. As Conture (1990) suggests, a shortening in the duration of stuttering (even though the frequency
may not change) is a sign of progress. The client is stuttering, to be sure, but
it is speech that is produced with less effort and is much easier to listen to.
Certainly, this new form of speech is not the old helpless, reflexive stuttering.
It is, most certainly, progress.

Decreasing the Frequency and Duration of Motoric Fluency Breaks

Decreasing the frequency of motoric fluency breaks is an obvious goal of treatment and a commonly used indicator of progress. As the speech becomes more
open and flowing, both the frequency and, especially, the duration of stuttering moments should show some obvious change. It may be that the frequency of brief stuttering events may even increase somewhat if the speaker
is successful in changing his patterns of avoidance and word substitution. However, if the duration and associated tension, in terms of both the degree and
the sites of physical tension, decreases, real progress is being accomplished.
Again, this progress will be more likely to be recognized by the speaker if
self-monitoring is maintained.

Bloodstein (1987) suggests that successful treatment should result in speech
that sounds, not only natural, but also spontaneous, and that subjects should
be free of the need to monitor their speech. St. Louis and Westbrook (1987)
suggest that clients should be free from stuttering before being dismissed from
treatment. Whether it is realistic to expect adults who have stuttered for most
of their lives to be completely fluent before being dismissed from formal treatment is questionable. While it is possible that this level of nonmonitored fluency may be a realistic goal for some clients, it is not often the case for the
typical adult developmental stutterer. Obviously, there should be relatively
few stuttering moments as formal treatment is concluded, but there are still
likely to be occasions where some form of stuttering takes place. It may take
the form of either overt stuttering, or, even more likely, unstable stuttering
that is just under the surface, as described in Chapter 1. There may also continue to be some degree of avoidance and word substitution. These responses
to the possibility of stuttering are extremely powerful and overlearned. They
will not simply go away in response to a few months or even years of treatment. In addition, there are likely to be several attitudinal and cognitive aspects of the syndrome still operating.

A decrease in the number of stuttering moments is a sign of progress to be sure. Most important, however, changes in the frequency and, especially, the form of stuttering moments reflect the ability of the speaker to take charge and both monitor and self-manage his speech. He is gradually beginning to take control of previously uncontrollable behavior. Underlying the successes of these surface changes is the management of the cognitive and affective aspects of the syndrome. As the speaker becomes able to take charge of his speech during these events, which previously were associated with fear and helplessness, he comes to see that there are alternatives other than struggling with the old, maladaptive behaviors and cognitions. As the techniques of fluency modification become practiced in gradually more stressful speaking situations, the success expands and self-efficacy will gradually increase. If these techniques are practiced by the client between formal treatment sessions, they tend to become automatic in the presence of stress. However, it takes *overpractice* to achieve such automaticity.

One way for the clinician to illustrate her understanding of this process is to use an analogy that involves learning another activity that also possesses elements of balance, possible loss of control, and even anxiety or fear. She could use a variety of speech- or nonspeech-related challenges. I have chosen the experience of paddling a boat in white water (opposite page).

As a result of practice, persons who stutter succeed as well. The speaker gains ability and confidence, and he is more likely to successfully repair his mistakes in the stream of speech. He begins to realize that he is not helpless. He comes to understand that it is possible for him to successfully use well-practiced responses to previously feared situations. Moreover, he is free to move ahead and achieve new success in increasingly more difficult speaking situations.

Increasing the Frequency of Formulative Fluency Breaks

Nearly all clinicians would agree that progress during treatment is reflected by decreases in the occurrence of motoric fluency breaks. However, as Goldman-Eisler (1961) and Starkweather (1987) have indicated, fluency breaks are an important aspect of normal speech formulation. Adults who stutter, while they obviously produce more motoric fluency breaks, also demonstrate significantly fewer formulative fluency breaks (Manning & Monte, 1981). If speech is to be normalized for people who stutter, one important aspect of that process, aside from a decrease in motoric breaks, may well be an increase to near-normal levels of formulative fluency breaks (Manning & Monte, 1981).

As the speaker in treatment experiences fewer motoric fluency breaks, there are less opportunities for him to consider alternative ways of expressing what he wants to say. In order to have an opportunity to formulate his ideas, he will need to include some formulative breaks in order to express himself. As with normal speakers, the breaks provide the chance to organize and reorganize his thoughts. Many speakers who stutter will be unwilling to voluntarily stop to use a formulative fluency break because they fear that beginning speech again may precipitate

VIGNETTE Kayaking in white water requires a high level of balance and confidence. It is easy to lose control, to find yourself under the water in a threatening situation. Early in the process of learning this activity, anxiety and fear are often present. The novice tends to be rigid and inflexible, especially as the stress associated with a series of difficult rapids approaches. Not surprisingly, the likelihood of a mistake is high. With continued practice, however, the paddler's skill increases. He becomes better at paddling accurately and smoothly with less effort. Progress is seen as the paddler's strokes become integrated and blended together. A crucial step takes place when he learns how to repair a mistake by rolling back to the surface when he finds himself upside down in the rapids.

Learning to roll takes practice. Practice begins in the safe confines of a pool or lake—and the paddler practices, first with assistance, and then on his own. The instructor explains the details of the rolling technique and, together, the instructor and paddler go over the sequence of events that must take place if the roll is to be successful. The techniques are done deliberately and slowly, in a preplanned manner. The paddler learns to roll to both the left and the right, to roll with the kayak filled with water, and to roll without a paddle using only his hands. He learns to roll without first setting up in a roll position in order to approximate the unexpected situations found on the river. Finally, it is time to move from the safety of the flat water to the reality and tumult of the river.

Depending on a number of factors, such as water temperature, turbulence, and obstacles that appear in the boater's path, the first attempts of the paddler to roll in a moving stream are not likely to be successful. The likelihood of success decreases dramatically when the stresses of time pressure, distraction, and especially fear enter the picture. A paddler's initial reaction to being upside down for the first time in white water is apt to be similar to the first time he was upside down in flat water—one of anxiety, fear, or even panic. The techniques that worked so well in the safety of the pool are quickly forgotten, and the reaction of the paddler is to panic, exit the boat, and swim to the surface. It is not until the paddler is able to overlearn the techniques that they can be counted on. They must be automatic to the degree that the paddler does not have to think about them. If he has to think about each of several movements, they will not occur. If he has to think about what to do, he will panic. What is required is reaction to the situation in the form of an overlearned sequence of procedures.

Once the paddler learns to react to the situations on the river in this manner, some positive things begin to take place. Paddling skills begin to increase geometrically. The paddler becomes more flexible, and his style becomes one of working with, rather than against, the power of the water. If he makes a mistake, he can repair it. He gradually becomes less rigid, and he begins to paddle with greater flexibility. Because he is more flexible, he is less apt to make mistakes—and the best part is that he gains confidence in his ability to correct errors and right himself. After a time, he finds that he is looking around for more challenging rapids to paddle and new rivers to negotiate.

another moment of stuttering. Accordingly, if treatment has been successful, the speaker will be more likely to be willing to make use of formulative breaks, being less concerned about his ability to continue once he has organized his thoughts. He does not have to be concerned about pauses, especially pauses that allow the formulation of thought. Because many clients have not had the opportunity to practice using formulative breaks for formulating speech, during the later stages of treatment it may be helpful for them to practice sequencing or branching activities. It is an opportunity to speak "without putting on the brakes" and to free-associate. Once a reasonably high degree of fluency is achieved, the client needs to practice speaking in a less inhibited manner, slowly freeing himself from scanning ahead for feared words and pretasting feared sounds.

Even for those speakers who demonstrate a nearly total absence of stuttering moments in all speaking situations, investigators have shown that many are not necessarily perceived as normal (Ingham & Onslow, 1985; Onslow & Ingham, 1987; Runyan, Hames, & Proseck, 1982; Sacco, Metz, & Schiavetti 1992). One reason for the unnaturalness of such posttreatment speech may be the lack of normal, effortless, formulative breaks. Manning and Monte (1981) suggested the possible prognostic value of promoting an *increase* in the number of formulative fluency breaks as one way to determine the stability of fluency. Given the presence of formulative breaks even in accomplished adult speakers, a lack of these breaks suggests something other than normal fluency. Possibly the increase of formulative fluency breaks to near-normal levels may be one of the surface behaviors that could be used to predict relapse. Although there are no data yet available to support this suggestion, it may be that an increase in such fluency breaks could serve as one of several criteria for making the decision to terminate formal treatment.

Increasing the Naturalness of Fluent Speech

As discussed earlier, there are several aspects of change during formal treatment other than the frequency of stuttering that influence the long-term success and the associated handicap. One of these is the clinical research beginning in the late 1970s concerning the naturalness of speech. Much of the impetus for studying the naturalness of speech of treated stutterers came from observations that many individuals who had undergone successful treatment using fluency-modification strategies continued to sound less than satisfactory. That is, listeners found the speech of these clients unnatural and distracting. Even with an absence of abnormal, constricted, tension-filled breaks in fluency, the client's speech may not sound normal or natural. The speech may be nonstuttered but still not flowing and not comfortable to listen to. There are still aspects of the speech that will prevent the listener from attending to the content of the message.

Development of a Naturalness Rating Scale. In an early attempt to investigate this effect, Ingham and Packman (1978) studied the normalcy of speech following treatment by comparing nine stutterers undergoing treatment with a prolonged speech procedure. These subjects were compared with nine normally fluent speakers matched for age and sex. The stutterers, seven males and two females, were adolescents and adults ranging in age from thirteen to twenty-four years old. Listeners rated whether one-minute speech samples were either natural or unnatural. Ingham and Packman found that the listeners' ratings of naturalness of the posttreatment stutterers were not significantly different from those of normal speakers.

In 1984, Martin, Haroldson, and Triden developed a reliable scale for rating speech naturalness. The scale was a nine-point Likert scale with 1 equivalent to highly natural-sounding speech and 9 equivalent to highly unnatural-sounding speech. The authors had thirty listeners use the scale to assess the speech naturalness of ten adult stutterers (ages 20–53) speaking without delayed auditory feedback, ten stutterers (ages 20–51) speaking under delayed auditory feedback, and a group of ten nonstutterers (ages 21–45). They found that both groups of stuttering speakers (those with and without delayed auditory feedback) sounded significantly less natural than the non-stuttering samples. The mean naturalness ratings for the speakers who stuttered (without delayed auditory feedback) was 6.52. The stuttering speakers under delayed auditory feedback received a naturalness rating of 5.84. The speech of the nonstuttering speakers (without delayed auditory feedback) received a score of 2.12. Based on interrater agreement and rater consistency, Martin et al. concluded that observers are able to quantify speech naturalness.

Following the introduction of this scaling technique there was interest by a variety of researchers on this topic. Using the same nine-point scale, Ingham, Gow, and Costello (1985) studied the speech naturalness of fifteen fluent speakers and fifteen treated stutterers who had completed the initial phases of a prolonged speech treatment program. Listeners judged the stutterers' speech to be significantly more unnatural than the nonstutterers' speech. The listeners were also asked to identify whether or not the samples came from "normal speakers." Interestingly, listeners judged an equal amount of samples from both the stutterers and the nonstutterers to be from "normal speakers."

Ingham and Onslow (1985) used the same nine-point scale for assessing the speech naturalness of stutterers during a treatment program. They conducted a two-part investigation in which they first described the speech naturalness of clients enrolled in a prolonged speech treatment program. The subjects for this investigation were adolescent speakers (three males and twenty-one females) ranging from ten to fourteen years of age. One-minute speech samples taken at different phases of the treatment program (instatement, transfer, and maintenance phase) were presented to a practicing clinician. The clinician used the nine-point scale to rate naturalness. The speakers were all found to improve their speech naturalness, but not at the same rate.

Three of the subjects who took part in the first part of the study participated in a second study (Ingham & Onslow, 1985). These speakers were chosen for the follow-up study based on their speech naturalness scores during the final stages of the instatement phase of treatment. All three subjects had a speech naturalness score of 4 or higher. Each of these subjects spoke spontaneously while maintaining a targeted speaking rate. Every fifteen seconds, a clinician made a naturalness rating of between 1 and 9. The ratings were displayed so that the speaker could see them. The subjects were told that they would be given their naturalness rating score at the end of a five-minute period. The results indicated that feedback about their ratings resulted in an improvement in speech naturalness ratings during treatment.

Onslow, Adams, and Ingham (1992) considered the reliability of the nine-point scale in a clinical situation. Their intent was (1) to determine the reliability of listeners' repeated ratings of one subject's speech, (2) to compare the reliability of sophisticated and unsophisticated judges' speech naturalness, and (3) to evaluate the influence of the duration of the speech sample. Speech samples were obtained from ten adults and adolescents who were receiving treatment in a prolonged speech program. The listeners were thirty sophisticated and thirty unsophisticated judges. Subgroups of listeners rated speech samples of fifteen, thirty, or sixty seconds in duration. The results indicated that the judges were inconsistent in their ratings, suggesting that procedures for rating naturalness need to be developed. There were no important differences between sophisticated and unsophisticated raters. Ratings made for thirty and sixty seconds resulted in the highest agreement and intraclass correlations.

The Effect of Feedback. Ingham, Martin, Haroldson, Onslow, and Leney (1985) also considered the effect of feedback on the improvement of speech naturalness. In this case, the subjects were six male stutterers between the ages of sixteen and fifty-five. The speakers had either never received treatment or had not received treatment for at least two years. The subjects varied widely in their frequency of stuttering. Each subject spoke spontaneously while monitored by two clinicians. One clinician counted stuttered and non-stuttered syllables or words, while the other clinician made naturalness ratings of between 1 and 9. Every thirty seconds, the clinician displayed a naturalness rating that the subject could see. Each subject was instructed to keep the naturalness ratings low and to sound as natural as possible. The speakers were not told, however, how to accomplish this task. The results indicated that five of the six subjects improved their speech naturalness scores when receiving feedback.

Ingham, Ingham, Onslow, and Finn (1989) analyzed the effects of instructions to stutterers to rate and change their own speech naturalness. Three male stutterers between the age of twenty-two and thirty who were in a treatment program volunteered for this study. Two experimenters listened to each subject as he spoke for five minutes for a series of two- to four-hour sessions. One experimenter counted stuttered and nonstuttered syllables, while the other experimenter made naturalness ratings of between 1 and 9 every thirty seconds. The stutterers also rated their own speech naturalness.

The results indicated that when the subjects were asked to make their speech sound more unnatural, both the subjects' and judges' ratings were similar. When the stutterers were asked to improve their speech naturalness ratings, they judged their speech to be more natural, but the judges did not note the same improvements. Differences in the stutterers' and judges' speech naturalness ratings suggested that stutterers are able to recognize features of their naturalness better than listeners. The authors suspected that the two groups of listeners were using different criteria for making the judgment of speech naturalness. The listeners who stuttered indicated that they listened for unusual prolongations or prosody in their speech to help them rate their naturalness.

Runyan, Bell, and Proseck (1990) considered whether there was a difference between the speech naturalness of nonstutterers and stutterers who had been successfully treated in six different treatment programs. They investigated whether the identification of stuttering was related to speech naturalness. Finally, they considered if pretreatment severity (mild, moderate, or severe) was related to posttreatment naturalness scores.

Tape-recorded samples of speech from treated stutterers and normal speakers were used. The recorded samples were the same as those described by Runyan and Adams (1978). The clinicians who supplied the speech samples also supplied the pretreatment severity ratings of these subjects. The stutterers had participated in several different treatment programs (Van Riperian, metronome-conditioned speech retraining, delayed auditory feedback, operant conditioning, precision fluency shaping, or holistic treatment).

Ten graduate students in speech-language pathology who had received training in fluency and fluency disorders served as judges. These listeners identified whether each speech sample was from a stutterer or nonstutterer. Once this was decided, they again listened to the sample and rated each speaker's naturalness using Martin, Haroldson, & Triden's (1984) nine-point scale. Listener responses were examined and speech samples were divided into two groups: easily identified, treated stutterers and difficult-to-identify stutterers.

The results indicated that significant differences were found between speech naturalness ratings of treated stutterers and fluent speakers. Listeners judged the treated stutterers' speech as being more unnatural than that of normal speakers. Moreover, (the difficult-to-identify stutterers were rated as sounding significantly more natural than the easily identified stutterers (p < .003). The difficult-to-identify stutterers' mean speech naturalness score (2.38) was not significantly different from the normal speakers' mean score (2.79). Finally, the authors found that posttreatment naturalness ratings of all stutterers were similar despite differences in pretreatment severity ratings. Posttreatment scores were 4.26 for subjects judged to be mild, 3.82 for subjects judged to be moderate, and 3.68 for subjects judged to be severe.

Onslow, Hayes, Hutchings, and Newman (1992) also considered the effect of pretreatment severity on both pre- and posttreatment naturalness ratings. Thirty-six subjects between nine and fifty years of age (mean of twenty-one years) were studied. Fifteen listeners rated the naturalness of a thirty-second speech sample from each subject. The results indicated that the most severe stutterers prior to treatment had naturalness scores that were more than two values higher (less natural) than the least severe stutterers. These results differed from those of Runyan, Bell, and Prosek (1990), who found similar post-treatment speech naturalness rating of all stutterers, regardless of pretreatment severity.

Acoustic Features of Speech Naturalness. Metz, Schiavetti, and Sacco (1990) examined the speech of nonstutterers and treated stutters for acoustic features related to naturalness. Twenty stutterers (fifteen males and five females) were seen following treatment. These adolescent subjects ranged in age from 9 to 20 years old with a mean age of 14.5 years. Using the Stuttering Severity Instrument (SSI) (Riley, 1972) prior to treatment, seven subjects were rated, as moderate stutterers, eleven were rated as severe, and two were determined to be very severe. Twenty nonstuttering subjects were matched with the stuttering speakers for the factors of sex and age (within one year). Subjects read a passage and described a picture.

Results indicated that the stutterers were perceived as sounding more unnatural than the nonstutterers. This was true for both the read and spontaneous speech samples. Voice onset time (VOT) and sentence duration were found to be significantly related to, and predictive of, speech naturalness with the VOT values being most predictive of naturalness during spontaneous speech. Sentence duration was the primary predictor of naturalness during reading.

The Effect of Speaking Task. Nearly all investigations of speech naturalness have used monologue speech or some combination of monologue and oral reading. Some authors failed to specify the speech task. Onslow, Adams, and Ingham (1992) first studied the effect of speaking task by comparing the influence of monologue and conversational speech. Subjects were seven males ranging in age from fourteen to thirty-six years (average age of twenty-one) who had received treatment. The subjects were matched in age (within six months) with seven nonstuttering male speakers.

All subjects were recorded during conversation and monologue on three different occasions. Ninety-six speech samples were selected for analysis by listeners. Using the nine-point scale developed by Martin, Haroldson, and Triden (1984), a group of twenty-nine undergraduate university students assigned naturalness scores. The results showed no significant differences in the naturalness scores of conversation or monologue for either stutterers or nonstutterers. The results confirmed the external validity of previous studies that were based only on monologue speech or failed to make the speech task clear.

Audio and Video Samples. All the studies discussed thus far used audio-recordings of speech samples. There are, of course, many visual components of stuttering that are related to judgments of speech naturalness in the everyday world. In the first attempt to distinguish possible visual components, Martin and Haroldson (1992) studied six male and four female stutterers (ages 20–62) and six male and four female nonstutterers (ages 21–64). Twenty-four undergraduate college students made speech naturalness ratings of one-minute speech samples. Using the nine-point scale by Martin, Haroldson, and Triden (1984), subjects rated both audio and audiovisual speech samples. Another group of thirty undergraduate students rated stuttering *severity* of the stuttered speech samples. Stuttering severity was also rated using a nine-point scale, with 1 representing very mild stuttering and 9 representing very severe stuttering.

The results indicated that the naturalness judgments of nonstutterers were not significantly different for audio and audiovisual samples. However, for the stuttering subjects, the audiovisual samples were consistently judged as being more unnatural than audio only samples. The rating of stuttering severity influenced the naturalness ratings. These results may have been influenced by the fact that the speech samples of the stuttering subjects in this study were not stutter free.

Kalinowski, Nobel, Armson, and Stuart (1994) determined the pre- and posttreatment speech naturalness of five mild (0–4% disfluency) stutterers and five severe (23% or greater disfluency) stutterers. Sixty-four naive listeners rated these adult male speakers using the Martin, Haroldson, and Triden (1984) nine-point scale. The listeners rated both pre- and posttreatment one-minute videotape recordings of conversational speech. All subjects took part in the Precision Fluency Shaping Program (Webster, 1975).

Following treatment, small amounts of stuttering were present in all but three of the ten speakers, and there was a substantial decrease in stuttering for all subjects. However, despite the reduction in the frequency of stuttering for mild as well as severe subjects, the speakers were rated as being less natural sounding following treatment. As with several previous studies, the five subjects with severe stuttering were rated with significantly higher (less natural) naturalness scores than those with mild stuttering.

These results indicate that the goal of treatment may be considerably more complex than just producing perceptually fluent speech. It may even be that some moments of stuttering do not significantly detract from speech naturalness, particularly if they are open, forward moving, and relatively effortless. Such fluency breaks may indicate greater spontaneity to the listener and be more desirable than controlled speech devoid of any breaks. Starkweather (1992) suggested that successful therapies often tend to diminish the quality of a person's speech, even with increased fluency.

In summary, the naturalness of speech fluency appears to be an important consideration in determining the success of treatment. Martin, Haroldson, and Triden's nine-point scale appears to be reliable for either oral reading or spontaneous speech. Furthermore, pre- and posttreatment severity ratings will influence judgments of naturalness; clients improve naturalness as a result of treatment, but at their own rate; and subjects who differ on naturalness ratings at the outset of treatment may be rated much the same after treatment. Moreover, feedback about naturalness during treatment appears to enhance that quality, listeners and clients rate naturalness differently, voice onset time and sentence duration appear to be important acoustic features of speech naturalness, and audiovisual ratings of naturalness tend to be rated somewhat less natural than audio only.

Although several studies have included adolescents (Ingham & Onslow, 1985; Ingham & Packman, 1978; Metz, Schiavetti, & Sacco, 1990; Onslow, Adams, & Ingham, 1992; Onslow, Hayes, Hutchins, & Newman, 1992), there are no naturalness data concerning children who stutter. It may be that the naturalness of a speaker's speech posttreatment may provide some indication of relapse. In addition, there may be other acoustic features that could be considered beyond voice onset time and sentence duration such as formant transition measures (particularly the second formant), that have been found to be useful in predicting the status of other (nonstuttering) speakers.

There is a wide range of performance that is possible, but fluency without ease of listening represents something short of a complete therapeutic success. If the client's nonstuttered speech is something less than fluent—if it sounds unnatural or if the fluency is tenuous—this may also be one of the surface behaviors with some value in forecasting relapse. Adams and Runyan (1981) state that the stutterer who is ready for dismissal should have speech that is objectively and perceptively indistinguishable from that of normal speakers. The client's speech should not only be free of stuttering but should be produced at an acceptable rate, sound natural, and be free of perceptible signs of *tenuous* fluency. As suggested earlier in this chapter, these are lofty and, perhaps, unrealistic goals for many adults who stutter. Nonetheless, such changes certainly can be viewed as signs of progress.

Metalinguistic Changes

As people progress through effective treatment, they begin to think and talk differently about themselves and their speech. The intrinsic features of affective and cognitive change are reflected in the words the client uses to describe himself, his speech, and his interactions with others. How the client talks about himself and his speech provides a window for viewing these intrinsic features.

Early in treatment the client typically feels helpless. He believes he is unable to do much to change his speech or himself. There is a high degree of mystery associated with stuttering. He will say such things as "When *it* happens I feel helpless," or "When I'm in a block I feel lost and I don't know what to do." As treatment progresses, clients slowly begin to develop the "language of fluency" (Blodgett & Cooper, 1988; Cooper & Cooper, 1985), as well as use more appropriate self-talk (Daly, 1986; Emerick, 1988; Maxwell, 1982). As the client begins to successfully change his previously uncontrollable behavior, he will begin to change the way he observes himself and his speech. Moreover, he will begin to describe his behavior and actions in more objective, specific, and realistic ways. The client will begin to interpret stuttering as something that he is *doing* rather than something that is happening to him. He will begin to say such things as:

"When I stutter sometimes I stop the airflow at the vocal folds. I was able to change the way I repeated that syllable into a smoother and easier way of stuttering. Even though that was a difficult telephone call, I was able to make the call and successfully achieve most of my fluency targets."

These metalinguistic changes provide the clinician with important evidence of change and indicate that the client is beginning to take charge of the problem. Such utterances may be used as a way to monitor cognitive change, or in some cases, the clinician can take a more active role and point out to the client how he is describing himself and his problem. It may be possible for the client to begin talking about his problem in a different way in order to, in turn, facilitate new and better ways of thinking about himself and his speech (Daly, 1986; Emerick, 1988; Maxwell, 1982). One adult female client related how she approached a feared speaking situation she had previously avoided. Afterwards she related to her clinician that "I stuttered as much as I always have but this time I didn't feel ashamed." As discussed in Chapter 6, facilitating these cognitive changes is similar to the cognitive-restructuring activities, as advocated by several others in the field of fluency disorders (Curlee, 1984; Fransella, 1972; Hayhow & Levy, 1989; Johnson, 1946; Williams, 1979).

Increasing Open Decision Making

Coinciding with the client's gradual reinterpretation of himself and his speech is his increasing ability to make choices that are based on information other than the possibility of stuttering. The client begins to open his focus beyond the influence of stuttering and consider other, more expansive, possibilities and options. With this wider focus comes the adjustment to new responsibilities and challenges. Furthermore, once a new way of viewing life becomes available to the client, he has the obligation, if he is to be true to himself, to act on this new information. If his hard-won progress is to continue, he must make new choices and accept new challenges. There will be many opportunities for open decision making during daily work and social activities. Years of avoidance and less-than-complete interpersonal involvement will gradually change. However, it is important for the clinician as well as the client to recognize that what is changing is not only the surface behavior of the client's speech but a way of living.

Decreased Avoidance. As avoidance decreases, the frequency of fluency breaks may increase. Early in treatment, less avoidance and greater participation in speaking activities may yield a slight increase in the frequency of stuttering. There may even be an increase in the duration and tension of stuttering events. Although these changes may not be pleasant to the client, if a stuttering-modification strategy is being used, they can be viewed as progress within the context of the overall treatment process. The good news is that decreased avoidance translates directly into decreased handicap. Taking part in (speaking) activities and making better choices may not be the first step for each client, but it is always a critical step. Furthermore, a decrease in avoidance behavior permits the client to go directly at the problem and the associated fear. It is not simply the stuttering that comprises the problem, but uncontrolled and helpless stuttering. As experienced clinicians have pointed out for decades, much of the handicapping effect of stuttering is the result of maladaptive efforts to avoid any type of overt stuttering. A temporary increase in the frequency and duration of stuttering may be viewed as a small and often necessary price to pay for increased approach behavior and assertiveness.

Increased (Speech) Assertiveness. With a decrease in avoidance behavior there is likely to be a corresponding increase in overall assertiveness. In reality, being more assertive about one's speaking behavior is likely to translate into increased assertiveness in general. There may be changes in roles and relationships as the person no longer plays the primary role of a stutterer (Sheehan, 1970). It is a distinctive indicator of progress when the speaker begins to decrease his reflexive censorship and beings to consider many speaking situations he once considered unimaginable. This is not to say that he will now take part in these situations with ease or idyllic fluency, but choosing to take part nonetheless and thus to consider new opportunities is a significant measure of progress.

Increased Risk Taking. Closely associated to an increase in speech assertiveness is an increase in risk taking. Just as an athlete, in order to improve his skills, reaches to the edge of his ability (or sometimes, for a moment, just beyond), the speaker is extending the envelope of his experience and performance. Each time he extends himself into positions of responsibility for organizing social or work-related activities, he is expanding his world. He is risking failure, of course, and sometimes degrees of failure will occur. Taking on these challenges is more indicative of progress for some clients than others. However, for many clients, this expansion of risk-taking activities provides evidence of the cognitive changes that are part of long-term success.

Improved Self-Concept, Improved Self-Esteem, and Role Changes. Self-concept and self-esteem have been referred to many times in the literature on fluency disorders. According to Peck (1978), self-esteem is the cornerstone of psychological change. Although persons who stutter have not been found to have a unique self-concept or to be lacking in self-esteem, this concept has frequently been mentioned as an aspect of treatment programs (Van Riper, 1973, see pp. 364–367).

Self-esteem is not something that can be given to you. Nonetheless, the stage can be set by loving parents and friends as well as by a competent clinician. As the clinician provides a secure and stable therapeutic environment, growth will be likely to occur. When the client experiences success in the self-management of surface and intrinsic aspects of his fluency disorder, self-esteem and the self-concept begin to shift in a positive direction. This is certainly the case with children who are still in the process of developing their self concept. Of course, this is a major reason why intervention for fluency problems is much more likely to result in long-term success with this group of clients. However, adults are also able to make big changes that are reflected in a changed view of themselves during and following treatment. They are able to redefine themselves and create an altered paradigm of their lives. Such changes can be quantified by self-reports during individual and group treatment sessions as well as by measures such as the locus of control (Kuhr & Rustin, 1985).

Success also can be observed through the reports of others in the speaker's environment, such as teachers, parents, a spouse, or friends, who indicate to the client or the clinician the changes both in fluency and participation in activities. For example, Conture (1990) indicates that early signs of improvement often take the form of others reporting that they are noticing an improvement in speech or related behavior. These reports may appear spontaneously or may be elicited from those in the client's environment who are able to provide candid feedback. This feedback should be taken seriously and regarded as a valid indicator of change.

Increased Distancing and Objectivity through Humor. With the client's development of greater objectivity, self-monitoring, and modification abilities, he learns to generate the ability to back up and distance himself from his problem. Such cognitive change may be reflected in the presence of humor. As discussed in Chapter 1, in most cases the clinician must lead the way in identifying and appreciating the humorous aspects of the situation, providing the "new eyes" for viewing this old problem. However, once the process has been initiated, surprising results often occur. This is especially true during group treatment sessions, where one humorous story by a client often leads to a change in perspective by others. The question, "What humorous thing occurred this week because of your stuttering?" may elicit incredulous looks from new members of the group. Experienced members, however, often provide wonderfully humorous stories that, more often than not, allow the new members of the group to summon equally amusing stories from their past. With the distance afforded by the passage of time, the client is able to release the damaging effects of the experience and see the incident with new eyes. The entire group can share the experience and participate in a new interpretation of an old predicament. Here are three examples of the many stories we have heard over the years (vignettes across the next two pages):

VIGNETTE One of the men in the group, James, related how, during his college years, he finally worked up the courage to call a young woman for a date. In those days, there was only a single telephone on each floor of the women's dorm, and it was located in the hallway. The coed's name was Harriet, and rather than risk saying the entire sentence, "Can I speak to Harriet?" he decided to simply say "Harriet," to whoever happened to answer the telephone. When someone did answer the telephone, the only sound James could produce was several repetitions of the initial "H" sound, resulting in a series of breathy utterances. After a momentary pause, he heard the coed partially cover the phone and say to the other women in the hall, "It's him again!"

VIGNETTE Two clinicians described taking a client to a shopping mall to practice some voluntary stuttering and analyzing the reactions of several listeners. Entering a book store, one of the clinicians performed some realistic (voluntary) stuttering as she asked for a book on physical therapy. The clerk checked the computer and indicated that this particular book was not available. The clinician continued to stutter and asked for something on the topic of occupational therapy. This time, when the clerk searched the computer records for such a book, he said: "I don't seem to have anything on occupational therapy. But I do have several books on speech therapy!"

The various types of listener reactions, from mildly inappropriate to obviously patronizing, can be painful to endure at the moment they occur, but they lose some of their bite when distance and objectivity are applied to the wound. The appreciation of the humorous perspective is one way to deal with such experiences. The ability of the clients to respond to these situations with humor provides a way to gauge progress in terms of objectivity, distancing, and mastery.

CRITERIA FOR THE TERMINATION OF FORMAL TREATMENT

There are few guidelines concerning the termination of formal treatment. For children, the decision may be clearer. Once the child is able to maintain easy, fluent speech in a variety of situations at home and in school for several months, the decision to conclude treatment is reasonable.

> **VIGNETTE**   Another adult male who had just graduated from college was in the early stages of treatment. As part of a group therapy session, he was required to walk into town and ask several strangers where the police station was located. Still highly disfluent at this stage of treatment, his task was a daunting one. In an attempt to find the easiest possible subject for his task, he spied the best of all possible listeners. He saw what appeared to be a grandmother walking in his direction less than a block away. He approached her and positioned himself so that, even if he stuttered, she would have to stop. She was the prototypical grandmother. She wore a cloth coat and a hat with a veil, and she was carrying a shopping bag in each hand along with an umbrella. As the client stood in front of her and began to ask her for directions, she looked up at him and placed the two shopping bags on the ground. He stuttered his way through the required question about the location of the police station. Yes, she did know where the police station was, and she began to respond. The client attempted to focus on her face, a feat made difficult because of the veil she was wearing. Her lipstick-red mouth seemed to move even slower than the words she was so carefully and slowly articulating. "See . . . that . . . big . . . red . . . light?" she asked as she pointed to a stop light about a block behind her. "When . . . you . . . get . . . to . . . that . . . light . . . turn (a pause here as she held his right arm at the elbow) . . . left." To emphasize her instructions, she spun him around to his left. Somewhat mortified for the moment, he shared the experience back in the group session minutes later. His humorous telling of the story to the other clients in the group resulted in laughter all around as they all recognized a classic example of the well-meaning but overly helpful response.

For adults, the issue is more complex. After all, the adult who stutters has had lots of practice, and the behavioral and cognitive aspects are resistant to change. If the process of change for adults is viewed as a continuum of formal-informal treatment, it will never be quite complete. Van Riper (1973) provided guidelines for terminating treatment. He suggested, for example, that if the client becomes bored and unexcited about treatment or even about maintaining fluency, it may be time to terminate formal treatment. Certainly it is better to anticipate the end of treatment and to schedule a final exit meeting or two rather than have the client simply cease attending treatment. Such lack of closure leaves the clinician feeling at a loss about the final outcome.

Discussing the criteria for termination from the outset of treatment is one solution to this dilemma. It is probably never too soon for the clinician to begin asking the client to address the issue of termination. Often the client will respond with, "You're the expert, you tell me." Of course, the clinician is the expert about fluency disorders in a generic sense, but the client must become an expert about his own situation, and requesting him to operationally define when he will be able to be on his own is a valid issue from the outset of treatment.

If the clinician and the client agree that termination is appropriate, it makes sense to schedule a meeting to review the progress. The clinician can make it clear that she is available for consultation and that group treatment on an informal basis is also possible. Referral to a support group such as a local chapter of the National Stuttering Project can serve to keep the client's momentum going and assist in keeping him desensitized and assertive concerning his fluency.

Although clients sometimes leave treatment before we deem it desirable, it is also possible to err in the direction of keeping the client in treatment for too long. Continued treatment beyond what is necessary or helpful may serve to reinforce the client's dependency. In addition, there is a law of diminishing returns whereby at a certain point, the cost, financial or otherwise, is no longer worth the effect. Ideally, during an exit meeting, both the client and the clinician can recognize and agree that, for now at least, they have each done their best.

On occasion, termination from formal treatment may be temporary. If the client has reached a plateau and little progress is noted for several weeks, it may suggest that the client, not to mention the clinician, needs a break. A break from treatment may be indicated if the client becomes bored or other issues such as financial constraints or the logistics of attending treatment become preeminent. Just as in the case of attending graduate school or beginning a period of arduous athletic training, pushing ahead at full speed is not always the best strategy. Sometimes it is best to back away for a while. A break may provide the opportunity to reassess priorities and evaluate and regain motivation. Perhaps the clinician needs to assist the client in backing away from the treatment process. It may be that a vacation from treatment is the best investment for future growth. Temporary dismissal from treatment may not be an easy decision, for there is the chance that we will lose the clients and progress will cease. Nonetheless, forgoing treatment for a time can be an essential step in overall success.

CONCLUSIONS

Clinicians must be able to recognize success when it occurs, often in the form of small victories. Certainly, change during treatment is far from linear, with many plateaus, successes, and failures. Some change may even occur prior to initiating formal treatment as clients regress toward the mean following acceptance into a program. Although some adult clients achieve spontaneous fluency, many others do not, particularly those who drop out of treatment prior to dismissal. There is no behavioral or standard assessment measure that allows the clinician to predict which clients will be successful. The probability of success varies across many factors, including age, motivation, and intensity of treatment. Progress may be noted in either a decrease or an increase in the frequency of stuttering, an increase in formulative breaks, and especially the presence of shorter and less effortful stuttering events. Progress is also seen in more open decision making in the form of decreased avoidance, greater speech assertiveness, and greater objectivity about the stuttering experience.

It is never too early in treatment to begin considering criteria for termination; what will it take for this client to be on his own and to manage his speech without the assistance of the clinician? Planning for termination and possible relapse will bring closure to formal treatment. A return to treatment as needed may be a good option, and such a decision should not be viewed as failure but rather an opportunity for continued growth.

RECOMMENDED READINGS

DiClemente, C. C. (1993). Changing addictive behaviors: A process perspective. *Current Directions in Psychological Science* 2(4), 101–106.

Hillis, J. W. (1993). Ongoing assessment in the management of stuttering: A clinical perspective. *American Journal of Speech-Language Pathology*, 2 (1), 24–37.

Prochaska, J. O., DiClemente, C. C., & Norcross, J. C. (1992). In search of how people change: Applications to addictive behaviors. *American Psychologist*, 47 (9), 1102–1114.

Sheehan, J. G. (1980). Problems in the evaluation of progress and outcome. In W. H. Perkins (Ed.), *Strategies in stuttering therapy for seminars in speech, language and hearing*. New York: Thieme-Stratton.

Determining Progress Following Treatment

INTRODUCTION

Is it realistic to think of adults recovering as a result of treatment for fluency disorders? Alternatively, is it more reasonable to think of treatment as an evolving process of recovery? Although investigators of treatment efficacy indicate that substantial changes take place during treatment for the majority of clients, a review of this literature also suggests that, with sporadic exceptions, few people who stutter into adulthood will ever fully recover. That is, following treatment there are likely to be some residual aspects of the syndrome, even for those speakers who have become highly fluent. Furthermore, these speakers will need to, at times, activate techniques that allow them to achieve smooth and flowing speech production.

Stuttering is a syndrome made up of a complex combination of attitude, behavioral, and cognitive features and, particularly in adults, it is resistant to long-term change. In a number of ways, altering this syndrome is similar to other areas of clinical intervention where relapse is a common phenomenom, such as marital problems, drug addiction, alcoholism, weight reduction, and quitting smoking (Lefcourt, 1976). For example, one-year success rates for intensive smoking-cessation programs range from 20 percent to 40 percent; they range from 10 percent to 20 percent for nonintensive interventions (DiClemente, 1993).

After formal treatment is concluded, the client is on his own. It is then that the crucial process of informal treatment begins. This phase of the treatment process has most often been termed *maintenance* and typically lasts much longer than formal treatment. In many important ways, for the adult who stutters, this stage of treatment continues for the rest of the speaker's life. During maintenance, the stutterer must be able to accept the responsibility of self-management, a function he gradually begins to assume during the later stages of formal treatment.

OUR LIMITED VIEW OF CHANGE

Probably the major consideration throughout this period of informal treatment is the possibility of relapse. This is especially true during the first few months and years following the termination of formal intervention. Relapse may occur, not only in terms of fluency level, but more important, in the direction of the pretreatment attitude and cognitive features of the syndrome. Just as the assessment of this syndrome must be multidimensional, the maintenance of success is multidimensional as well. Concentration on a single feature, such as the level of fluency, excludes the cognitive features of the syndrome that those who are doing the stuttering perceive as critical (Prins, 1970). In any case, maintenance of the many changes that take place during formal treatment is difficult when the client is on his own, doing battle alone against a long history of stuttering. Therefore, a major portion of this chapter is devoted to understanding relapse and the strategies for dealing with this common problem.

As discussed in Chapter 1, student clinicians usually lack the opportunity to view more than a semester or two of the affective, behavioral, and cognitive changes that occur as a result of treatment. At best, clinicians are usually able to see a only small window of this progress. To some degree, this is also the case for professional clinicians. Although the professional clinician will likely follow a client through the entire period of formal treatment, there is often little or no interaction with the client during the long process of informal treatment. Some clients do maintain contact with the clinic, but mostly, as Van Riper (1973) points out, these are clients who need additional help. The majority of clients go off on their own, leaving the clinician with no idea about their progress over the many years of informal treatment. Comprehensive clinical programs should have a system for assisting the client in the maintenance of clinical gains as well as refresher programs emphasizing the client self-management of cognitive and attitudal changes (Boberg, 1986).

MAINTENANCE AND TRANSFER

Of the three stages of treatment—establishment of fluency, transference of new abilities to extratreatment speaking situations, and maintenance of the new abilities following formal treatment—maintenance has come to be regarded as the most challenging aspect of the treatment process (Boberg, 1986). Maintenance is burdensome for the client, for he is working against many forces that are pulling in the direction of pretreatment performance and cognition.

Furthermore, maintenance is enigmatic for the clinician, for it is typically difficult to maintain contact with the client. Even when contact is continued, there are many practical, and even some ethical, problems that make it difficult to obtain accurate data concerning posttreatment performance. Maintenance of the changes achieved during informal treatment will be more likely to occur if, during the period of formal treatment, the clinician has enabled the client to focus on the *transfer* of cognitive, affective, and behavioral changes to a variety of extratreatment settings. Gregory states, "The essence of effective therapy is transfer" (1995, p. 199). As mentioned earlier, transfer refers to the generalization of gains made in the treatment environment to extratreatment situations. Rather than wait until partial or complete fluency is achieved in treatment before beginning these transfer activities, most clients can benefit from such activities from the outset of treatment. During the first treatment sessions, the speaker can begin the process of desensitization to a large variety of environmental stimuli that have had a powerful handicapping effect. The clinician can assist in extending the victories of identification and self-monitoring to real-world speaking situations. Activities, objects, and individuals that are brought to the treatment setting can serve as powerful discriminative stimuli that will cue the client for achieving a similar performance outside the treatment environment. Even something as basic as an audiotape recorder can function as a discriminative stimulus in extratreatment speaking situations (Howie, Woods, & Andrews, 1982).

As discussed in both Chapters 6 and 7, the lack of homogeneity among clients is a major variable that contributes to the inconsistent effects of treatment. This lack of client and environmental homogeneity may also provide a good explanation for the difficulty of successful client maintenance following treatment. For example, Boberg (1986) suggested that differences in long-term progress are as likely to be due to personality factors and the ability of the clients as they are to the treatment program or even the clinician. During informal treatment, there is little or no direct influence by the clinician concerning the fluency-disrupting stimuli in the client's world. The client is on his own as he responds to the stimuli and attempts to alter the old roles and expectancies of those in his environment. Clearly, his success, or lack thereof, will have a critical impact on long-term effects of intervention.

THE NATURE OF RELAPSE

By discussing the nature of relapse with the client and preparing him for the possibility of regression, is the clinician creating a self-fulfilling prophecy? If the topic of regression is never mentioned is relapse less apt to occur, or does the clinician have an obligation to prepare the client for something that, in some form at least, is likely to happen? Certainly, the literature indicates that for adult clients, the possibility of relapse is real. Thus, understanding the nature of this experience and the likelihood of its occurrence is one of the clinician's responsibilities.

The Possibility of Relapse

Many authors have recognized relapse as a common event following treatment for adults who stutter (Bloodstein, 1987; Kuhr & Rustin, 1985; Perkins, 1979; Silverman, 1981; Van Riper, 1973). Prins (1970) found that about 40 percent of clients taking part in an intensive residential program experienced some regression following treatment. In addition, the clients perceived maximum regression to occur within six months after the termination of formal treatment. Cooper (1977) asserts that relapse is part of the human condition. Silverman (1981) suggests that relapse is likely to occur with a 40 to 90 percent probability. Van Riper states, "Relapses and remissions are the rule, not the exception for the adult stutterer if long-term follow-up investigations are conducted" (1973, p. 178). St. Louis and Westbrook report that "relapse is a ubiquitous and familiar problem in stuttering therapy" (1987, p. 252). Perkins states that "maintenance of fluency is the perennial weak link in the therapeutic chain" (1979, p. 119) of stuttering treatment. Finally, as Bloodstein (1995) maintains, although we are adept at making stutterers fluent, we know little about how to keep them that way.

Thus, for most clients, some type of follow-up is necessary. The learning curve is long, and the old habits are the strongest. Clients should at least have the option of continuing treatment in some form for as long as they need it. This, of course, is not likely to happen if coming back to the center is viewed, by the clinician or the client, as an indication of failure. If changing the syndrome of stuttering in adults is viewed as a long-term process, which in the majority of cases it surely is, for the client to return for follow-up sessions is not a sign of failure. Rather, it is a natural and acceptable part of the process of change. Additional treatment, more than anything else, simply means that those involved are intelligent enough to recognize that they are likely to benefit from further effort and growth. Fortunately, many clients do not require a return to intensive individual treatment. Often, group treatment sessions or support group meetings once or twice a month will enable the client to either get back on track or continue making progress.

Defining Relapse

Defining relapse following formal treatment is nearly as difficult as determining the severity of the stuttering at the outset. Of course, the frequency of overt stuttering events is one indicator, but usually it is far from the only and typically not the initial indicator of regression. As Van Riper stated: "Stuttering does not mean relapse. Another moment of fear is no catastrophe" (1973, p. 209). The attitude and cognitive aspects of the problem, often in the form of negative self-talk, are likely to take the lead in the progression of relapse. As elements of avoidance and fear begin to multiply and increasingly influence the speaker's decision making, overt stuttering will not be far behind.

Relapses may take many forms and may range from brief periods that are mildly irritating to long episodes that are extremely handicapping. The clinician may be able to determine that the client has reached the threshold of a relapse based on observable affective, behavioral, and cognitive aspects of the syndrome. However, the presence and degree of relapse are probably best determined by the client himself. When the client gets to the point where he believes he is no longer confident of managing his speech on his own or that his decisions are increasingly based on the possibility of stuttering, relapse has reached a clinical level. If he is making choices because of the *possibility* of a stuttering event, the problem has again become significant. At that point, it is both reasonable and desirable to seek additional professional help.

POSSIBLE CAUSES OF RELAPSE

Silverman (1981) suggested a number of possible reasons for relapse. Clients who are especially likely to relapse are those who, following treatment, believe themselves to be cured. Believing they have experienced a cure, they are less likely to continue the rigorous process of self-management. Other clients may regress as they come to lose confidence in the treatment program. This is more apt to occur if they have experienced relapse following previous treatment experiences. As Silverman points out, people tend to expect events to replicate themselves.

Other possible causes of relapse include the clinician or the client having thresholds for fluency breaks that are too liberal; in this case, small fluency breaks are accepted and left unmodified. Relapse is also more likely to occur if clients are released from treatment too soon, although how soon is too soon may be difficult to assess. It may be worthwhile seeing the client through one relapse while the support of the clinician is immediately available. The presence of stuttering can provide an escape from responsibilities or work. This probably does not occur enough to explain relapse in most people, but no doubt, it is one force that can push the client back into his old pattern of avoidance. We all make use of excuses to avoid performing unpleasant tasks. For any client, but perhaps especially for adolescents, an emotional crisis resulting in loss of self-esteem may negatively influence fluency (Daly, Simon, & Burnett-Stolnack, 1995). As Daly et al. indicate, adolescent clients are likely to see many negative events, be they social, academic, or treatment related, as catastrophic.

Neurophysiological Loading

Several authors who have gathered and studied data concerning etiology, spontaneous recovery, and relapse for subjects with fluency disorders suggest that some of these speakers possess an underlying physiological or neurophysiological condition (Boberg, 1986; Moore & Haynes, 1980; Perkins, Kent, & Curlee, 1990; Zimmerman, 1980, 1981). This may be especially likely for clients with "genetic loading," who have a family history of stuttering. Boberg (1986) suggests that just as recovery from stuttering may be related to a family history of stuttering (Sheehan & Martyn, 1966), there also may be a greater chance of relapse for such speakers (Cooper, 1972; Neavers, 1970).

If these findings are accurate, there are some important implications for the treatment process. That is, the treatment techniques acquired by the client may be thought of as providing skills necessary to *compensate* for an innate deficiency (Boberg, 1986). This, in turn, implies that the maintenance of these skills is best viewed as a lifelong process. This would be the case even if the speaker were not seen as having a deficiency. If, as Starkweather and Gottwald (1990) and Conture (1990) suggest, the demands placed on the speaker consistently exceed the person's capacities to produce speech, fluency breaks will be apt to occur. The treatment techniques then would provide a response to the discrepancy between the demands placed on the speaker and his individual capacities. In any case, the person must maintain appropriate self-management abilities to compensate for this situation.

Continued Effort Is Required

Changing the surface and intrinsic features of the stuttering syndrome takes considerable effort. This is apparent throughout the often arduous process of formal treatment. However, for some people, the continuing effort and vigilance that are required for long-term change are not perceived as worth the effort. As Cooper (1977) has pointed out, it takes a good deal of psychic energy to initiate and maintain all the necessary changes in the stuttering syndrome. As with most things, it does become easier with practice and success. However, if, as a result of treatment, the problem itself becomes less handicapping to the client, the continued effort may not be worth the effect. The problem will no longer be a major one for the person, and he may decide to devote his finite time and energies to issues in his life that he considers more important. Whether clinicians like it or not, this is the scenario that often occurs. Progress can continue in the direction of enhanced fluency and improved self-management, but the curve of success is never linear and does not always travel in an upward direction.

CLIENT ADJUSTMENT TO A NEW ROLE

Joseph Sheehan often suggested that for treatment to be successful, the client must eventually make the adjustment of viewing himself as something beyond an individual who stutters. In many important ways, he must evolve as a person and form a new paradigm, a new view of himself and his possibilities (Boberg, Howie, & Woods, 1979; Emerick, 1988; Hayhow & Levy, 1989). Kuhr and Rustin (1985) noted, for example, that following treatment, those clients who were most satisfied with their fluency also made changes in their lifestyle, which Kuhr and Rustin attributed to the maintenance of fluency. Unfortunately, it takes some time to change decades of expectancies in the face of many old and powerful stimuli. Near the end of successful treatment, some clients may express some anxiety, and even vague feelings of guilt, concerning their new fluency. Kuhr and Rustin (1985) found evidence of minor depression in several fluent speakers during maintenance following formal treatment. Clients may state that they are not as comfortable as they thought they would be with their fluency. They may even have the vague feeling that they are deceiving others. They do not feel like themselves. Their new fluency and all the responsibility for self-management that goes with it have changed the self they had grown used to. In addition, though the speaker may be fluent and feel that his fluency is earned, there may be the feeling of waiting for the other shoe to fall. He may be afraid of losing his fluency, thinking, "Yes, I'm fluent for the moment, but what happens if I lose it?"

While the new fluency may be nice, it will not always feel immediately comfortable. It will take some time before the client, as well as others in the environment, can adjust to the speaker's new way of communicating and interacting with others. Of course, the client's fluency may not be something that others in their lives are used to, either. If treatment has been successful, many aspects of the syndrome have changed, and not just the speaker's fluency. It takes some time for everyone, speakers and listeners alike, to adjust to the many implications of these changes.

LISTENER ADJUSTMENT TO A NEW SPEAKER

Related to the demands for continued effort and adjustment by the client is the need for the adjustment of other people in the client's daily environment to this altered speaker. Successful treatment of the client who stutters will impact others. If these other people in the client's life fail to understand and recognize the nature of progress, they will be less likely to provide positive reinforcement for these changes, and to some degree, long-term progress will be less likely to occur. If treatment has genuinely been successful, there will have been some important changes in the client's thinking about himself and others. As discussed in Chapter 6, for some clients, changes in speech assertiveness and risk taking are likely to influence ways of interacting and communicating with others. Not only must the client adjust to a new role beyond that of a person who stutters, others may have to shift their position in order to establish a new equilibrium. The other people in the clients's life must recognize that they may also need to readjust their roles. Of course, these other people may not want to change. Following treatment, there will be forces brought about by others in their expectations that the client will continue playing his old role. Kuhr and Rustin provide an example of just such a response. They described a wife who felt uncomfortable when her husband returned home with fluent speech, following successful in-patient treatment. His wife's reaction was a negative one: she accused the clinician, saying, "You took him away and made him fluent" (1985, p. 234).

Related to these old expectancies of others is the pressure that is often placed on the speaker to exhibit fluency following treatment. This may be particularly true if the speaker has attended an intensive program away from his home and family. Upon returning home, there may be expectancy and pressure to demonstrate much-improved or even perfect fluency. The occurrence of stuttering will likely be viewed as an immediate sign of failure: "How awful, after all this time and effort and money and he still stutters!" Although many clients can show much-improved fluency, the fear of even a single fluency break can be immense. One good response to the pressure of others to be fluent when they say such things as, "Your speech is wonderful now that you've had therapy. You don't stutter at all any more, do you," might be to say something such as, "Wwwwell, I'm do, do, doing my best!" (Van Riper, personal communication, October, 1971).

Speaking in a Nonhabitual Manner

It has been argued by several writers and clinicians that treatment programs that bring about increased fluency by encouraging the stutterer to speak in a nonhabitual manner tend to have only a temporary impact on a speaker's fluency (Bloodstein, 1949, 1950; Boberg, 1986; Van Riper 1973, 1990). Altering an individual's habitual rate and manner of articulation is obviously possible for relatively short periods of time, and without question, such altered ways of speaking can result in rapid and obvious increases in fluency. However, such changes in habitual speech production are difficult to change in the long term. It takes concentration and a great deal of effort to maintain what are clearly nonhabitual respiratory, phonatory, and articulatory patterns. Without question, some speakers are able to maintain these altered ways of producing speech. For others, however, the use of these altered patterns eventually wears off. Kalinowski, Nobel, Armson, and Stuart (1994) obtained reading passages from five adults with mild stuttering and five adults with severe stuttering. The subjects were randomly selected from clients who had undergone an intensive fluency-shaping program. Reading passages of one minute each from both pre- and posttreatment recordings were rated by sixty-four listeners for speech naturalness. Despite the fact the pretreatment samples contained several instances of stuttering and the posttreatment audio samples were largely free from stuttering events, the listeners indicated that posttreatment recordings resulted in a significant decrease in speech naturalness for both mildly and severely stuttering clients. The authors suggested that perhaps one reason why many individuals who stutter may fail to conscientiously use target behaviors following their discharge from treatment is because of the unsatisfactory therapeutic effects of unnatural-sounding speech.

Starke (1994) points out that the use of artificial speech often results in prosodic distortion. Although the altered ways of producing speech may promote fluency in a traditional sense, they may also result in messages being misperceived. Because of the altered prosody, there is a distinct possibility of a distortion in the speaker's communicative intentions and the relationship between the speaker and the listener, an effect Starke terms "message incompatibility conflict" (1994). Although the speaker may no longer be stuttering in his typical manner, the pragmatics of human communication may suffer unless the listener is able to understand that artificial speech is being used.

Failure to Follow Maintenance Procedures

Boberg (1986) suggests that, in many ways, the requirements of practicing self-management techniques (regardless of whether the techniques involve stuttering modification or fluency modification) can be a highly punishing experience. As we have indicated, the use of nearly all modification techniques carries with it a loss of spontaneity and an emphasis on how the speech is produced rather than what is being said. As Boberg (1986) suggests, being accountable for using the speech modification techniques may be more internally punishing for many speakers than hoping for the periods of normal speech that occur. Boberg suggests that most treated stutterers will continue to practice these techniques "only if the perceived positive consequences of practice outweigh the perceived negative consequences" (1986, p. 498).

The Cyclical Nature of Fluency

In Chapter 3 we discussed how the cyclical nature of fluency in children and adults contributes to the difficulty of diagnosing stuttering and predicting future levels of fluency. This characteristic of fluency also continues following treatment. Kamhi (1982) points out that some stutterers have to work harder than others to achieve and maintain fluency due to the natural variability of their speech-production systems. For some speakers, such variability as well as relapses are more common and perhaps more severe. Kamhi suggests that knowing the stimuli that are likely to produce stress, the speaker can learn to predict and work through these occurrences. The higher the level of fluency desired, the more work is usually required to maintain that level.

OVERT AND COVERT MEASURES OF LONG-TERM CHANGE

One of the difficulties in determining how clients are performing following treatment involves the method of assessment. That is, if speakers are aware of the assessment, will they respond differently than they might otherwise? Howie, Woods, and Andrews (1982) compared the effect of overt and covert measures, both prior to and following treatment. Twenty-two adult male stutterers were assessed before, and fifteen were contacted after, intensive fluency treatment. Howie et al. found no difference between overt and covert measures in terms of percent syllables stuttered (%SS) before treatment. However, following treatment, there were significantly more stuttering events noted following treatment when the speakers were measured covertly. Both overt and covert samples consisted of two (one monologue and one face-to-face conversation with a stranger) three-minute samples of speech, which were audiotaped. All but three of the fifteen subjects assessed posttreatment stuttered more during covert assessment than during overt assessment.

There is some evidence that such differences in percent syllables stuttered between overt and covert measures become less pronounced with increased time posttreatment (Ingham, 1975; Howie, Tanner, & Andrews, 1981). Andrews and Craig (1982) suggest that after approximately eighteen months posttreatment, covert assessment may no longer be necessary.

PREDICTING SUCCESS FOLLOWING TREATMENT

To date, researchers have had little success predicting the long-term success of treatment. It is difficult to know what features to monitor as predictors. It is also difficult to know which features of the syndrome should be used as criterion measures. The results of Andrews and Craig (1988) provide support for a multidimensional approach for predicting long-term success. Using a combination of three factors, they found that 97 percent of the subjects who maintained high skill mastery (0% syllables stuttered), normal speech attitudes as indicated by such measures as the Modified Erickson Scale of Communication Attitudes (S-24) (Andrews & Cutler, 1974), and an internal locus of control as indicated by the Locus of Control of Behavior Scale (LCB) (Craig, Franklin, & Andrews, 1984) were able to maintain success. Perhaps more telling is the fact that none of the subjects who failed to achieve any of these goals was able to maintain his posttreatment fluency level. In a related study, Madison, Budd, and Itzkowitz (1986) found that pretreatment locus of control (LOC) measures corresponded to the degree of change in stuttering following treatment for a group of seven- to sixteen-year-old children. That is, those children who had a more internal LOC prior to intervention tended to achieve more fluent speech during treatment. However, no significant relationship was found between pretreatment LOC scores and fluency levels during evaluations conducted at both two and six months following treatment.

Another recent attempt to predict long-term success was conducted by deNil and Kroll (1994). They considered the extent to which adult stutterer's scores on the Locus of Control of Behavior Scale (Craig, Franklin, & Andrews, 1984) are predictive of their ability to maintain speech fluency both immediately following intensive treatment and approximately two years later. Twenty-one subjects participated in a three-week intensive treatment program based on the Precision Fluency Shaping Program (Webster, 1975). Thirteen subjects who were contacted again two years later participated in a follow-up evaluation, which consisted of the administration of several scales, the reading of a brief passage, and a conversation with a research assistant. All subjects were seen by an assistant who was unknown to the subjects and unaware of their previous performance. Furthermore, the assessment took place in a new and unfamiliar location. While subjects showed a significant long-term improvement in fluency no predictive relationship was found between scores on the LCB scale and level of fluency, as measured in percent words stuttered, either posttreatment or follow-up. However, LCB scores were found to be predictive of the subjects' fluency self-evaluation measured posttreatment and at follow-up. The study suggests that while the LCB may contribute to the prediction of the long-term treatment outcome, particularly as perceived by the client, other client and process variables will need to be considered.

Using a measure such as the locus of control is intuitively appealing. Early in treatment, clients typically express the feeling that stuttering is something that happens to them. When they stutter, they feel helpless and have no control (Van Riper, 1982). In one way or another, all treatment programs place a major emphasis on the client's self-management of his speech behavior and his cognitive interpretation of his circumstances (Adams, 1983; Kuhr & Rustin, 1985). As treatment progresses, speakers must gradually internalize cognitive and behavioral changes. If they do not, these speakers are more likely to relapse once formal treatment is completed (Boberg, Howie, & Woods, 1979). Other researchers (Craig, Franklin, & Andrews, 1984; Andrews and Craig, 1985) have demonstrated that changes in clients' LCB scores toward more internal control during treatment are related to the long-term treatment outcome. On the other hand, Ladouceur, Caron, and Caron (1989) found no relationship between LCB scores and fluency improvement in nine adults. Surprisingly, they found that some clients became more externally oriented during treatment while also acquiring increased fluency. Although Ladouceur et al. suggested that the changes in fluency, internal control, at least as gauged by the LCB, and behavior may have to do with the treatment strategy used. Obviously, the association is far from a simple one.

SUPPORT GROUPS

One of the more important influences on the long-term maintenance of treatment gains may be the client's involvement in support groups (see Appendix B). Whether these groups are referred to as support, self-help, or advocacy groups, they all can provide sources of information and motivation for those who stutter as well as their families and friends. The meetings of the local chapters of such organizations also furnish important opportunities to practice techniques and stabilize cognitive changes following formal treatment. The encouragement of the other members is apt to enhance increases in motivation and assertiveness. The meetings can also provide an important social function for some of the members, fostering interaction in an accepting, penalty-free environment. It is a place where members can continue the process of coming to terms with the problem. Appendix B provides the addresses, telephone, fax, and internet numbers for a variety of such groups.

The development of self-help groups is closely related to the development and growth of consumerism (Hunt, 1987; Ramig, 1993b). As Hunt (1987) describes (citing Katz & Bender, 1976), support groups are volunteers who come together for mutual assistance with common problems, handicaps, or chronic complaints. They provide face-to-face contact among members and stress members' personal responsibility. The groups provide a variety of members' needs including the facilitation of personal change, fostering of personal responsibility by members, provision of information and advice, discussion of alternative treatments, fund-raising, and political activities relating to the goals of the group. Most often, however, the majority of the activities relate to providing members with support and information.

Hunt (1987) reported that the greatest virtue of support groups was providing the members with a sense of relief from the feeling of isolation and by providing others who understood their distress and frustration. A survey conducted by Krass-Lehrman and Reeves (1989) of 600 National Stuttering Project (NSP) members (141 questionnaires returned) indicated that the *least* important focus of the groups was to provide an adjunct to formal treatment. Ramig (1993b), in a survey of 62 support group participants, found that 49 indicated that their fluency had improved "at least somewhat" as a direct result of their involvement in such groups. Interestingly, there was also some indication that group members had to attend something approaching twenty meetings for this to be the case. More importantly, 55 of the 62 respondents indicated that support group involvement resulted in "at least somewhat positive" or "very positive" impact on their daily life.

In order to appreciate the nature of such groups we will provide a brief history of two of them, the British Stammering Association (BSA) and the U.S.-based National Stuttering Project (NSP). The BSA was founded in 1968. As is often the case, the initial development of such groups results from the efforts of one person (in this case, Robin Harrison) who is willing to dedicate many years of administrative, public relation, and fund-raising activities in order to get the group off the ground. A review of the BSA membership by Hunt (1987) indicated that a small proportion of the total population of people with fluency disorders belonged to the group. The age range for the membership is generally from twenty-five to forty, with few teenagers. The average age of people in groups was higher than those in treatment, where few clients over the age of fifty are found (Manning & Shirkey, 1981). The size of most local groups was four to six members. It ranged from as small as two to a rarely exceeded upper limit of twelve. The most common goal reported by individual chapters was to transfer and maintain techniques learned in formal treatment. Although group members often practiced treatment techniques during the meetings, much of the discussion centered on adjusting to the cognitive aspects of the fluency disorder, including fears, anxieties, and feelings of inferiority, powerlessness, and frustration. Hunt (1987) reports that this was especially true for groups with "more mature members" who have had success in controlling their speech.

Most of the local chapters tended to be short-lived, lasting for only one or two years. In order for a local group to continue for any length of time, strong leadership is essential. In addition, from time to time, the group needs to elicit the support of local speech-language pathologists for referrals as well as advice. Finally, as Hunt suggests, the group must discipline itself so that it will be more than a social group. It must have specific guidelines and objectives that focus on the self-management of fluency disorders.

A second group, well known in the United States, is the National Stuttering Project. This was founded in 1977 by Michael Sugarman and Bob Goldman for the purpose of providing information and support to children and adults who stutter, their families, as well as professional clinicians. The guiding principle of this group is their statement, "If you stutter, you are not alone." Participation in the NSP group expanded during the leadership of John Albach and at this writing is composed of more than 4,000 members throughout the United States and more than fifty local support groups. The current Director of Development and Administration is Annie Braberry. Their monthly publication, *Letting Go*, is sent to all members and provides information and support in the form of articles, letters, stories, and reflections written by members. The activities include the monthly newsletter as well as brochures, books, tapes, the local group meetings, and regional workshops. All these activities as well as an annual national convention are designed to educate, advocate, and instill a sense of solidarity and confidence in the members. The specific goals of NSP are to provide an opportunity for members to share with others their fears, frustrations, and triumphs, practice therapeutic techniques in a safe and supportive environment, take part in speaking experiences they would otherwise be likely to avoid; develop positive cognitive and affective strategies for managing their fluency disorder; and assist other members in achieving these goals.

There are, as Hunt (1987) points out, some potential difficulties in the functioning of support groups. Some groups tend to see themselves as treatment groups without the therapist. Of course, there is the potential in such situa-

VIGNETTE

Adult male, age fifty-three: basically, I want to share that striving for perfection impeded my improvement. I read about William Jennings Bryan (The Golden Tongued orator) and he was my goal. When I readjusted my sights to become "as fluent as my motor system would allow," then I started to make progress. Gradual progress over a three- or four-year period, with occasional relapses and real breakdowns (like when three people very close to me—one my mother—died within a two-week period). My speech suffered tremendously, but even then I knew that I was grieving and when I grew strong again, and focused attention to my speech again, that I would regain my fluency. I never doubted that. My belief system remained positive that I would speak fluently again, as fluently as my timing system or motor coordination abilities would allow. But striving for perfection was abandoned as unrealistic and really as unnecessary for success and happiness.

Also, when I took my stuttering out from under the microscope and saw that disfluencies were only a part of me, that helped. When I saw that other qualities (like being a good friend, listener, and caring person to others) was also a part of who and what I was—then I put speech (stuttered or fluent) in a proper perspective. I worked on using light pressure on my first sounds, sure, but also on improving tennis or sailing skills, too. And becoming a better administrator and writer, etc. Putting disfluencies in perspective helped—I realized that our Creator may have more challenges in store for me other than just becoming a perfect speaker. So I decided to work not only on fluency but on other "talents" I might have too. That thinking seemed to send me in a more positive direction.

tions for inappropriate or counterproductive attitudes, information, and techniques to be promoted. Furthermore, Hunt (1987) suggests that many people who could benefit from participation do not belong to such groups because they refuse to define themselves as persons who stutter. Cooper (1987), Silverman (1996), and Ramig (1993b) have all pointed out that many clinicians have a skeptical view of support groups, generally because they fail to understand the positive potential of this process. Overall, however, these groups play an important, often critical role, in providing individuals with an opportunity for support and encouragement that is essential for long-term success following treatment.

REPORTS OF SUCCESS

There are many individuals who, following formal treatment for what were moderate-to-severe fluency disorders, are able to achieve a high level of flu-

VIGNETTE   *Adult male, age fifty-two:* I completed an intensive program of treatment in my mid-twenties. That was twenty-eight years ago at this writing. I made obvious progress during the twenty-week period of formal treatment. I learned how to slowly decrease my avoidance behaviors and change the way I was stuttering. Very slowly, I began to take charge of my speech, especially my moments of stuttering. I also began to make some preliminary changes in the way I thought about my speech, both my stuttering as well as my fluent speech. But these cognitive changes, what I was telling myself about myself and my speech, came along at a much slower pace. Following my dismissal from treatment, I continued to expand my new ways of speaking, of stuttering, and thinking in ever expanding speaking situations. I slowly continued to make progress but it certainly wasn't linear. It was many years, at least fifteen, before the handicap of stuttering decreased to the point where it was insignificant.

Now, nearly three decades following my dismissal from formal treatment I find that I do something that could be classified as stuttering (including both overt stuttering and avoidance behaviors) less than ten times a year. I continue to think of myself as someone who stutters. It is just that I don't do it very often. It is no big deal to be a stutterer, and it can actually be quite helpful if you're working with others who stutter. You have taken the "rite of passage," and you have insight into the deep structure of the problem. It is a little easier to tune into the decision-making process of others who stutter because you've been there, making those same decisions. Although I still may stutter on a few occasions, I make sure that it is easy, open stuttering. And most important, the fact that I might stutter has absolutely no influence on my choices.

ency, perhaps even spontaneous fluency. Most likely, these are speakers who do not possess the high level of neurophysiological loading discussed earlier. There are few, if any, other individuals in the family who have stuttered and they received treatment during their adolescent or young adult years.

TRANSFER AND MAINTENANCE ACTIVITIES

A basic theme in changing human behavior is that the individual must gradually take the major responsibility for identifying and modifying his own behavior and attitudes concerning his situation (DiClemente, 1993; Egan, 1990). In the case of fluency disorders, the client must become sophisticated about stuttering in general, and his own stuttering in particular. The speaker must be able to recognize his errors and assign activities for confronting and changing his mistakes. Moreover, in order for change to take place, the speaker must do the majority of his practice outside the context of the treatment set-ting. Formal training takes place for only a few hours each week, and changes are not likely to occur unless the individual is disciplined enough to practice on his own. To the degree that a person does well in extratreatment settings during formal treatment, he will be likely to do well in those same situations during the months and years of informal treatment.

The following is a compilation of suggestions presented by St. Louis and West-brook (1987) and includes activities suggested by Van Riper (1958, 1973); Boberg (1983); Boberg and Kelly (1984); Boberg and Sawyer (1977); Ryan (1979, 1980); Daly (1987); Dell (1980); Shames and Florance (1980); Howie, Tanner, and An-dress (1981); St. Louis (1982); Williams, (1983); and the current author.

- The clinician can make it clear to the client that continued consultation and support are available following the termination of formal treatment. Returning to treatment is not only acceptable, it is expected.

- Treatment intensity can vary and decrease gradually, with individual meetings gradually occurring less often. Individual treatment sessions can gradually be supplemented with group meetings.

- Treatment can be transformed from face-to-face meetings to contact via the telephone or postcards. Audio- or videotape recordings of self-prac-tice sessions can be mailed to the clinician, who can mail back critiques.

- Videotapes made in treatment can be used on a home VCR, enabling the client to demonstrate techniques learned in treatment and to record ex-amples of the client's ability to use the techniques in extratreatment speaking situations.

- Prior to dismissal from formal treatment, the clinician and client can dis-cuss the reasons for relapse and plan specific client responses at the first indications of relapse (e.g., design voluntary stuttering activities in order to decrease the fear and avoidance of specific sounds, words, and speak-ing situations).

- Following formal treatment, the client can continue to seek new, as-sertive speaking situations where the envelope of comfort can gradually be expanded. If professional or social contacts do not provide such op-portunities, the client may consider taking part in groups such as Toast-masters or Dale Carnegie.

- The client can expand his assertive and risk-taking behaviors for both speech and nonspeech activities, expanding and cultivating other talents and interests.

- The client may contact local groups and organizations to talk about his or her interests and professional experiences. Libraries are often interested in finding such speakers.

- The client may consider contacting local agencies that need volunteers to read newspapers or books on tape to older people who cannot read or to the blind.

- The client can continue to reassess opportunities for changes in his lifestyle, including possible alteration of interpersonal, vocational, and social roles.

- The client can continue to improve and expand on a variety of nonspeaking skills that are likely to enhance his participation in life and his interaction with others.

- The client can join and take an active part in a local self-help or support group, possibly assuming a leadership role.

- The client can continue to monitor and evaluate his positive-negative self-talk, using the stopping and positive redirection activities (see Chapter 6).

- The client can practice the use of positive affirmations on a regular basis.

- The client can volunteer to work in a formal treatment setting with adults and children who have fluency disorders.

CONCLUSION

Although change occurs throughout formal treatment, progress must continue long after formal intervention has been completed. Unfortunately, as with other complex human problems, relapse is not unusual, particularly for adult clients. Emphasis on transfer and maintenance activities that include extra-treatment performance will help decrease the possibility of relapse. Following formal treatment, continued vigilance and effort are required for long-term success. It is important to realize that many others beside the client must also adjust, not only to new fluency but to new roles as well. Family members and friends must adapt to the speaker, who may be more assertive than previously. Membership in a support group following treatment is highly recommended for maintaining both behavioral and attitudinal changes. If treatment is truly successful, the client should be able to gradually assume the responsibility for self-evaluating and systematically altering both the surface and intrinsic features of stuttering.

Throughout this text I have tried to be true to the goals stated in the preface. However, if there is one goal that rises above all the others, it is the need to create enthusiasm in clinicians for helping children and adults with fluency disorders. Enthusiasm is enhanced by exploration. The clinician must continually seek new information and consider new strategies and techniques. Knowing the possibilities and choices of intervention, the experienced clinician will be free to focus on the needs of the person who has come for help. The professional must be able to make clinical decisions that are based on experience and perception of the client's needs at a moment in time, not so much on the doctrine of any particular method or technique.

Magnificent changes are possible in the speech and the lives of those who come to us for help. Following treatment, some clients will become fluent. Others will continue to stutter but in a smoother and effortless form, and some, for now at least, will make little change. Nearly all speakers have the potential to develop to the point where they have very little, and in some cases, essentially no, handicap because of their speech.

Not every speech-language pathologist is equipped to work in the area of fluency disorders for, as in each of the specialty areas of the field, it takes some unique abilities. However, for those who do choose to come to the assistance of these clients, there are exciting and rewarding victories to be shared and marvelous colleagues who are willing to help.

RECOMMENDED READINGS

Boberg, E. (1983). Behavioral transfer and maintenance programs for adolescent and adult stutterers. pp. 41–61. In J. Fraser Gruss (Ed.) *Stuttering therapy: Transfer and maintenance* (Publication No. 19) Memphis, TN: Stuttering Foundation of America.

Boberg, E., Howie, P., & Woods, L. (1979). Maintenance of fluency: A review. *Journal of Fluency Disorders*, 4, 93–116.

Manning, W. H. (1991). Making progress during and after treatment. In W. H. Perkins (Ed.), *Seminars in speech and language* 12:349–354. New York: Thieme Medical Publishers.

Appendix A: Annotative Listing of Assessment Procedures

1. Adams, M.R. (1977a). "A Clinical Strategy for Differentiating the Normal Nonfluent Child and the Incipient Stutterer." *Journal of Fluency Disorders*, 2, 141–148.

This measure is designed for preschool children. The clinician first obtains a 300–500 word sample of conversational speech. The following five behaviors are used to identify nonnormal speech: (1) more than ten fluency breaks per 100 words, (2) occurrences of part-word repetitions and prolongations, (3) part-word repetitions of four or more units, (4) cessation of airflow/voicing, and (5) schwa vowel substitutions. The analysis can be somewhat time-consuming and the clinician must be certain that one or more representative samples of the child's speech can be obtained.

2. Ammons, R., & Johnson, W. (1944). Iowa Scale of Attitudes toward Stuttering. In Studies in the psychology of stuttering. *Journal of Speech Disorders*, 9, 39–49.

This five-point rating scale consists of forty-five statements about stutterers and what they should or should not do or feel in various speaking situations. The stutterer's intolerance (avoidance) may indicate the need for counseling therapy or modification of attitudes through hierarchial practice.

3. Andre, S., & Guitar, G. (1979). The A-19 Scale for Children Who Stutter. See Guitar, B. & Grimes, S. (1979). *Developing a scale to assess communication attitudes in children who stutter.* Paper presented to the annual meeting of American Speech-Language-Hearing Association. See also Peters, T., & Guitar, B. (1991). *Stuttering, an integrated approach to its nature and treatment* (p. 179). Baltimore, MD: Williams & Williams.

This nineteen-item scale was designed to assess communication attitudes in children who stutter. The child responds by saying "yes/no" to each of the questions (e.g., Do you like to talk on the phone?) As with the S-scale mentioned above (Erickson, 1969), the scale is obtained by comparing the subject's responses to the way a stutterer would respond. Nonstuttering children typically respond as a stutterer would to an average of 8.17 items. Stuttering children respond as a stutterer to an average of 9.07 items (SD = 2.44).

4. Andrews, G., & Cutler, J. (1974). S-24 Scale. "Stuttering therapy: The relations between changes in symptom level and attitudes." *Journal of Speech and Hearing Disorders*, 39, 312–319.

This popular measure is a shortened version of the thirty-nine-item Erickson S-Scale (1969). Using regression analysis, the authors developed a more efficient twenty-four-item version of the original scale, which may be used for repeated measures (e.g., during treatment). This scale contains twenty-four true–false items that the speaker completes. It is designed for use with older teenagers and adults and contains items such as "I usually feel that I am making a favorable impression when I talk." Nonstuttering adults typically respond as a stutterer would to an average of 9.14 of the items (SD = 5.38). Stuttering adults respond as a stutterer to an average of 19.22 of the items (SD = 4.24). The S–24 is quickly and easily administered.

5. Brutten, G. J., & Dunham, S. L. (1989). The Communication Attitude Test: A normative study of grade school children. *Journal of Fluency Disorders*, 14, 371–377.

This thirty-five-item questionnaire, called the CAT-D, is designed to assess the speech-associated beliefs of children. The children who stutter circle true or false about negative or positive attitudes toward speech. Sample items include: "I like the way I talk. Talking is easy for me. I am afraid the words won't come out when I talk." Scoring is done by assigning a 0 to all responses that reflect a positive attitude toward speech and a 1 for responses that reflect a negative attitude. Brutten and DeNill (1991) studied sixty-three stuttering children from Belgium (7–14 years of age) who scored an average of 15.95 (SD = 7.28), compared with 134 control subjects, who averaged 8.57 (SD = 5.22).

6. Brutton, E., & Shoemaker, D. (1974). Fear Survey Schedule. In *The Southern Illinois Behavior Checklist*. Carbondale, IL: Southern Illinois University. This is an adaptation of the Fear Survey Schedule developed by J. Wolpe and P. Lang, Educational and Industrial Service, San Diego, CA.

This schedule is designed for both children (eighty items) and adults (fifty-one items). The subject responds by circling a point on a 1 (no fear) to 5 (great fear) scale indicating the amount of fear associated with a variety of things (sharp objects, being criticized, death, being misunderstood, meeting with someone in authority). Average scores for nonstuttering children were 162.5, but no scores were given for stuttering children. Average scores for nonstuttering adults were 70.45, and average scores for stuttering adults were 108.08.

7. Brutten, E., & Shoemaker, D. (1974). Speech Situation Checklist. In *The Southern Illinois Checklist*. Carbondale, IL: Southern Illinois University.

This checklist is designed for both children (fifty-five items) and adults (fifty-one items). The checklist was developed to assess speech-related anxiety and speech disruptions. The subject is asked to respond to typical speaking situations (talking on a telephone, giving your name, making introductions, asking for help with homework) by using an interval scale from 1 (no anxiety; no disruptions) to 5 (much anxiety; many disruptions). Average scores for nonstuttering children were 96.90 (anxiety level) and 86.92 (disruption level). Average scores for stuttering adults were 100.74 (anxiety level) and 105.40 (disruption level). Average scores for stuttering adults were 100.74 (anxiety level) and 105.40 (disruption level).

8. Cooper, E. B. (1973). Cooper Chronicity Prediction Checklist for School-Age Stutterers: A Research Inventory for Clinicians. *Journal of Speech and Hearing Disorders*, 38, 215–223. Also in E. Cooper. Personalized fluency control therapy. *DLM Teaching Resources*, 1 DLM Park, Allen, Texas 75002.

This inventory utilizes questions and clinical observations regarding case history, child attitudes, parental attitudes, and behavioral symptomology to predict the likelihood of a child "outgrowing" stuttering. The clinician completes the checklist after sampling the child's speech and interviewing the parent(s). There are a total of twenty-seven questions covering "historical," "attitudinal," and "behavioral" indicators of chronicity. The clinician scores each question by indicating, "yes, no, not available, or unknown." "Yes" responses may indicate that stuttering is likely to become a chronic problem. A total score of 0–6 suggests possible recovery; 7–15 indicates continued vigilance, and 16–27 is predictive of chronicity. Longitudinal data needs to be obtained and weighing of items needs to be done before this potentially useful inventory will yield helpful assessment information.

9. Cooper, Eugene. Client and Clinician Perceptions of Stuttering Severity Ratings. In *Personalized Fluency Control Therapy*. DLM Teaching Resources, 1 DLM Park, Allen, Texas 75002.

The client is asked for a self-rating of global severity which may then be compared to the clinician's perception of the client's severity. The clinician rates four aspects of severity: frequency, duration, tension, and concomitant behaviors.

10. Cooper, Eugene. Concomitant Stuttering Behavior Checklist. In *Personalized Fluency Control Therapy*. DLM Teaching Resources, 1 DLM Park, Allen, Texas 75002.

Clinical observations are recorded on this assessment form. Thirty-two behaviors that may accompany moments of stuttering are observed in five categories: posturing, respiratory, facial, syntactic/semantic, and vocal behaviors. These may be monitored during reevaluations.

11. Cooper, Eugene. Parent Attitudes toward Stuttering Checklist. In *Personalized Fluency Control Therapy*. DLM Teaching Resources, 1 DLM Park, Allen, Texas 75002.

Parental attitudes and feelings may be identified with this twenty-five-item checklist. Areas of parental concern or misperceptions may then be targeted in counseling sessions.

12. Cooper, Eugene. Situation Avoidance Behavior Checklist. In *Personalized Fluency Control Therapy*. DLM Teaching Resources, 1 DLM Park, Allen, Texas 75002.

Fifty common speech situations are listed to ascertain those that are avoided. The score is the total number of situations avoided and may be useful in monitoring progress during treatment or to establish a hierarchy of tasks during treatment.

13. Cooper, Eugene. (1985). Stuttering Attitudes Checklist. In *Personalized Fluency Control Therapy*. DLM Teaching Resources, 1 DLM Park, Allen, Texas 75002.

Twenty-five statements are used to assess a client's own feelings and attitudes toward stuttering. This pencil-and-paper checklist is claimed useful with children and adults, although modifications will be necessary for young or poor readers. The total score may be useful for pre-, during, and posttreatment assessments. Individual statements may indicate topics for counseling and discussion of feelings.

14. Cooper, Eugene. Stuttering Frequency and Duration Estimate Record. In *Personalized Fluency Control Therapy*. DLM Teaching, 1 DLM Park, Allen, Texas 75002.

The severity of stuttering, based on only frequency (percentage) and duration, is assessed with this instrument. Severity is assessed under the conditions of answering questions that elicit a one- to two-word response, recitation of the alphabet, and reading of a 200-syllable passage.

15. Craig, A. R., Franklin, J. A., & Andrews, G. (1984). [Locus of Control of Behavior (LCB) Scale.] A scale to measure locus of control behavior. *British Journal of Medical Psychology*, 57, 173–180.

This seventeen-item, Likert-type scale was constructed to measure the degree to which a person perceives events as being a consequence of his own behavior and subsequently takes responsibility for maintaining new (desired) behavior. Designed for adults, the scale has been shown to have good internal reliability and is not influenced by sex, age, or social desirability of subject responses. The scale appears to differentiate between individuals with and without chronic behavioral conditions. Items 1, 5, 7, 8, 13, and 16 are reverse-scored. Higher scores on the LCB Scale reflect greater self-perception of external control (chronic stutterers averaged 31.01), while lower scores indicate greater internal control (control subjects averaged means of 27.9 and 28.3). The scale may help predict those stutterers who will relapse after treatment and those who have the ability to maintain change in behavior they previously believed to be uncontrollable.

16. Daly, D. A. (1992–93). Daly's Checklist for Possible Cluttering. *Clinical Connection,* Winter, 6.

This checklist consists of thirty-three descriptive statements on a four-point scale (1 = not at all, 2 = just a little, 3 = pretty much, 4 = very much). Adults and/or children answer by reflecting how well the statements describe them. Preliminary evidence suggests that a score of 60 or above indicates the diagnosis of cluttering. A score between 30 and 60 may be indicative of a clutterer-stutterer. Daly also suggests that the following items may be particularly critical: 2, 3, 7, 9, 10, 12, 14, 20, 25, 33.

17. DeVore, J., Nandur, M., & Manning, W. (1984). Projective drawings and children who stutter. *Journal of Fluency Disorder*, 9, 217–226.

These authors provide preliminary information indicating significant differences between the drawings of children (ages five to ten years) who stuttered and those who did not. Children who did not stutter drew significantly larger drawings that were placed nearer to the center of the page. Significant changes were found for the drawings of the children who stuttered after treatment. That is, the clients drew larger figures and began to place them more toward the center of the page as treatment progressed. No significant differences were found between the groups of children after the stutterers received treatment. These preliminary results suggest that projective drawings may provide a means of assisting personality dynamics of young stutterers and personality change that might otherwise go undetected and unrewarded.

18. Erickson, R. (1969) [Scale of Communication Attitudes (S-Scale)]. *Journal of Speech and Hearing Research, 12,* 711–724.

Designed for older adolescents and adults, this scale consists of thirty-nine statements ("I find it easy to talk with almost anyone"; "Some words are harder than others for me to say."). The subject responds by indicating true or false. Stutterers tend to answer an average of thirty items, while nonstutterers typically answer no more than four items in this fashion.

19. Erickson, R. (1969) [Severity Scale and Adjective Checklist]. In Assessing communication attitudes among stutterers. *Journal of Speech and Hearing Research, 12,* 711–724.

Eighty adjectives that are descriptive of various feelings and types of behaviors potentially experienced during interpersonal communication are included in the Adjective Checklist (ACL).

20. Goldberg, Stanley A. (1981). The Child Fluency Assessment Instrument; The Adolescent Fluency Assessment Instrument; The Adult Fluency

Assessment Instrument. In *Behavioral Cognitive Stuttering Therapy*, C. C. Publication, Inc., P.O. Box 23699, Tigard, Oregon 97223.

These three assessment instruments are extensive systems for appraising the many facets of stuttering. Included are case history questions, frequency counts, situational rating scales, self-perception questionnaires, and, in the child and adolescent version, questions for assessing parental attitudes.

21. Gough, H. G., & Heilbrun, A. B. Adjective Checklist. *The Adjective Checklist*. Palo Alto, CA: Consulting Psychologists Press.

This all-purpose checklist of favorable adjectives has been used with stuttering to monitor attitudinal shifts as a function of therapy. The checklist consists of twenty-four scales covering areas such as self-confidence, personal adjustment, and achievement.

22. Hanson, B. R., Gonhoud, K. D., & Rice, P. L. (1981). Speech Situation Checklist. *Journal of Fluency Disorders*, 6, 351–360.

These authors used discriminative analysis to select the most discriminating items in the original SSC (Brutton & Shoemaker, 1974). The resulting twenty-one items provide a screening device for identifying stutterers who experience a high level of speech-related anxiety.

23. Johnson, W., Darley, F., & Spriestersbach, D. (1952). Stutterer's Self Ratings of Reactions to Speech Situations (SSR). In *Diagnostic Manual in Speech Correction*. New York: Harper & Row.

The measure provides a comprehensive view of the client's reactions to forty extratreatment speaking situations. The client uses a 1–5 scale to indicate a self-measurement in each of four categories: Frequency (how often he encounters the situation), Avoidance (how likely he would be to avoid the situation), Reaction (how much he would like or dislike speaking in this situation), and Stuttering (the estimated severity of stuttering in each situation). Total scores are computed by averaging the scaled totals for each of the four categories.

24. Johnson, W., Darley, F., & Spriestersbach, D. (1963). [Iowa Scale of Attitudes Toward Stuttering.] In *Diagnostic Methods in Speech Pathology*. New York: Harper & Row.

This forty-five-item scale is designed to assess the attitudes toward stuttering of older children and adult stutterers and their listeners. The subject responds to each item (e.g., "A stutterer should not try out for the debating team.") by circling one of five points on an ordinal scale ranging from strongly agree to strongly disagree. The lower the score the better the attitude of the respondent. Average group scores on the data obtained by these authors ranged from an 1.36 (clinicians) to 11.73 (controls). Scores for a group of 63 stutterers averaged 1.53.

25. Johnson, W., Darley, F., & Spriestersbach, D. (1963). Iowa Scale for Rating the Severity of Stuttering. In *Diagnostic Methods in Speech Pathology*. New York: Harper & Row.

This scale provides the clinician with descriptive categories of stuttering behavior ranging from (1) very mild–stuttering on less than 1 percent of words, very little tension, disfluencies generally less than one second in duration, patterns of disfluency simple, no associated body movements, to (7) very severe–stuttering on more than 25 percent of words, very conspicuous tension, disfluencies average more than four seconds in duration, very conspicuous distorting of sounds, facial grimaces, and conspicuous associated movements.

26. Lanyon, R. (1967). Stuttering Severity Scale (SS). *Journal of Speech and Hearing Research*, *10*, 836–843.

This paper-and-pencil scale is designed to evaluate the overt behaviors and attitudes of older teens and adults who stutter. The sixty-four items ("I worry about the fact that I'm a stutterer. When I talk I often become short of breath.") are answered as true or false. The scores on the sixty-four items are converted to ratings on a 1 (mild) to 7 (severe) scale.

27. Lewis, D., & Sherman, D. (1951–52). Sherman-Lewis Scale. *Journal of Speech and Hearing Disorders*, *16*, 320–326, and *Journal of Speech and Hearing Disorders*, *17*, 316–320.

For clients displaying overt struggle behaviors, this five-point scale rates the frequency of overt struggle, degree of tension present, duration of blocks, pattern of blocking, and distracting movements of the body. Using a nine-point equal-interval scale (1 = least severe; 9 = most severe), the speech-language pathologist listens to a sample of conversational speech and directly assigns a value. Intra- and interjudge reliability scores were good using this approach. A correlation of +.98 was obtained between groups of undergraduate students, and a correlation of +.97 was obtained between women and men.

28. Luper, Harold L. and Mulder, R. L. (1964). Stuttering Diagnostic and Evaluative Checklist. In *Stuttering therapy for children* (pp. 207–211). Englewood Cliffs, NJ: Prentice-Hall.

This checklist includes features of stuttering: case history descriptions, disfluency symptoms (regarding repetitions, prolongations, hard attacks, interjections), consistency and adaptation, secondary mannerisms, and concealment devices.

29. Manning, W. (1994). *The SEA-Scale: Self-efficacy scaling for adolescents who stutter*. Paper presented to the annual meeting of the American Speech-Language-Hearing Association, New Orleans.

Based on the work of Bandura (1977), this technique is designed to measure the confidence that an adolescent stutterer can (1) enter into speaking situations typically found outside of treatment and (2) achieve a predetermined level of fluency in the speaking situation. Using a decimal scale the subject assigns a whole number value (1 to 10) to each situation, and these scores are then averaged across all one-hundred speaking situations in order to obtain a total score for the approach and performance items. The scale is composed of thirteen subscales (after Watson, 1988). The overall alpha level for all 100 items was 0.98, with subscale alphas ranging from 0.74 to 0.94. Forty adolescents who stuttered scored significantly ($p < 0.001$) lower (mean = 7.21; SD = 1.8) than a matched group of nonstuttering controls subjects (mean = 8.65; SD = 1.2). The technique is likely to be most helpful in assessing extra-treatment performance during and following treatment.

30. Martin, R. R., Haroldson, S. K., & Woessner, G. L. (1988). Perceptual Scaling of Stuttering Severity. *Journal of Fluency Disorders, 13,* 27–47.

After observers judged stuttering severity on a seven-point scale with equal-appearing intervals, observers judged "on line" the severity of stutterers' speech under normal circumstances and under delayed auditory feedback.

31. McDonough, A., & Quesal, R. W. (1988). Locus of control orientation of stutterers and nonstutterers. *Journal of Fluency Disorders, 13,* 97–106.

This task is used to determine whether an adult or adolescent client believes in an internal or external locus of control for speech. It consists of eight questions or statements that are answered yes or no.

32. Ornstein, A., & Manning, W. (1985). Self-efficacy scaling by adult stutterers. *Journal of Communication Disorders, 18,* 313–320.

Based on the work of Bandura (1977), this technique is designed to measure the confidence that an adult stutterer can (1) enter into speaking situations typically found outside treatment and (2) achieve a predetermined level of fluency in the speaking situation. Using a decile (10–100) scale, the subject assigns a value to each situation and these scores are then averaged across the fifty speaking situations in order to obtain a total score for both approach and performance sections. The technique is likely to be most helpful in assessing extratreatment performance during and following treatment. (See also Hillis, 1993.)

33. Pindzola, Rebekah H., & White, Dorenda T. (1986). A protocol for differentiating the incipient stutterer. *Language Speech and Hearing Services in Schools, 17* (1), 2–15.

This protocol assesses behaviors such as type, size, frequency, and duration of the disfluencies, level of effort, rhythm, use of avoidance tactics, visual (secondary) mannerisms, and historical and psychological indicators. A unique feature of this protocol is a normal-versus-abnormal rating grid for interpreting each behavior.

34. Riley, G., A Stuttering Severity Instrument for Children and Adults. (1972). *Journal of Speech and Hearing Disorders, 37,* 314–322. Also available from C. C. Publications, Inc., P.O. Box 23699, Tigard, OR 97223.

This instrument was designed in order to provide scale values for stuttering severity for both children and adults. Speakers who can read are asked to (1) describe their job or school and (2) read a short passage. Nonreaders are given a cartoon picture task to which they respond. Scoring is accomplished across three areas. The frequency of the fluency breaks tabulated and the percentage of stuttering is converted to a task score (range, 4–18). The duration of the three longest stuttering moments (fleeting to more than sixty seconds) is tabulated and converted to a task score (range, 1–7). Last, physical concomitant across four categories are scaled on a 0-to-5 scale (0 = none, 5 = severe and painful looking) and totaled (range, 0–20). The total overall score ranges from 0 to 45 points.

35. Riley, G. (1981). *Stuttering Prediction Instrument for Young Children*. C. C. Publications, Inc., P.O. Box 23699, Tigard, OR 97223. Rev. ed., Austin, TX: Pro-Ed, 1981.

Designed to predict chronicity of stuttering in young children (ages 3–8), this instrument is divided into five sections: (1) history, (2) parent's reactions, (3) part-word repetitions, (4) prolongations, and (5) frequency. After interviewing the parents, the conversational speech of the child is elicited using pictures and tape recordings. The speech samples are then analyzed for the behaviors and scored by assigning numerical values to the child's behavior. The total possible score is 40. The average score of 22.2 (standard deviation of 7.01) was obtained by children who continued to stutter, whereas those children who did not become chronic stutterers had an average score of 6.17 (standard deviation of 3.13).

36. Riley, G., & Riley, J. (1986). [Oral Motor Assessment Scale (OMAS).] *Oral Motor Assessement and Treatment*. Tigard, OR: C. C. Publications.

This scale provides norms for assessing the accuracy of target speech sounds, the even flow of articulatory sequences of syllables, and rate of production. This scale is designed to provide a comprehensive and quantitative measure of a child's neuromotor development.

37. Riley, G. and Riley, J. (1989). Physician's Screening Procedure for Children Who May Stutter. *Journal of Fluency Disorders, 14*, 57–67.

This screening is designed to assist clinicians in making diagnostic decisions in preschool children. It is devised as a data-based screening protocol and can be used by physicians and speech-language pathologists for assessing degree of abnormality of a child's disfluency and reactions to it.

38. Ryan, B. (1980). Stuttering Interview (SI, Form A). In *Programmed Therapy for Stuttering Children and Adults*. Springfield, IL: Charles C. Thomas.

The format for this twenty-item interview ranges from "automatic" (saying the alphabet) to "conversational" speech. Intended for young children, speech is elicited by using a variety of materials (pictures, puppets, reading material). Scoring is accomplished by relating the frequency scores and types of fluency breaks to a scale. Scale values range from 0 (normal) to 3 (severe).

39. Ryan, B. (1974). [Stuttering Interview (SI, Form B)]. In *Programmed Therapy for Stuttering Children and Adults*. Springfield, IL: Charles C. Thomas.

Scoring for this fourteen-item interview is similar to that of Form A described in (38). This form is designed to be used with upper elementary and high school students as well as adults.

40. Sherman, D. (1952). Clinical and Experimental Use of the Iowa Scale of Severity of Stuttering. *Journal of Speech Hearing Disorders*, *17*, 316–320.

This scale has a range from 0 to 7 (with 0 indicating "no stuttering"). Each point is associated with stuttering frequency and duration, amount of muscle tension, and facial grimaces and general body movement. This scale is used for rating the severity of stuttering and utilizing information about behaviors that occur during moments of stuttering.

41. Shine, Richard E. (1980). Assessment Form: Systematic Fluency Training for Young Children. In *Systematic Fluency Training for Children*. C. C. Publications, Inc., P.O. Box 23699, Tigard, OR 97223.

This assessment form covers history of the stuttering problem, rate of stuttering (during assorted speaking tasks), severity rating, a speech sample, and a checklist of affected physiological speaking processes.

42. Shumak, I. C. (1955). A speech situation rating sheet for stutterers. pp. 341–347, In Johnson, W. and Leutenegger, R. R. (Eds.) *Stuttering in Children and Adults*. Minneapolis: University of Minnesota Press.

Forty common speech situations are rated on four aspects of adjustment: avoidance, reaction, stuttering, and frequency. Pre-, during, and posttreatment administrations of this scale may monitor attitudinal improvements. The scale also may assist in hierarchy ranking of speaking situations for practice.

43. Silverman, F. H. (1980). Stuttering Problem Profile (SPP). *Journal of Speech and Hearing Disorders*, *45*, 119–123.

The SSP was created with the idea of assisting the clinician and the client in identifying treatment goals for adults who stutter. The profile consist of eighty-six first-person statements ("I am usually willing to stutter openly. I now rarely anticipate stuttering."). The profile is not scored but rather the stutterer indicates those statements that he or she would like to be able to make at the termination of treatment but could not honestly be made at the outset. The list may be added to in order to make the statements more relevant to the client's interests and goals.

44. Stocker, B. (1980). *The Stocker Probe*. Tulsa, OK: Modern Education Corporation.

This procedure is designed to differentiate the chronic young stutterer from the child whose stuttering is temporary. The procedure is based on the assumption that the more novel the message, the greater the communication demand is on the speaker. Two common objects are used and the clinician asks the child a total of ten questions across five "levels of demand." The levels of demand range from Level I (The clinician hands the child a ball and asks "Is it hard or is it soft?") to Level V (The clinician says, "Make up a story about the ball."). At any level of demand, the frequency of disfluencies are associated with clinical levels of severity: 1–10 (mild), 11–20 (moderate), 21–30 (severe), and 31 (very severe).

45. Van Riper, C. (1982). [Profile of Stuttering Severity.] In *The Nature of Stuttering*. Englewood Cliffs, NJ: Prentice-Hall.

This profile provides a quick assessment of severity across four behavior areas: frequency, duration, tension/struggle, and postponement/avoidance. The clinician uses a 1–7 scale for each behavior, with a scale value of 1 representing less than 1 percent of stuttered words and no postponement avoidance behavior. A scale value of 7 represents stuttering on 25 percent or more words, excessive tension and struggle in the trunk of the body, duration of breaks lasting five seconds or more, and postponement/avoidance occurring more than 70 percent of the time. This is one of the few behavioral scales that includes the important factor of avoidance behavior and can be used with both children and adults.

46. Watson, J. B. (1987). Profiles of stutterers' and nonstutterers' affective, cognitive, and behavioral communication attitudes. *Journal of Fluency Disorders, 12*, 389–405.

This self-report inventory for adults obtains ratings of different types of speaking situations, using five response scales reflecting behavioral, affective, and cognitive aspects of attitudes. Examination of profile characteristics revealed two significant discriminators, classification as a stutterer or nonstutterer, and an overall speech rating. Nondiscriminatory characteristics include sex, age, education, therapy experiences, stuttering severity self-rating, onset of stuttering, total therapy time, current therapeutic status, and familial history.

47. Williams, D. (1978). Stutterers' Self-Ratings of Reactions of Speech Situations. In F. Darley and D. Spriestersbach, *Diagnostic methods in speech pathology* (2nd ed.), New York: Harper & Row.

This self-rating scale was created to determine specific speaking situations that a speaker was having difficulty adjusting to outside the treatment setting as well as the possible need for continued counseling. It is appropriate for use with the adolescents (fourteen years and above) and adults. The stutterer rates his reaction to forty speaking situations (e.g., ordering in a restaurant, saying hello to a friend, telephoning to make an appointment) using a 1 to 5 scale. Four categories of reactions are scored for each question: avoidance, reaction, stuttering, and frequency. For example, a scale value of 1 indicated that the speaker would never avoid the situation and a scale value of 5 indicated that the speaker would avoid the situation whenever possible. The scale values for all situation are averaged over all forty speaking situations for each of the four reaction categories.

48. Williams, D., Darley, F., & Spriestersbach, D. (1978). Measures of Disfluency of Speaking and Oral Reading (Form 5). In F. Darley & D. Spriestersbach, *Diagnostic methods in speech pathology*, (2nd ed.), New York: Harper & Row.

Designed for the older adolescent and adult, this measure consists of two speaking tasks (job description and description of the pictures from the The-matic Apperception Test and two oral reading tasks). The examiner calculates a disfluency index and types of disfluencies as a percentage of breaks per one hundred words. These disfluency types considered are: interjections, part-word repetitions, word repetitions, phrase repetitions, revisions, incomplete phrases, broken words, prolonged sounds, dysrhythmic phonation in words, and tension-pauses.

49. Woods, C., & Williams, D. (1976). Bi-Polar Adjective Scale. In "Traits attributed to stuttering and normally fluent males." *Journal of Speech and Hearing Research, 19*, 267–278.

This scale consists of twenty-five paired adjectives (open-guarded, tense-relaxed, daring-hesitant) organized in a 7-point semantic differential format. It may be used by clinicians or others (including the stutterer) in an attempt to describe the perceived personality characteristics of children or adults. Rather than a measure for differentiating stutterers from nonstutterers, it may be best applied as an indication of cognitive and attitude change for the client during treatment.

50. Woolf, G. (1967). Perception of Stuttering Inventory (PSI). In "The Assessment of Stuttering as Struggle, Avoidance and Expectancy." *British Journal of Disorders of Communication, 2*, 158–171.

This inventory is intended to determine the avoidance, struggle, and expectancy of older adolescent and adult stutterers. The subject responds to sixty behavioral and attitude characteristics by indicating whether they are characteristic themselves. Those items that are not typical of their behavior are left unmarked. Examples of inventory items include: "Avoiding talking to people in authority" (avoidance), "Having extra and unnecessary facial movement" (struggle), and "Adding an extra sound in order to get started" (expectancy).

Appendix B: Resources and Support Groups in Fluency Disorders

American Speech-Language-Hearing Association (ASHA)
10801 Rockville Pike
Rockville, MD 20852
Phone: 301–897-5700
Fax: 301–471-0457
Net: none

The British Stammering Association (BSA)
15 Old Ford Road
London, England E2 9PJ
Phone: 0181-983 1003
Fax: 0181-983 3591
Net: none

Canadian Association for People Who Stutter (CAPS)
2269 Lakeshore Boulevard, West
Etobikoke, Ontario, Canada M8V 3X6
Phone: 416–252-0842
Fax: 416–252-0720
Net: http://chat.carleton.ca/~dblock/caps.html

International Fluency Association (IFA)
Box 870242
Tuscaloosa, AL 35487-0242
Phone: 205–348-7131
Fax: 205–348-1845
Net: ECOOPER@UA1VM.UA.EDU

National Council on Stuttering
558 Russell Road
DeKalb, IL   60115
Phone: 815–756-6986
Fax: none
Net: none

National Stuttering Project (NSP)
5100 E. La Palma Avenue
Suite 208
Anaheim Hills, CA 92807
Phone: 800–364-1677
Fax: 714–693-7554
Net: NSPMAIL@AOL.COM

Speak Easy International
233 Concord Drive
Paramus, NJ 07652
Phone: 201–262-0895
Fax: none
Net: none

Stuttering Foundation of America (SFA)
3100 Walnut Grove Road
Suite 603
Memphis, TN 38111-0749
Phone: 800–992-9392 / 901–452-7343
Fax: 901–452-3931
Net: STUTTERSFA@AOL.COM

Stuttering Resource Foundation
Ellen Rind, Director
123 Oxford Road
New Rochelle, NY 10804
Phone: 800–232-4772 / 914–632-3925
Fax: 914–235-0615
Net: ESR1@IONA.BITNET

International Stuttering Association (ISA)
c/o Mel Hoffman
811 Nisqually Drive
Sunnyvale, CA 94087
Phone: 408–245-5654
Fax: 408–730-8154
Net: JAAN_PILL@SBE.SCARBOROUGH.ON.CA

ELECTRONIC NETWORK SYSTEMS

Stutt-L:

Listserv Address:	LISTSERV@TEMPLEVM.BITNET or
	LISTSERV@UM.TEMPLE.EDU
List Address:	STUTT-L@TEMPLVM
Owner:	C. W. Starkweather

Stut-Hlp:

Listserv Address:	LISTPROC2BGU.EDU
List Address:	STUT-HLP@BGU.EDU
Owner:	Bob Quesal

Stutt-X:

Listserv Address:	LISTSERV@ASUVM.INRE.ASU.EDU
List Address:	STUTT-X@ASUVM.INRE.ASU.EDU
Owner:	Don Mower

UseNet Discussion Group: ALT.SUPPORT.STUTTERING

Gopher Information System, Mankato State University:
GOPHER.MANKATO.MSUS.EDU
Note: follow the path: academic colleges and departments/communication disorders/stuttering.

The Mankato State University Gopher Site information is also available on the World Wide Web:
http://www.mankato.msus.edu/dept/comdis/kuster/stutter.html

Appendix C: Useful Pamphlets and Videotapes

FOR GENERAL USE

Cooper, E. G. (1990). *Understanding Stuttering. Information for parents*. Chicago, IL: National Easter Seal Society. This booklet describes the nature and possible causes of stuttering. Also discussed are diagnostic signs of stuttering, suggestions for parents of stuttering children, and the nature of treatment programs (28 pages.)

Selmar, J. W. (1991). *Help! This child is stuttering*. Austin, TX: Pro-Ed. Written for parents and teachers of school-age children who stutter, this booklet provides suggestions concerning selecting a speech-language pathologist and the nature of a treatment programs (41 pages.)

National Stuttering Project. *A guide for parents of children who stutter*. Designed as a brief guide for parents of stuttering children by three experts in the field (15 pages.)

Stuttering Foundation Publications

These booklets are edited by Malcolm Fraser, founder of SFA, or his daughter Jane. They are inexpensive ($1.00–$2.00) and contain concise information for clinicians, parents, teachers, and interested others.

To the stutterer (Publication No. 9). Practical advice by twenty-four men and women speech-language pathologists who have been stutterers (116 pages.)

If your child stutters: A guide for parents (Publication No. 11, 3rd rev. ed.) Suggestions for parents when helping the young stuttering or disfluent child (56 pages.)

Self-therapy for the stutterer (Publication No. 12, 7th ed.). Written for adults who are unable to obtain formal treatment, the booklet describes self-therapy activities (192 pages.)

Do you stutter: A guide for teens (Publication No. 21). Written by seven speech-language pathologists who give practical advice to teens on coping with stuttering (80 pages.)

Stuttering and your child: Questions and answers (Publication No. 22). Written for parents, teachers, and day care personnel to help young children who stutter (64 pages.)

FOR PROFESSIONAL USE:

Stuttering words (Publication No. 2). A glossary of terms associated with fluency and fluency disorders (64 pages.)

Therapy for stutterers (Publication No. 10). Outlines a program of treatment for clinicians who are working with adult or older adolescents (120 pages.)

Treating the school age stutterer, a guide for clinicians (Publication No. 14). Written by Carl Dell, Ph.D., this booklet describes a large variety of clinical procedures for young stutterers (112 pages.)

Stuttering: An integration of contemporary therapies (Publication No. 16). Describes combining the treatment strategies of stuttering modification and fluency modification for stutterers of all ages (80 pages.)

Counseling Stutterers (Publication No. 18). This booklet discusses the counseling aspects of treatment for adults and parents of children undergoing treatment (80 pages.)

Stuttering therapy: Transfer and maintenance (Publication No. 19). Discusses the importance of transfer and maintenance procedures during and following the final stages of formal treatment (112 pages.)

Stuttering therapy: Prevention and intervention with children (Publication No. 20). A discussion of prevention and early intervention strategies and techniques with young children (152 pages.)

Brief Informational Pamphlets from the Stuttering Foundation of America

If You Think Your Child is Stuttering;
Turning On to Therapy;
The Child Who Stutterers at School: Notes to the Teacher;
How to React When Speaking with Someone Who Stutters.

VIDEOTAPES

Adult Stuttering Therapy. Charles Van Riper, Ph.D. (1977). A series of eight videotapes demonstrating Van Riper's version of the stuttering-modification treatment strategy. Jeff, a young adult client, is taken through the stages of treatment from the initial diagnostic interview through variation, modification, stabilization and a one-year followup. Recently added to this series is a ninth tape, *Adult stuttering therapy: A twenty year followup with Jeff* (1995). This video is a 28-minute interview with Jeff, discussing his continued treatment success two decades following formal treatment.

Childhood stuttering: A videotape for parents. Conture, E., Guitar, B., & Williams, D. (1994). Stuttering Foundation of America. A thirty-minute tape that describes the nature of stuttering in children and helpful ways for parents to respond.

Prevention of stuttering part I: Identifying the danger signs. (1975). This thirty-three-minute video demonstrates the early signs of stuttering behavior in young children.

Speaking of Courage. (1992). A one-hour video of three children who describe their stories of living with stuttering. The video stresses the importance of understanding by parents, family members, and professionals for both the detection and support of a child who stutters. In the United States, order from Suncoast Media, Inc., 12551 Indian Rocks Road, No. 15, Largo, Florida 34644; Tel: 813–596-1112, 800–899-1008; Fax: 813-596–3939.

Voices to Remember. (1992). A one-hour video of four adults as seen through the eyes of an eleven-year old child. The video discusses the effects of stuttering on the educational, social, and professional lives of four adults. The effects of treatment and support group groups are stressed. In the United States, order from Suncoast Media, Inc., 12551 Indian Rocks Road, No. 15, Largo, Florida 34644; Tel: 813–596-1112, 800–899-1008; Fax: 813–596-3939.

References

Ackoff, R. (1974). *Redesigning the future*. New York: Wiley.

Adams, M. R. (1977a). A clinical strategy for differentiating the normal nonfluent child and the incipient stutterers. *Journal of Fluency Disorders, 2,* 141–148.

Adams, M. R. (1977b). The young stutterer: Diagnosis, treatment and assessment of progress. *Seminars in Speech, Language and Hearing, 1,* 289–299.

Adams, M. R. (1983). Learning from negative outcomes in stuttering therapy: Getting off on the wrong foot. *Journal of Fluency Disorders, 8,* 147–153.

Adams, M. R. (1984). The differential assessment and direct treatment of stuttering, In J. Costello (Ed.), *Speech disorders in children* (pp. 260–295). San Diego, CA: College-Hill Press.

Adams, M. R. (1993). The home environment of children who stutter. In *Seminars in Speech and Language, 14*(3), 185–191.

Adams, M. R. (1990). The demands and capacities model I: Theoretical elaborations. *Journal of Fluency Disorders, 15,* 135–141.

Adams, M. R., & Hayden, P. (1976). The ability of stutters and nonstutterers to initiate and terminate phonation during production of an isolated vowel. *Journal of Speech and Hearing Disorders, 19,* 290–296.

Adams, M. R., & Runyan, C. (1981). Stuttering and fluency: Exclusive events or points on a continuum? *Journal of Fluency Disorders, 6,* 197–218.

Agnello, J. G. (1975). Voice onset and voice termination features of stutterers. In L. M. Webster & L. C. Furst (Eds.), *Vocal tract dynamics and disfluency*. New York: Speech and Hearing Institute. Ainsworth, S. (Ed.). (1992). *Counseling stutterers* (4th ed. Publication No. 18), 171–186. Memphis, TN: Speech Foundation of America.

Albach, J., & Benson, V. (Eds.). (1994). *To say what is ours. The best of 13 Years of letting GO.* (3rd Ed.). San Francisco, CA: National Stuttering Project.

Allen, G. (1975). Speech rhythm: Its relation to performance universals and articulatory timing. *Journal of Phonetics, 3,* 75–86.

Alport, G. W. (1937). *Personality, a psychological interpretation*. New York: Hold.

Alport, G. W. (1961). *Pattern and growth in personality*. New York: Holt, Rinehart & Winston.

Ambrose, N. G., & Yairi, E. (1995). The role of repetition units in the differential diagnosis of early childhood incipient stuttering. *American Journal of Speech-Language Pathology, 4*(3), 82–88.

American Academy of Neurology. (1990). Assessment: The clinical usefulness of botulinum toxin-A in treating neurologic disorders. *Neurology, 40,* 1332–1336.

American Psychiatric Association. 1987. *Diagnostic and statistical manual of mental disorders* (3rd ed.–rev. [DSM-III-R]). Washington, DC: American Psychiatric Association.

American Psychiatric Association. 1994. *Diagnostic and statistical manual of mental disorders* (4th ed.–rev. [DSM-IV]). Washington, DC: American Psychiatric Association.

Amman, J. O. C. (1700/1965). *A dissertation on speech* (reprint). New York: Stechert-Hafner, 1965.

Andrews, G. (1984). Epidemiology of stuttering. In R. F. Curlee & W. H. Perkins (Eds.), *Nature and treatment of stuttering: New directions* (pp. 1–12). San Diego, CA: College Hill Press.

Andrews, G., & Craig, A. (1982). Stuttering: Overt and covert assessment of the speech of treated subjects. *Journal of Speech and Hearing Disorders, 47,* 96–99.

Andrews, G., & Craig, A. R. (1985). The prediction and prevention of relapse in stuttering. The value of self-control techniques and locus of control measures. *Behavior Modification, 9,* 427–442.

Andrews, G., & Craig, A. R. (1988). Prediction of outcome after treatment for stuttering. *British Journal of Psychiatry, 153,* 236–240.

Andrews, G., Craig, A., & Feyer, A. M. (1983). *Therapist's manual for the stuttering treatment programme.* Sydney, Australia: Prince Henry Hospital, Division of Communication Disorders.

Andrews, G., Craig, A., Feyer, A., Hoddinott, S., Howie, P., & Neilson, M. (1983). Stuttering: A review of research findings and theories circa 1982. *Journal of Speech and Hearing Disorders, 48,* 226–246.

Andrews, G., & Cutler, J. (1974). Stuttering therapy: The relation between changes in symptom level and attitudes. *Journal of Speech and Hearing Disorders, 39,* 312–319.

Andrews, G., Guitar, B., & Howie. P. (1980). Meta-analysis of the effects of stuttering treatment. *Journal of Speech and Hearing Disorders, 45,* 287–307.

Andrews, G., & Harris, M. (1964). *The syndrome of stuttering* (Clinics in Developmental Medicine No. 17). London: Spastics Society Medical Education and Information Unit, in association with W. Heinemann Medical Books.

Andrews, G., & Harvey, R. (1981). Regression to the mean in pretreatment measures of stuttering. *Journal of Speech and Hearing Disorders, 46,* 204–207.

Andrews, G., & Neilson, M. (1981). *Stuttering: A state of the art seminar.* Paper to the annual meeting of the Speech-Hearing Association, Los Angeles, CA.

Andrews, G., Yates-Morris, A., Howie, P., & Martin, N. G. (1991). Genetic factors in stuttering confirmed. *Archives of General Psychiatry, 48*(11), 1034–1035.

Arnold, G. E. (1960). Studies in tachyphemia: I. Present concepts of etiologic factors. *Logos, 3,* 25–45.

Arnott, N. (1928). *Elements of physics.* Edinburgh, Scotland: Adams.

Aronson, A. E. (1973). *Psychogenic voice disorders: An interdisciplinary approach to detection, diagnosis, and therapy.* New York: W. B. Saunders.

Aronson, A. E. (1992). *Clinical voice disorders. An interdisciplinary approach.* New York: Thieme.

Aronson, A. E., Brown, J., Litin, E. M., & Pearson, J. S. (1968). Spastic dysphonia. I: Voice, neurological and psychiatric aspects. *Journal of Speech and Hearing Disorders, 33,* 219–231.

Attanasio, J. (1987). The dodo was Lewis Carroll you see: Reflections and speculations. *Journal of Fluency Disorders, 12,* 107–118.

Azrin, N. H., Nunn, R. G., & Frantz, S. E. (1979). Comparison of regulated breathing versus abbreviated desensitization on reported stuttering episodes. *Journal of Speech and Hearing Disorders, 44,* 331–339.

Backus, O. (1947). Intensive group therapy in speech rehabilitation. *Journal of Speech Disorders, 12,* 39–60.

Backus, O. (1957). Group structure in speech therapy. In L. E. Travis (Ed.), *Handbook of speech pathology,* 1025–1064. New York: Appleton-Century-Crofts, Inc.

Baken, R. J. (1987). *Clinical measurement of speech and voice.* Boston: Little, Brown, & Co.

Bamberg, C., Hanley, J., & Hillenbrand, J. (1990). Pitch and amplitude perturbation in adult stutterers and nonstutterers. Paper presented to the annual meeting of the American Speech-Language-Hearing Association, Seattle, WA.

Bandura, A. (1977). Toward a unifying theory of behavior change, *Psychological Review, 1,* 191–215.

Barbara, D. A. (Ed.) (1965) *New Directions in Stuttering: Theory and Practice.* Springfield, IL: Charles C. Thomas.

Barbara, D. A. (1982). *The psychodynamics of stuttering.* Springfield, IL: Charles C. Thomas.

Beech, H., & Fransella, F. (1968). *Research and experiment in stuttering.* Oxford, England: Pergamon Press.

Bell, A. M. (1853). *Observations on defects of speech, the cure of stammering, and the principles of elocution.* London: Hamilton-Adams.

Berenson, B. G., & Carkhuff, R. R. (1967). *Sources of gain in counseling and psychotherapy,* New York: Holt, Rinehart & Winston.

Berenson, B. G., & Mitchell, K. M. (1974). *Confrontation: For better or worse.* Amherst, MA: Human Resource Development Press.

Berkowitz, M., Cook, H., & Haughey, J. (1994). Fluency program developed for the public school setting. *Language, Speech and Hearing Services in Schools, 25,* 94–99.

Berry, M. F. (1938). Developmental history of stuttering children. *Journal of Pediatrics, 11,* 209–217.

Black, J. W. (1951). The effect of delayed sidetone upon vocal rate and intensity. *Journal of Speech and Hearing Disorders, 16,* 56–60.

Blanton, S., & Blanton, M. G. (1936). *For stutterers.* New York: Appleton-Century.

Bloch, E. L., & Goodstein, L. D. (1971). Functional speech disorders and personality: A decade of research. *Journal of Speech and Hearing Disorders, 36,* 295–314.

Blodgett, E. G., & Cooper, E. B. (1988). Talking about it and doing it: Metalinguistic capacity and prosodic control in three to seven year olds. *Journal of Fluency Disorders, 13,* 283–290.

Blood, G. (1995). POWER 2: Relapse management with adolescents who stutter. *Language, Speech, and Hearing Services in Schools, 26,* 169–179.

Blood, G. W., & Blood, I. M. (1982). A tactic for facilitating social interacting with laryngectomees. *Journal of Speech and Hearing Disorders, 47,* 416–419.

Blood, G. W., & Hood, S. B. (1978). Elementary school-age stutterers' disfluencies during oral reading and spontaneous speech. *Journal of Fluency Disorders, 3,* 155–165.

Blood, G., & Seider, R. (1981). The concomitant problems of young stutterers. *Journal of Speech and Hearing Disorders, 46,* 31–33.

Bloodstein, O. (1949). Conditions under which stuttering is reduced or absent: A review of literature. *Journal of Speech and Hearing Disorders, 14,* 295–302.

Bloodstein, O. (1950). Hypothetical conditions under which stuttering is reduced or absent. *Journal of Speech and Hearing Disorders, 15,* 142–153.

Bloodstein, O. (1958). Stuttering as anticipatory struggle reaction. In J. Eisenson (Ed.), *Stuttering: A symposium,* 1–69. New York: Harper & Row.

Bloodstein, O. (1960). The development of stuttering I. Changes in nine basic features. *Journal of Speech and Hearing Disorders, 25,* 219–237.

Bloodstein, O. (1961). The development of stuttering III. Theoretical and clinical implications. *Journal of Speech and Hearing Disorders, 26,* 67–82.

Bloodstein, O. (1974). The rules of early stuttering. *Journal of Speech and Hearing Disorders, 39,* 379–394.

Bloodstein, O. (1987). *A handbook on stuttering* (4th ed). Chicago: National Easter Seal Society.

Bloodstein, O. (1992). Response to Hamre: Part I. *Journal of Fluency Disorders, 17,* 29–32.

Bloodstein, O. (1993). *Stuttering: The search for a cause and cure,* Needham Heights, MA: Allyn & Bacon.

Bloodstein, O. (1995). *A handbook on stuttering* (5th ed). San Diego: Singular Publishing Group.

Bloodstein, O., & Grossman, M. (1981). Early stutterings: Some aspects of their form and distribution. *Journal of Speech and Hearing Research, 24,* 298–302.

Bloodstein, O., & Shogun, R. (1972). Some clinical notes on forced stuttering. *Journal of Speech and Hearing Disorders, 37,* 177–186.

Bluemel, C. S. (1932). Primary and secondary stammering. *Quarterly Journal of Speech, 18,* 187–200.

Bluemel, C. S. (1957). *The riddle of stuttering.* Danville, IL: Interstate.

Boberg, E. (1983). Behavioral transfer and maintenance programs for adolescent and adult stutterers. In J. Fraser Gruss (Ed.), *Stuttering therapy: Transfer and maintenance* (Publication No. 19), 41–61. Memphis, TN: Stuttering Foundation of America.

Boberg, E. (Ed.). (1986). *Maintenance of fluency.* New York: Elsevier.

Boberg, E., Howie, P., & Woods, L. (1979). Maintenance of fluency: A review. *Journal of Fluency Disorders, 4,* 93–116.

Boberg, E., & Kully, D. (1984). Techniques for transferring fluency. In W. H. Perkins (Ed.), *Current therapy of communication disorders: Stuttering disorders,* 178–201. New York: Thieme-Stratton.

Boberg, E., & Sawyer, L. (1977). The maintenance of fluency following intensive therapy. *Human Communication, 2,* 21–28.

Bonfanti, B. H., & Culatta, R. (1977). An analysis of the fluency patterns of institutionalized retarded adults. *Journal of Fluency Disorders, 2,* 117–128.

Bordeau, L. A., & Jeffrey, C. H. (1973). Stuttering treated by desensitization. *Journal of Behavior Therapy and Experimental Psychiatry, 4,* 209–212.

Borden, G. D., Kim, D. H., & Spiegler, K. (1991). Acoustics of stop consonant-vowel relationships during fluent and stuttered utterances. *Journal of Fluency Disorders, 12*(3), 175–184.

Bosshardt, H. (1990). Subvocalization and reading rate differences between stuttering and nonstuttering children and adults. *Journal of Speech and Hearing Research, 33,* 776–785.

Bosshardt, H., & Nandyal, I. (1988). Reading rates of stutterers and nonstutterers during silent and oral reading. *Journal of Fluency Disorders, 13,* 407–420.

Breitenfeldt, D. H., & Lorenz, D. R. (1989). *Successful stuttering management program.* Cheney: Eastern Washington University.

Brill, A. A. (1923). Speech disturbances in nervous and mental diseases. *Quarterly Journal of Speech, 9,* 129–135.

Brodnitz, F. S. (1976). Spastic dysphonia. *Annals of Otorhinolaryngology, 85,* 210–214.

Brown, G., & Cullinan, W. L. (1981). Word-retrieval difficulty and disfluent speech in adult anomic speakers. *Journal of Speech and Hearing Research, 24,* 358–365.

Brutten, G. J., & Shoemaker, D. J. (1967). *The modification of stuttering.* Englewood Cliffs, NJ: Prentice-Hall.

Bryngleson, B. (1935). Method of stuttering, *Journal of Abnormal Psychology, 30,* 194–198.

Bryngleson, B., Chapman, B., & Hansen, O. (1944). *Know yourself: A guide for those who stutter.* Minneapolis: Burgess Publishing.

Bullen, A. K. (1945). A cross cultural approach to the problem of stuttering. *Child Development, 16,* 1–88.

Burton, A. (1972). *Interpersonal psychotherapy*. Englewood Cliffs, NJ: Prentice-Hall.

Cabanas, R. (1954). Some findings in speech and voice therapy among mentally deficient children. *Folia Phoniatrica, 6*, 34–39.

Cannito, M. P., & Sherrard, K. C. (1995). *Fluency in spasmodic dysphonia I: Oral reading rate and disfluency occurrence*. Unpublished manuscript.

Carkhuff, R. R., & Berenson, B.·G. (1967). *Beyond counseling and psychotherapy*. New York: Holt, Rinehart & Winston.

Carlise, J. A. (1985). *Tangled tongue: Living with a stutter*. Toronto, Canada: University of Toronto Press.

Caruso, A. J. (1988). Childhood stuttering: A review of behavioral, acoustical, and physiological research. *ASHA, 30*, 73 [abstract].

Caruso, A., Conture, E., & Colton, R. (1988). Selected temporal parameters of coordination associated with stuttering in children. *Journal of Fluency Disorders, 12*, 67–82.

Cerf, A., & Prins, D. (1974). *Stutterers' ear preference for dichotic syllables*. Paper presented to the annual meeting of the American Speech-Language-Hearing Association, Las Vegas.

Clark, H. (1971). The importance of linguistics for the study of speech hesitations. In D. Horton & J. Jenkins (Eds.), *The perception of language: Proceedings of the symposium, University of Pittsburgh*. Columbus, OH: Charles E. Merrill.

Colburn, N. (1985). Clustering of disfluency in stuttering children's early utterances. *Journal of Fluency Disorders, 10*, 51–58.

Cole, L. (1986). The social responsibility of the researcher. In F. H. Bess, B. S. Clark, & H. R. Mitchell (Eds.), *Concerns for minority groups in communication disorders* (pp. 93–100). (ASHA Reports No. 16, ISSN 0569–8553), 93–100. Rockville, MD: American Speech-Language-Hearing Association.

Cole, L. (1989). E pluribus pluribus: Multicultural imperatives for the 1990s and beyond. *Journal of the American Speech-Language-Hearing Association, 31*, 65–71.

Collins, C. R., & Blood, G. W. (1990). Acknowledgement and severity of stuttering as factors influencing nonstutterers' perceptions of stutterers. *Journal of Speech and Hearing Disorders, 55*, 75–81.

Combs, A., & Snygg, D. (1959). *Individual behavior*. New York: Harper.

Conture, E. G. (1982). Stuttering in young children. *Journal of Developmental and Behavioral Pediatrics, 3*, 163–169.

Conture, E. G. (1990). *Stuttering* (2nd Ed.). Englewood Cliffs, NJ: Prentice-Hall.

Conture, E., & Caruso, A. (1987). Assessment and diagnosis of childhood disfluency. In L. Ruskin, D. Rowley, & H. Purser (Eds.), *Progress in the treatment of fluency disorders* (pp. 57–82). London, England: Taylor & Francis.

Conture, E., Colton, R., & Gleason, J. (1988). Selected temporal aspects of coordination during fluency speech of young stutterers. *Journal of Speech and Hearing Research, 31,* 640–653.

Conture, E., & Guitar, B. (1993). Evaluating efficacy of treatment of stuttering: School-age children. *Journal of Fluency Disorders, 18,* 253–287.

Conture, E., & Kelly, E. (1988). *Nonverbal behavior of young stutterers and their mothers.* Paper presented to the annual meeting of the American Speech-Language-Hearing Association, Boston, MA.

Conture, E., Louko, L., & Edwards, M. L. (1993). Simultaneously treating stuttering and disordered phonology in children: Experimental therapy, preliminary findings. *American Journal of Speech-Language Pathology, 2*(3), 72–81.

Conture, E., Rothenberg, M., & Molitor, R. (1986). Electroglottographic observations of young stutterers' fluency. *Journal of Speech and Hearing Research, 29,* 384–393.

Conture, E., & Schwartz, H. (1984). Children who stutter: diagnosis and remediation. *Communication Disorders, 9:* 1–18.

Conture, E. G., & Zebrowski, P. M. (1992). Can child speech disfluencies be mutable to the influences of speech-language pathologists, but immutable to the influence of parents? *Journal of Fluency Disorders, 17,* 121–130.

Cooper, E. B. (1968). A therapy process for the adult stutterer. *Journal of Speech and Hearing Disorders, 33,* 246–260.

Cooper, E. B. (1972). Recovery from stuttering in a junior and senior high school population. *Journal of Speech and Hearing Research, 15,* 632–638.

Cooper, E. B. (1973). The development of a stuttering chronicity prediction checklist: A preliminary report. *Journal of Speech and Hearing Disorders, 38,* 215-223.

Cooper, E. B. (1975a). *Clinician attitudes toward stutterers: A study of bigotry?* Paper presented at the annual meeting of the American Speech-Language-Hearing Association, Washington, DC.

Cooper, E. B. (1975b). *Clinician Attitudes Toward Stuttering Inventory (CATS).* Allen, TX: DLM.

Cooper, E. B. (1977). Controversies about stuttering therapy. *Journal of Fluency Disorders, 2,* 75–86.

Cooper, E. B. (1979a). Intervention procedures for the young stutterer. In H. Gregory (Ed.), *Controversies about stuttering,* 63–96. Baltimore, MD: University Park Press.

Cooper, E. B. (1979b). *Understanding stuttering: Information for parents.* Chicago: National Easter Seal Society for Crippled Children and Adults.

Cooper, E. B. (1985). *Cooper personalized fluency control therapy—revised.* Allen, TX: DLM.

Cooper, E. B. (1986a). The mentally retarded stutterer. In K. O. St. Louis (Ed.), *The atypical stutterer,* 123–154. San Diego, CA: Academic Press.

Cooper, E. B. (1986b). Treatment of dysfluency: Future trends. *Journal of Fluency Disorders, 11,* 317–327.

Cooper, E. B. (1987). The chronic perseverative stuttering syndrome: incurable stuttering. *Journal of Fluency Disorders, 12,* 381–388.

Cooper, E. B. (1990). *Understanding stuttering: Information for parents.* Chicago: National Easter Seal Society.

Cooper, E. B., Cady, B. B., & Robbins, C. J. (1970). The effect of the verbal stimulus words wrong, right and tree on the disfluency rates of stutterers and nonstutterers. *Journal of Speech and Hearing Research, 13,* 239–244.

Cooper, E. B., & Cooper, C. S. (1965). Variations in adult stutterer attitudes towards clinicians during therapy. *Journal of Communication Disorders, 2,* 141–153.

Cooper, E. B., & Cooper, C. S. (1985a). Clinician attitudes toward stuttering: A decade of change (1973–1983). *Journal of Fluency Disorders, 10,* 19–33.

Cooper, E. B., & Cooper, C. S. (1985b). The effective clinician. Chapter 3 in E. B. Cooper and C. S. Cooper, *Personalized fluency control therapy—revised (handbook).* Allen, TX: DLM.

Cooper, E. B. (1993). Red herrings, dead horses, straw men, and blind alleys: Escaping the stuttering conundrum. *Journal of Fluency Disorders, 18,* 375–387.

Cooper, E. B., & Cooper, C. S. (1991a). A fluency disorders prevention program for preschoolers and children in the primary grades. *American Journal of Speech-Language Pathology, 1,* 28–31.

Cooper, E. B., & Cooper, C. S. (1991b). *Multicultural considerations in the assessment and treatment of fluency disorders.* Paper presented at the American Speech-Language-Hearing Association Annual Convention, Atlanta, GA.

Cooper, E. B., & Cooper, C. S. (1992). *Clinician attitudes toward stuttering: two decades of change.* Paper presented to the annual meeting of the American Speech-Language-Hearing Association, San Antonio, TX.

Coriat, I. H. (1943). Psychoanalytic concept of stammering. *Nervous Child, 2,* 167–171.

Costello, J. M. (1983). Current behavioral treatment of children. In D. Prins & R. J. Ingham (Eds.), *Treatment of stuttering in early childhood: Methods and issues* (pp. 69–112). San Diego, CA: College-Hill Press.

Cousins, N. (1979). *Anatomy of an illness.* New York: Norton.

Covey, S. (1989). *The seven habits of highly effective people.* New York: Simon & Schuster.

Cox, J. J., Seider, R. A., & Kidd, K. K. (1984). Some environmental factors and hypotheses for stuttering in families with several stutterers. *Journal of Speech and Hearing Research, 27,* 543–548.

Craig, A., & Andrews, G. (1985). The prediction and prevention of relapse in stuttering. The value of self-control techniques and locus of control measures. *Behavior Modification, 9,* 427–442.

Craig, A., Franklin, J., & Andrews, G. (1984). A scale to measure locus of control of behavior. *British Journal of Medical Psychology, 57,* 173–180.

Cross, D. E., & Luper, H. L. (1983). Relation between finger reaction time and voice reaction time in stuttering and nonstuttering children and adults. *Journal of Speech and Hearing Research, 26,* 356–361.

Cross, D. E., Shadden, B. B., and Luper, H. L. (1979). Effects of stimulus ear presentation on the voice reaction time of adult stutterers and non-stutterers. *Journal of Fluency Disorders, 4,* 45-58.

Crowe, T. A., & Cooper, E. B. (1977). Clinician attitudes toward and knowledge of stuttering. *Journal of Communication Disorders, 10,* 343–357.

Crystal, D. (1987). Towards a "bucket" theory of language disability: Taking account of interaction between linguistic levels. *Clinical Linguistics and Phonetics, 1,* 7–22.

Culatta, R., & Goldberg. S. A. (1995). *Stuttering therapy: An integrated approach to theory and practice.* Boston: Allyn & Bacon.

Curlee, R. (1984). Counseling with adults who stutter. In W. Perkins (Ed.) *Stuttering Disorders.* New York: Thieme-Stratton.

Curlee, R. (1985). Training students to work with stutterers. In E. Boberg (Ed.), *Stuttering: Part one. Seminars in speech and language* 6(2), 131–144. New York: Thieme-Stratton.

Curry, F., & Gregory, H. (1969). The performance of stutterers on dichotic listening tasks thought to reflect cerebral dominance. *Journal of Speech and Hearing Research, 12,* 73–81.

Daly, D. A. (1981). Differentiation of stuttering subgroups with Van Riper's developmental tracks: A preliminary study. *Journal of the American Student Speech and Hearing Association.*

Daly, D. A. (1986). The clutterer. In Kenneth O. St. Louis (Ed.), *The atypical stutterer,* 155–192. Orlando, FL: Academic Press.

Daly, D. (1987). Use of the home VCR to facilitate transfer of fluency. *Journal of Fluency Disorders* 12, 103–106.

Daly, D. A. (1988). *Freedom of fluency.* Tucson, AZ: LingaSystems.

Daly, D. A. (1992). Helping the clutterer: Therapy considerations. In F. Myers & K. St. Louis (Eds.), *Cluttering: A clinical perspective,* 27–41. San Diego, CA: Singular Publishing Group, Inc.

Daly, D. A. (1993). Cluttering: Another fluency syndrome. In R. Curlee (Ed.), *Stuttering and related disorders of fluency,* 151–175. New York: Thieme Medical Publishers.

Daly, D. A. (1994). Practical techniques that work with children and adolescents who stutter. Paper presented to the annual meeting of the American Speech-Language-Hearing Association, New Orleans.

Daly, D. A., & Kimbarow, M. L. (1978). Stuttering as operant behavior: Effects of the verbal stimuli wrong, right, and tree on the disfluency rates of school-age stutterers and nonstutterers. *Journal of Speech and Hearing Research, 21,* 589–597.

Daly, D., Simon, C., & Burnett-Stolnack, M. (1995). Helping adolescents who stutter focus on fluency. *Language, Speech, and Hearing Services in Schools, 26,* 162–168.

Davis, J. M., & Farina, A. (1970). Appreciation of humor: An experimental and theoretical study. *Journal of Personality and Social Psychology, 15*(2), 175–178.

DeBuck, A. (1970). *Egyptian readingbook, exercises and Middle Egyptian tests.* Leiden, Holland: Nederlands Instituut Voor Nabije Oosten.

Dell, C. (1970). *Treating the school age stutterer: A guide for clinicians* (Publication No. 14). Memphis, TN: Speech Foundation of America.

deNil, L. F., & Brutten, G. J. (1991). Speech-associated attitudes of stuttering and nonstuttering children. *Journal of Speech and Hearing Research, 34,* 60–66.

deNil, L. F., & Kroll, R., M. (1995). The relationship between locus of control and long-term stuttering treatment outcome in adult stutterers. *Journal of Fluency Disorders, 20,* 345–364. Copyright © Elsevier Science Publishing Co. Reprinted with permission.

DeVore, J., Nandur, M., & Manning, W. (1984). Projective drawings and children who stutter. *Journal of Fluency Disorders, 9,* 217–226.

Dewar, A., Dewar, A. D., & Anthony, J. F. K. (1976). The effect of auditory feedback masking on concomitants of stammering. *British Journal of Disorders of Communication, 11,* 95–102.

DiClemente, C. C. (1993). Changing addictive behaviors: A process perspective. *Current Directions in Psychological Science 2* (4), 101–106.

Doopdy, I., Kalinowski, J., Armson, J. (1993) Stereotypes of stutterers and nonstutterers in three rural communities in Newfoundland. *Journal of Fluency Disorders, 18,* 363–373.

Douglass, E., & Quarrington, B. (1952). The differentiation of interiorized and exteriorized secondary stuttering. *Journal of Speech and Hearing Disorders, 17,* 377–385.

Dunlap, K. (1917). The stuttering boy. *Journal of Abnormal Psychology, 12,* 44–48.

Dunlap, K. (1932). *Habits: Their making and unmaking.* New York: Liveright.

Dykes, R., & Pindzola, R. (1995). Racial/ethnic differences in the prevalence of school-aged stutterers. Paper presented to the annual meeting of the American Speech-Language-Hearing Association, Orlando.

Egan, G. (1990). *The skilled helper: A systematic approach to effective helping* (4th ed.), Pacific Grove, CA: Brooks/Cole Publishing Co.

Eisenson, J., & Ogilvie, M. (1963). *Speech correction in the schools* (2nd ed.) New York: Macmillan.

Ellis, A. (1977). The basic clinical theory of rational-emotive therapy. In A. Ellis & R. Grieger (Eds.), *Handbook of rational-emotive therapy,* 218–250. New York: Springer.

Emerick, L. (1988). Counseling adults who stutter: A cognitive approach. *Seminars in Speech and Language* (Thieme Medical Publishers), 9(3), 257–267.

Erickson, R. L. (1969). Assessing communication attitudes among stutterers. *Journal of Speech and Hearing Research, 12,* 711–724.

Fairbanks, G. (1954). Systematic research in experimental phonetics–I. A. A theory of the speech mechanism as a servomechanism. *Journal of Speech and Hearing Disorders, 19,* 133–139.

Fant, G. (1960). *The acoustic theory of speech production.* The Hague, Holland: Mouton.

Farrelly, F., & Brandsma, J. (1974). *Provocative therapy*. Cupertino, CA: Meta Publications.

Faulkner, R. O. (1962). *A concise dictionary of Middle Egyptian*. Oxford, England: University Press.

Fenichel, O. (1945). *The psychoanalytic theory of neurosis*. New York: Norton.

Filmore, C. J. (1979). On fluency. In *Individual differences in language ability and language behavior*. New York: Academic Press.

Fisher, R., & Ury, W. (1981). *Getting to yes: Negotiating agreement without giving in*. Boston: Houghton Mifflin.

Fowler, C. (1978). Timing control in speech production. *Dissertation Abstracts International*, *38*, 3927–3928.

Fransella, F. (1972). *Personal change and reconstruction*. New York: Academic Press.

Freund, H. (1966). *Psychopathology and the problems of stuttering*. Springfield, IL: Charles C. Thomas.

Freud, S. (1905/1961). Jokes and their relation to the unconscious. In James Strachey (Ed.), *The complete psychological works of Sigmund Freud* (vol. 8), London: Hogarth Press.

Freud, S. (1928). Humor. *International Journal of Psychoanalysis*, *9*, 1–6.

Gaines, N., Runyan, C., & Meyers, S. (1991). A comparison of young stutterers' fluent versus stuttered utterances on measures of length and complexity. *Journal of Speech and Hearing Research*, *34*, 37–42.

Gay, T. (1978). Effect of speaking rate on vowel formant movements. *Journal of the Acoustical Society of America*, *63*, 223–230.

Gay, T., & Hirose, H. (1973). Effect of speaking rate on labial consonant production: a combined electromyographic high-speech motion picture study. *Phonetrica*, *27*, 203–213.

Gay, T., Ushijima, T., Hirose, H., & Cooper, F. S. (1974). Effect of speaking rate on labial consonant-vowel articulation. *Journal of Phonetics*, *2*, 47–63.

Geschwind, N., & Galaburda, A. M. (1985). Cerebral lateralization: Biological mechanisms, associations, and pathology: I. A hypothesis and a program for research. *Archives of Neurology*, *42*, 429–459.

Gildston, P. (1967). Stutterers' self-acceptance and perceived self-acceptance. *Journal of Abnormal and Social Psychology*, *72*, 59–64.

Gillespie, S. K., & Cooper, E. G. (1973). Prevalence of speech problems in junior and senior high schools, *Journal of Speech and Hearing Research*, *16*, 739–743.

Glasner, P. J., & Rosenthal, D. (1957). Parental diagnosis of stuttering in young children. *Journal of Speech and Hearing Disorders*, *22*, 288–295.

Glauber, I. P. (1958). The psychoanalysis of stuttering. In Jon Eisenson (Ed.), *Stuttering: A symposium* (pp. 71–119). New York: Harper & Brothers.

Glauber, I. P. (1982). *Stuttering: A psychoanalytic understanding*. New York: Human Sciences Press.

Goebel, M. (1989). *CAFET-for-kids*. Annandale, VA: Annandale Fluency Clinic.

Goldman-Eisler, F. (1958). The predictability of words in context and the length of pauses in speech. *Language and Speech, 1,* 226–231.

Goldman-Eisler, F. (1961). The continuity of speech utterance: Its determinants and its significance. *Language and Speech, 4,* 220–231.

Goldstein, J. H. (1976). Theoretical notes on humor. *Journal of Communication, 26,* 104–112.

Goleman, D. (1985). Switching therapists may be best. *Indianapolis News,* p. 9.

Goodstein, L. D. (1958). Functional speech disorders and personality: A survey of the research. *Journal of Speech and Hearing Research, 1,* 359–376.

Gordon, K. C., Hutchinson, J. M., & Allen, C. S. (1976). An evaluation of selected discourse characteristics in normal geriatric subjects. *Idaho State University Laboratory Research Reports, 1,* 11-21.

Gordon, P. (1991). Language task effects: A comparison of stuttering and non-stuttering children. *Journal of Fluency Disorders, 16,* 275–287.

Gordon, P., Luper, H., & Peterson, H. J. (1986). The effects of syntactic complexity on the occurrence of disfluencies in 5 year old nonstutterers. *Journal of Fluency Disorders, 11,* 151–164.

Gottwald, S. R., & Starkweather, C. W. (1995). Fluency intervention for preschoolers and their families in the public schools. *Language, Speech, and Hearing Services in Schools, 26,* 117–126.

Gregory, H. H. (1983a). *The clinician's attitudes in counseling stutterers* (Publication No. 18). Memphis, TN: Stuttering Foundation of America.

Gregory, H. H. (1989). *Stuttering therapy: A workshop for specialists.* Unpublished manuscript, Northwestern University and the Stuttering Foundation of American, Evanston, IL.

Gregory, H. H. (1991). Therapy for elementary school-age children. *Seminars in Speech and Language, 12,* 323–335.

Gregory, H. H. (1995). Analysis and commentary. *Language, Speech, and Hearing Services in Schools, 26*(2), 196–200.

Gregory, H. H., & Hill, D. (1980). Stuttering therapy for children. In W. Perkins (Ed.), *Stuttering Disorders,* 351–363. New York: Thieme-Stratton.

Gregory, H. H. (1972). An assessment of the results of stuttering therapy. *Journal of Communication Disorders, 5,* 320–334.

Gregory, H. H. (1979). Controversial issues: Statement and review of the literature. In H. H. Gregory (Ed.), *Controversies about stuttering therapy,* 1–62. Baltimore, MD: University Park Press.

Gregory, H. H. (1983b). Commentary. In J. Fraser Gruss (Ed.), *Stuttering therapy: Transfer and maintenance,* 99–107. Memphis, TN: Speech Foundation of America.

Gregory, H. H. (1984). Prevention of stuttering: Management of the early stages. In R. F. Curlee & W. H. Perkins (Eds.), *Nature and treatment of shuttering: New directions.* San Diego: College-Hill Press.

Guitar, B. (1976). Pretreatment factors associated with the outcome of stuttering therapy. *Journal of Speech and Hearing Research, 18,* 590–600.

Guitar, B., & Peters, T. J. (1980). *Stuttering: An integration of contemporary therapies* (Publication No. 16). Memphis, TN: Stuttering Foundation of America.

Guitar, B. E., & Bass, C. (1978). Stuttering therapy: The relation between attitude change and long-term outcome. *Journal of Speech and Hearing Disorders, 43,* 392–499.

Haefner, R. (1929). *The educational significance of left-handedness.* New York: Teachers College, Columbia University Press.

Hall, J. W., & Jerger, J. (1978). Central auditory function in stutterers. *Journal of Speech and Hearing Research, 21,* 324–337.

Hall, K. D., & Yairi, E. (1992). Fundamental frequency, jitter, and shimmer in preschoolers who stutter. *Journal of Speech and Hearing Research, 35,* 1002–1008.

Hall, P. K. (1977). The occurrence of disfluencies in language-disordered school-age children. *Journal of Speech and Hearing Disorders, 42,* 364–369.

Ham, R. (1986). *Techniques of stuttering therapy.* Englewood Cliffs, NJ: Prentice-Hall.

Ham, R. E. (1990). *Therapy of stuttering, preschool through adolescence.* Englewood Cliffs, NJ: Prentice-Hall.

Ham, R. E. (1992). I know the chapter, but what's the verse? *Journal of Fluency Disorders, 17,* 39–41.

Ham, R. E. (1993). Chronic perseverative stuttering syndrome: constructive or casuistic? *American Journal of Speech-Language Pathology, 2*(3), 16–20.

Hamre, C. (1992). Stuttering prevention I: Primacy of identification. *Journal of Fluency Disorders, 17,* 3–23.

Hanson, B. R., Gonhoud, K. D., & Rice, P. L. (1981). Speech situation checklist. *Journal of Fluency Disorders, 6,* 351–360.

Hastorf, A. H., Windfogel, J., & Cassman, T. (1979). Acknowledgement of handicap as a tactic in social interaction. *Journal of Personality and Social Psychology, 37,* 1790–1797.

Hayden, P. A., Scott, D. A., & Addicott, J. (1977). The effects of delayed auditory feedback on the overt behaviors of stutterers. *Journal of Fluency Disorders, 2,* 235–246.

Hayhow, R., & Levy, C. (1989). *Working with stuttering.* Bicester, Oxon, England: Winslow Press.

Healey, E. C. (1982). Speaking fundamental frequency characteristics of stutterers and nonstutterers. *Journal of Communications Disorders, 15,* 1, 21–29.

Healey, E. C., & Gutkin, B. (1984). Analysis of stutterers' voice onset times and fundamental frequency contours during fluency. *Journal of Speech and Hearing Research, 27,* 219–225.

Healey, E. C., & Scott, L. A. (1995). Strategies for treating elementary school-age children who stutter: An integrative approach. *Language, Speech, and Hearing Services in Schools, 26,* 151–161.

Heinze, B. A., & Johnson, K.L. (1985). *Easy does it–1: Fluency activities for young children.* East Moline, IL: LinguiSystems.

Heinze, B. A., & Johnson, K.L. (1987). *Easy does it–2: Fluency activities for school-aged stutterers.* East Moline, IL: LinguiSystems.

Helm, N. A., Yeo, R., Geschwind, M., Freedman, M., & Wenstein, C., (1986). Stuttering: Disappearance and reappearance with acquired brain lesions. *Neurology, 36,* 1109–1112.

Helm, N. A., Butler, R. B., & Canter, G. J. (1980). Neurogenic acquired stuttering. *Journal of Fluency Disorders, 5,* 269–279.

Helm-Estabrooks, N. (1986). Diagnosis and management of neurogenic stuttering in adults.In Kenneth O. St. Louis (Ed.), *The atypical stutterer,* 193–217. Orlando, FL: Academic Press.

Hillis, J. W. (1993). Ongoing assessment in the management of stuttering: A clinical perspective. *American Journal of Speech-Language Pathology, 2*(1), 24–37.

Hillman, R. E., & Gilbert, H. R. (1977). Voice onset time for voiceless stop consonants in the fluent reading of stutterers and nonstutterers. *Journal of the Acoustical Society of America, 61,* 610–611.

Howie, P., Woods, C., & Andrews, J. (1982). Relationship between covert and overt speech measures immediately before and immediately after stuttering treatment. *Journal of Speech and Hearing Disorders, 47,* 419–422.

Howie, P. M. (1981). Concordance for stuttering in monozygotic and dizygotic twin pairs. *Journal of Speech and Hearing Research, 24,* 317–321.

Howie, P. M., Tanner, S., & Andrews, G. (1981). Short and long term outcome in an intensive treatment program for adult stutterers. *Journal of Speech and Hearing Disorders, 46,* 104–109.

Hubbard, C. P., & Yairi, E. (1988). Clustering of disfluencies in the speech of stuttering and nonstuttering preschool children. *Journal of Speech and Hearing Research, 31,* 228–233.

Huggins, A. (1978). Speech timing and intelligibility. In J. Requin (Ed.), *Attention and performance VII,* 218–241. Hillsdale, NJ: Lawrence Erlbaum.

Hull, F., Mieke, P., Timmons, R., & Willeford, J. (1971). The National Speech and Hearing Survey: Preliminary Results, *ASHA, 13,* 501–509.

Hunt, B. (1987). Self-help for stutterers—Experience in Britain. In L. Rustin, H. Purser, K. D. Rowley (Eds.), *Progress in the treatment of fluency disorders,* 198–212. London: Taylor & Francis.

Hunt, H. (1861). *Stammering and stuttering, their nature and treatment.* Reprint, New York: Hafner Publishing Company, 1967.

Ingham, R. J. (1975). A comparison of covert and overt assessment procedures in stuttering therapy outcome evaluation. *Journal of Speech and Hearing Research, 16,* 246–254.

Ingham, R. J. (1980). *Stuttering therapy manual: Hierarchy control sched-*

ule. A clinician's guide. Sydney, Australia: Cumberland College of Health Sciences, School of Communication Disorders.

Ingham, R. J. (1982). The effects of self-evaluation and training and maintenance and generalization during stuttering treatment. *Journal of Speech and Hearing Disorders, 47,* 271–280.

Ingham, R. J. (1984). *Stuttering and behavior therapy: Current status and experimental foundations*. San Diego, CA: College-Hill Press.

Ingham, R. J. (1990). Commentary on Perkins (1990) and Moore and Perkins (1990): On the valid role of reliability in identifying "What is stuttering." *Journal of Speech and Hearing Disorders, 55,* 394–397.

Ingham, R. J., Andrews, G., & Winkler, R. (1972). Stuttering: A comparative evaluation of the short term effectiveness of four treatment techniques. *Journal of Communication Disorders, 5,* 91–117.

Ingham, R. J., Gow, M., and Costello, J. M. (1985). Stuttering and speech naturalness: Some additional data. *Journal of Speech and Hearing Disorders, 50,* 217–219.

Ingham, R. J., Ingham, J. C., Onslow, M., & Finn, P. (1989). Stutterers' self-ratings of speech naturalness: Assessing effects and reliability. *Journal of Speech and Hearing Research, 32,* 419–431.

Ingham, R. J., Martin, R. R., Haroldson, S. K., Onslow, M., & Leney, M. (1985). Modification of listener-judged naturalness in the speech of stutterers. *Journal of Speech and Hearing Research, 28,* 495–504.

Ingham, R. J., & Onslow, M. (1985). Measurement and modification of speech naturalness during stuttering therapy. *Journal of Speech and Hearing Disorders, 50,* 261–181.

Ingham, R. J., & Packman, A. C. (1978). Perceptual assessment of normalcy of speech following stuttering therapy. *Journal of Speech and Hearing Research, 21,* 63–73.

Ivy, A. E. (1983). *Intentional interviewing and counseling*. Pacific Grove, CA: Brooks/Cole.

Jacobs, M. K., & Goodman, G. (1989). Psychology and self-help groups: Prediction on a partnership. *American Psychologist, 44,* 536–545.

Johnson, W. (1930). *Because I stutter*. New York: Appleton-Century-Crofts.

Johnson, W. (1946). *People in quandaries*. New York: Harper Brothers.

Johnson, W. (1956). *Speech handicapped school children*. New York: Harper & Row.

Johnson, W. (1961). Measurement of oral reading and speaking rate and disfluency of adult male and female stutterers and nonstutterers. *Journal of Speech and Hearing Disorders* (Monograph Supplement 7), 1–20.

Johnson, W. (1962). *An open letter to the mother of a "stuttering" child*. Danville, IL: Interstate Printers and Publishers.

Johnson, W., & Associates. (1959). *The Onset of stuttering*. Minneapolis: University of Minnesota Press.

Johnson, W., Darley, F. L., & Spriestersbach, D. C. (1963). *Diagnostic meth-*

ods in speech pathology. New York: Harper & Row.

Johnson, W., & Leutenegger, R. R. (Eds.) (1955). *Stuttering in children and adults*. Minneapolis: University of Minnesota Press.

Jones, R. (1966). Observations on stammering after localized cerebral injury. *Journal of Neurology, Neurosurgery, and Psychiatry, 29,* 192–195.

Kalinowski, J., Nobel, S., Armson, J., & Stuart, A. (1994). Pretreatment and posttreatment speech naturalness ratings of adults with mild and severe stuttering. *American Journal of Speech-Language Pathology, 3*(2), 61–66.

Kamhi, A. G. (1982). The problem of relapse in stuttering: Some thoughts on what might cause it and how to deal with it. *Journal of Fluency Disorders, 7,* 459–467.

Kanfer, F. H. (1975). Self-management methods. In F. H. Kanfer & A. P. Goldstein (Eds.), *Helping people change,* 416–431. New York: Pergamon Press.

Kanfer, F. H., & Schefft, B. K. (1988). *Guiding therapeutic change*. Champaign, IL: Research Press.

Katz, A. H., & Bender, E. (1976). *The strength in us: Self-help groups in the modern world*. New York: Franklin Watts.

Kelly, E. M. (1994). Speech rates and turn-taking behaviors of children who stutter and their fathers. *Journal of Speech and Hearing Research, 37,* 1284–1294.

Kent, R. D. (1983). Facts about stuttering: Neurologic perspectives. *Journal of Speech and Hearing Disorders, 48,* 249–255.

Kent, R. D., & Read, C. (1992). *The acoustic analysis of speech*. San Diego, CA: Singular Publishing Group.

Kidd, K. K. (1977). A genetic perspective on stuttering. *Journal of Fluency Disorders, 2,* 259–269.

Kidd, K. K., Kidd, J. R., & Records, M. A. (1978). The possible causes of the sex ratio in stuttering and its implications. *Journal of Fluency Disorders, 3,* 13–23.

Kidd, K. K., Reich, T., & Kessler, S. (1973). *Genetics, 74* (Part 2), s137.

Kimmel, D. C. (1974). *Adulthood and aging*. New York: John Wiley & Sons.

Kirby, G., Delgadillo, J., Hillard, S., & Manning, W. (1992). *Visual imagery, relaxation, and cognitive restructuring integrated in fluency therapy*. Paper presented to the annual meeting of the American Speech-Language-Hearing Association, San Antonio.

Klich, R. J., & May, G. M. (1982). Spectrographic study of vowels in stutterers' fluent speech. *Journal of Speech and Hearing Research, 25*(3), 364–370.

Kline, M., & Starkweather, C. (1979). *Receptive and expressive language performance in young stutterers*. ASHA, 21, 797. Abstract.

Koszybski, A. (1941). *Science and sanity: An introduction to non-Aristotelian systems and general semantics* (2nd Ed.). New York: Int. Non-Aristotelian Library Publishing Co.

Kozhevnikov, V. A., & Chistovich, L. A. (1965). *Speech: Articulation and perception* (Joint Publications Research Service, 30, 543). Washington, DC: United States Department of Commerce.

Kramer, M. B., Green, D., & Guitar, B. (1987). A comparison of stutterers and nonstutterers on masking level differences and synthetic sentence identification tasks. *Journal of Communication Disorders*, 20, 379–390.

Krass-Lehrman, T., & Reeves, L. (1989). Attitudes toward speech-language pathology and support groups: Results of a survey of members of the National Stuttering Project. *Texas Journal of Audiology and Speech Pathology*, 15(1), 22–25.

Kubie, L. S. (1971). The destructive potential of humor on psychotherapy. *American Journal of Psychiatry*, 127, 861–866.

Kuhlman, T. (1984). *Humor and psychotherapy*. Homewood, IL. Dow: Jones-Irwin.

Kuhr, A., & Rustin, L. (1985). The maintenance of fluency after intensive inpatient therapy: Long-term follow-up. *Journal of Fluency Disorders*, 10, 229–236.

Ladouceur, R., Caron, C., & Caron, G. (1989). Stuttering severity and treatment outcome. *Journal of Behavior Therapy and Experimental Psychiatry*, 20, 49–56.

LaSalle, L. R., & Conture, E. G. (1991). Eye contact between young stutterers and their mothers. *Journal of Fluency Disorders*, 16(4), 173–199.

LaSalle, L. R., & Conture, E. G. (1995). Disfluency clusters of children who stutter: Relation of stutterings to self-repairs. *Journal of Speech and Hearing Research* 38, 5, 965–977.

Lass, N., Ruscello, D., Pannbaker, M., Schmitt, J., & Everly-Myers, D. (1989). Speech-language pathologists' perceptions of child and adult female and male stutterers. *Journal of Fluency Disorders*, 14, 127–134.

Lass, N. J., Ruscello, D. M., Schmitt, J. F., Pannbacker, M. D., Orlando, M. B., Dean, K. A., Ruziska, J. C., & Bradshaw, K. H. (1992). Teachers' perceptions of stutterers. *Language, Speech and Hearing Services in Schools*, 23, 78–81.

Lee, B. S. (1951). Artificial stutter. *Journal of Speech and Hearing Disorders*, 16, 53–55.

Lefcourt, H., & Martin, R. (1989). *Humor and life stress: Antidote to Adversity*. New York: Springer-Verlag.

Lefcourt, H., Sordoni, C., & Sordoni C. (1974). Locus of control and the expression of humor. *Journal of Personality*, 42, 130–143.

Lefcourt, H. M. (1976). *Locus of control: Current trends in theory and research*. Hillsdale, NJ: Erlbaum.

Lemert, E. M. (1953). Some indians who stutter. *Journal of Speech and Hearing Disorders*, 18, 168–174.

Lemert, E. M. (1962). Stuttering and social structure in two Pacific societies. *Journal of Speech and Hearing Disorders*, 27, 3–10.

Levine, J. (1977). Humour as a form of therapy. In A. J. Chapman & H. C. Foot (Eds.), *It's a funny thing, humour*. (127–137) Oxford, England: Pergamon.

Levy, C. (1983). Group therapy with adults. In P. Dalton (Ed.), *Approaches to the treatment of stuttering*, 150–171. London and Canberra, Australia: Croom Helm.

Lichtheim, M. (1973). *Ancient Egyptian literature, a book of readings: Volume 1. The Old and Middle Kingdoms*. Berkeley: University of California Press.

Lindaman, E. B., & Lippitt, R. O. (1979). *Choosing the future you prefer: Goal setting guide*. Washington, DC: Development Publications.

Loban, W. (1976). *Language development: Kindergarten through grade twelve*. Urbana, IL: National Council of Teachers of English.

Longhurst, T. M., & Siegel, G. M. (1973). Effects of communication failure on speaker-listener behaviors. *Journal of Speech and Hearing Disorders, 16*, 128–140.

Louko, L., Edwards, M. E., & Conture, E. (1990). Phonological characteristics of young stutterers and their normally fluent peers: Preliminary observations. *Journal of Fluency Disorders, 15*, 191–210.

Love, L. R., & Jefress, L. A. (1971). Identification of brief pauses in the fluent speech of stutterers and nonstutterers. *Journal of Speech and Hearing Research, 14*, 229–240.

Luchsinger, R., & Arnold, G. E. (1965). *Voice-speech-language clinical communicology: Its physiology and pathology*. Belmont, CA: Wadsworth.

Luper, Harold L., & Mulder, R. L. (1964). *Stuttering therapy for children*, Englewood Cliffs. NJ: Prentice-Hall.

Luterman, D. (1979). *Counseling parents of hearing impaired children*. Boston: Little, Brown, & Co.

Luterman, D. M. (1991). *Counseling the communicatively disordered and their families* (2nd ed.). Austin, TX: Pro-Ed. Reprinted with permission.

Madison, L. S., Budd, K. S., & Itzkowitz, J. S. (1986). Changes in stuttering in relation to children's locus of control. *Journal of Genetic Psychology, 147*, 233–240.

Malecot, A., Johnston, R., & Kizziar, P. A. (1972). Syllabic rate and utterance length in French. *Phonetica, 26*, 235–251.

Mallard, A. R., Gardner, L., & Downey, C. (1988). Clinical training in stuttering for school clinicians. *Journal of Fluency Disorders, 13*, 253–259.

Manders, E., & Bastijns, P. (1988). Sudden recovery from stuttering after an epileptic attack: A case report. *Journal of Fluency Disorders, 13*, 421–425.

Manning, W. (1977). In pursuit of fluency. *Journal of Fluency Disorders, 2*, 53–56.

Manning, W. H. (1991). Making progress during and after treatment. W. H. Perkins (Ed.). In *Seminars in speech and language*, (12:349–354). New York: Thieme Medical Publishers.

Manning, W. H. (1994). The SEA-Scale: Self-efficacy scaling for adolescents who stutter. Paper presented to the annual meeting of the American Speech-Language-Hearing Association, New Orleans.

Manning, W. H., & Beachy, T. S. (1994). *Humor as a variable in the treatment of fluency disorders*. Paper presented to the First World Congress on Fluency Disorders, Munich, Germany.

Manning, W., & Cooper, E. B. (1969). Variations in attitudes of the adult stutterer toward his clinician related to progress in therapy. *Journal of Communication Disorders, 2*, 154–162.

Manning, W., Dailey, D., & Wallace, S. (1984). Attitude and personality characteristics of older stutterers. *Journal of Fluency Disorders, 9*, 207–215.

Manning, W., & Monte, K. (1981). Fluency breaks in older speakers: Implications for a model of stuttering throughout the life cycle. *Journal of Fluency Disorders, 6*, 35–48.

Manning, W., Perkins, D., Winn, S., & Cole, D. (1984). *Self-efficacy changes during treatment and maintenance for adult stutterers*. Paper presented to the annual meeting of the American Speech-Language-Hearing Association, San Francisco.

Manning, W., & Shirkey, E. (1981). Fluency and the aging process. In D. S. Beasley and G. A. Davis (Eds.), *Aging: Communication Processes and Disorders* (175–189). New York: Grune & Stratton.

Manning W., & Shrum, W. (1973). The concept of control in stuttering therapy: A reappraisal. *Division for Children with Communication Disorders Bulletin, 9*(1), 32–34.

Market, K. E., Montague, J. C., Buffalo, M. D., & Drummond, S. S. (1990). Acquired stuttering: Descriptive data and treatment outcome. *Journal of Fluency Disorders, 15*, 21–34.

Martin, R., & Haroldson S. (1986). Stuttering as involuntary loss of speech control: Barking up a new tree. *Journal of Speech and Hearing Disorders, 51*, 187–190.

Martin, R., & Lefcourt, H. (1983). Sense of humor as a moderator of the relation between stressors and moods. *Journal of Personality and Social Psychology, 45*, 1313–1324.

Martin, R., & Lefcourt, H. (1984). Situational humor response questionnaire: Quantitative measure of sense of humor. *Journal of Personality and Social Psychology, 47*, 145–155.

Martin, R., & Lindamood, L. P. (1986). Stuttering and spontaneous recovery; Implications for the speech-language pathologist. *Language, Speech, and Hearing Services in Schools, 17*, 207–218.

Martin, R. R. (1981). Introduction and perspective: Review of published research. In E. Boberg (Ed.) *Maintenance of fluency,* 1–30. New York: Elsevier.

Martin, R. R., & Haroldson, S. K. (1982). Contingent self-stimulation for stuttering. *Journal of Speech and Hearing Disorders, 47*, 407–413.

Martin, R. R., & Haroldson, S. K. (1992). Stuttering and speech naturalness: Audio and audiovisual judgements. *Journal of Speech and Hearing Research, 35*, 521–528.

Martin, R. R., Haroldson, S. K., & Triden, K. A. (1984). Stuttering and speech naturalness. *Journal of Speech and Hearing Disorders, 49*, 53–58.

Maslow, A. (1968). *Towards a Psychology of Being* (2nd ed.). Princeton, NJ: Van Nostrand.

Masterson, J., & Kamhi, A. (1992). Linguistic trade-offs in school-age children with and without language disorders. *Journal of Speech and Hearing Research*, 35, 1064–1075.

Matkin, N., Ringle, R., & Snope, T. (1983). Master report of surveys discrepancies. In N. Rees & T. Snope (Eds.), *Proceedings of the Conference on Undergraduate, Graduate and Continuing Education* (ASHA Reports No. 13). Rockville, MD: American Speech-Language-Hearing Association.

Maxwell, D. (1982). Cognitive and behavioral self-control strategies: Applications for the clinical management of adult stutterers. *Journal of Fluency Disorders*, 7, 403–432.

McCall, G. N. (1974). Spasmodic dysphonia and the stuttering block: Commonalities or possible connections. In L. M. Webster & L. C. Furst (Eds.), *Vocal tract dynamics and dysfluency* (pp. 124–151). New York: Speech & Hearing Institute.

McCarthy, P., Culpepper, N., & Lucks, L. (1986). Variability in counseling experience and training among ESB accredited programs. *ASHA*, 28, 49–53.

McDearmon, J. R. (1968). Primary stuttering at the onset of stuttering: A reexamination of data. *Journal of Speech and Hearing Research*, 11, 631–637.

McGhee, P. E., & Goldstein, J. H. (1977). *Handbook of humor research: Volume 1, Basic issues*. New York: Springer-Verlag.

McLelland, J. K., & Cooper, E. B. (1978). Fluency-related behaviors and attitudes of 178 young stutterers. *Journal of Fluency Disorders*, 3, 253–263.

Merits-Patterson, R., & Reed, C. (1981). Disfluencies in the speech of language delayed children. *Journal of Speech and Hearing Research*, 24, 55–58.

Metz, D. E., Schiavetti, N., & Sacco, P. R. (1990). Acoustic and psychophysical dimensions of the perceived speech naturalness of nonstutterers and posttreatment stutterers. *Journal of Speech and Hearing Disorders*, 55, 516–525.

Meyers, S., Ghatak, L., & Woodford, L. (1990). Case descriptions of nonfluency and loci: Initial and follow-up conversations with three preschool children. *Journal of Fluency Disorders*, 14, 383–398.

Meyers, S., Hall, N. E., & Aram, D. M. (1990). Fluency and language recovery in a child with a left hemisphere lesion. *Journal of Fluency Disorders*, 15, 159–173.

Meyers, S., & Woodford, L. (1992). *The fluency development system for young children*. Buffalo, NY: United Educational Services.

Meyers, S. C., & Freeman, F. J. (1985). Mother and child speech rates as a variable in stuttering and disfluency. *Journal of Speech and Hearing Research*, 28, 436–444.

Moore, S. E., & Perkins, W. (1990). Validity and reliability of judgements of authentic and simulated stuttering. *Journal of Speech and Hearing Disorders*, 55, 383–391.

Moore, W. (1984). Hemispheric alpha asymmetries during an electromyographic biofeedback procedure for stuttering: A single-subject experimental design. *Journal of Fluency Disorders*, 9, 143–162.

Moore, W., & Haynes, W. (1980). Alpha hemispheric asymmetry and stuttering: Some support for a segmentation dysfunction hypothesis. *Journal of Speech and Hearing Research, 23,* 229–247.

Morgenstern, J. J. (1956). Socio-economic factors in stuttering. *Journal of Speech and Hearing Disorders, 21,* 25–33.

Morreall, J. (1982). *Taking laughter seriously.* Albany: State University of New York Press.

Murphy, A. T., & Fitzsimons, R. M. (1960). *Stuttering and personality dynamics.* New York: Ronald Press.

Murray, F. P., & Edwards, S. G. (1980). *A stutterer's story.* Danville, IL: Interstate Printers and Publishers.

Murray, H. L., & Reed, C. G. (1977). Language abilities of preschool stuttering children. *Journal of Fluency Disorders, 2,* 171–176.

Myers, F. L., & St. Louis, K. O. (1992). Cluttering: Issues and controversies. In F. L. Myers & K. O. St. Louis (Eds.), *Cluttering: A clinical perspective* (pp. 11–22). San Diego, CA: Singular Publishing Group, Inc.

Mysak, E. D. (1960). Servo theory and stuttering. *Journal of Speech and Hearing Disorders, 25,* 188–195.

Neaves, R. (1970). To establish a basis for prognosis in stammering. *British Journal of Disorders of Communication, 5,* 46–58.

Neeley, J. N. (1961). A study of the speech behavior of stutterers and non-stutterers under normal and delayed auditory feedback. *Journal of Speech and Hearing Disorders* (Monograph Supplement No. 7), 63–82.

Neilson, M., & Neilson, P. (1987). Speech motor control and stuttering: A computational model of adaptive sensory-motor processing. *Speech Communications, 6,* 325–333.

Newman, P. W., Harris, R. W., & Hilton, L. M. (1989). Vocal jitter and shimmer in stuttering. *Journal of Fluency Disorders, 14,* 87–95.

Nezu, A., Nezu, C., & Blissett, S. (1988). Sense of humor as a moderator of the relations between stressful events and psychological distress: A prospective analysis. *Journal of Personality and Social Psychology, 54,* 520–525.

Oates, D. (1929). Left-handedness in relation to speech defects, intelligence, and achievement. *Forum of Education, 7,* 91–105.

Ohman, S. (1965). Coarticulation in VCV utterances: Spectrographic measurements. *Journal of the Acoustical Society of America, 39,* 151–168.

Ojemann, R. (1931). Studies in sidedness: III. Relation of handedness to speech. *Journal of Educational Psychology, 22,* 120–126.

Onslow, M. (1992). Identification of early stuttering: Issues and suggested strategies. *American Journal of Speech-Language Pathology, 1*(4), 21–27.

Onslow, M., Adams, R., & Ingham, R. (1992). Reliability of speech naturalness ratings of stuttered speech during treatment. *Journal of Speech and Hearing Research, 35,* 994–1001.

Onslow, M., Hayes, B., Hutchins, L., & Newman, D. (1992). Speech naturalness and prolonged-speech treatments for stuttering: Further variables and data. *Journal of Speech and Hearing Research, 35,* 274–282.

Onslow, M., & Ingham, R. J. (1987). Speech quality measurement and the management of stuttering. *Journal of Speech and Hearing Disorders, 52,* 2–17.

Ornstein, A., & Manning, W. (1985). Self-efficacy scaling by adult stutterers. *Journal of Communication Disorders, 18,* 313–320.

Ost, L., Gotestam, K. G., & Melin, L. (1976). A controlled study of two behavioral methods in the treatment of stuttering. *Behavior Therapy, 7,* 587–592.

Otsuki, H. (1958). Study on stuttering: Statistical observations. *Otorhinolaryngology Clinic, 5,* 1150–1151.

Paden, E. P. (1970). *A History of the American Speech and Hearing Association 1925–1958.* Washington, DC: American Speech and Hearing Association.

Patterson, C. H. (1985). *The therapeutic relationship: Foundations for an eclectic psychotherapy.* Pacific Grove, CA: Brooks/Cole.

Patton, M. R., Montague, J. C., & Buffalo, M. D. (1996). A review of early data relating to the development of the Diagnosogenic theory of stuttering. *Journal of Fluency Disorders.* (In press.)

Pauls, D. L. (1990). A review of the evidence for genetic factors in stuttering ASHA Reports Series. *American Speech-Language-Hearing Association, 18,* 34–38.

Peck, M. S. (1978). *The road less travelled.* New York: Simon & Schuster.

Peins, M., McGough, W. E., & Lee, B. S. (1972). Evaluation of a tape-recorded method of stuttering therapy: Improvement in a speaking task. *Journal of Speech and Hearing Research, 15,* 364–371.

Perkins, W., Kent, R. D., & Curlee, R. F. (1990). A theory of neuropsycholinguistic function in stuttering. *Journal of Speech and Hearing Research, 34,* 734–752.

Perkins, W. H. (1973). Replacement of stuttering with normal speech: II. Clinical procedures. *Journal of Speech and Hearing Disorders, 38,* 295–303.

Perkins, W. H. (1979). From psychoanalysis to discoordination. In H. Gregory (Ed.), *Controversies about stuttering therapy,* 97–127. Baltimore, MD: University Park Press.

Perkins, W. H. (1983). The problem of definition: Commentary on stuttering. *Journal of Speech and Hearing Disorders, 48,* 246–249.

Perkins, W. H. (1990). What is stuttering? *Journal of Speech and Hearing Disorders, 55,* 370–382.

Peters, T. J., & Guitar, B. (1991). *Stuttering, an integrated approach to its nature and treatment.* Baltimore, MD: Williams & Wilkins.

Pickett, J. M. (1980). *The sounds of speech communication.* Baltimore, MD: University Park Press.

Pindzola, R. (1987). *Stuttering intervention program.* Austin, TX: Pro-Ed.

Postma, A., & Kolk, H. (1992). Error monitoring in people who stutter: Evidence against auditory feedback defect theories. *Journal of Speech and Hearing Research, 35,* 1024–1032.

Postma, A., & Kolk, H. (1993). The covert repair hypothesis: Prearticulatory repair processes in normal and stuttered disfluencies. *Journal of Speech and Hearing Research, 36,* 472–487.

Postma, A., Kolk, H. H. J., & Povel, D. J. (1990). Speech planning and execution in stutterers. *Journal of Fluency Disorders, 15,* 49–59.

Poulos, M. G., & Webster, W. G. (1991). Family history as a basis for subgrouping people who stutter. *Journal of Speech and Hearing Research, 34,* 5–10.

Preus, A. (1972). Stuttering in Down's syndrome. *Scandinavian Journal of Education Research 15,* 89–104.

Prins, D. (1970). Improvement and regression in stutterers following short-term intensive therapy. *Journal of Speech and Hearing Disorders, 35,* 123–135.

Prins, D., & Hubbard, C. (1988). Response contingent stimuli and stuttering: Issues and implications. *Journal of Speech and Hearing Research, 31,* 696–709.

Prochaska, J. O., DiClemente, C. C., & Norcross, J. C. (1992). In search of how people change: Applications to addictive behaviors. *American Psychologist, 47*(9), 1102–1114.

Quarrington, B., Seligman, J., & Kosower, E. (1969). Goal setting behavior of parents of beginning stutterers and parents of nonstuttering children. *Journal of Speech and Hearing Research, 12,* 435–42.

Ramig, P. R. (1993a). High reported spontaneous recovery rates: Fact or fiction? *Language, Speech, and Hearing in Schools, 24,* 156–160.

Ramig, P. R. (1993b). The impact of self-help groups on persons who stutter: A call for research, *Journal of Fluency Disorders, 18,* 351–361.

Ramig, P. R. (1993c). Parent-clinician-child partnership in the therapeutic process of the preschool and elementary-aged child who stutters. *Seminars in Speech and Language, 14,* 226–236.

Ramig, P., & Bennett, E. (1995). Working with 7- to 12-year-old children who stutter: Ideas for intervention in the public schools. *Language, Speech, and Hearing Services in Schools, 26,* 138–150.

Ratner, N. (1993). Parents, children, and stuttering. *Seminars in Speech and Language, 14*(3), 238–247.

Ratner, N., & Sih, C. (1987). The effects of gradual increases in sentence length and complexity on children's dysfluency. *Journal of Speech and Hearing Disorders, 52,* 278–287.

Ratner, N. B. (1995). Treating the child who stutters with concomitant language or phonological impairment. *Language, Speech, and Hearing in Schools, 26,* 180–186.

Reich, A., Till, J. A., & Goldsmith, H. (1981). Laryngeal and manual reaction times of stuttering and nonstuttering adults. *Journal of Speech and Hearing Research, 24,* (2), 192-196.

Riley, G. (1981). *Stuttering prediction instrument for young children* (rev. ed.) Austin, TX: Pro-Ed.

Riley, G., & Riley, J. (1979). A component model for diagnosing and treating children who stutter. *Journal of Fluency Disorders*, *4*, 279–293.

Riley, G., & Riley, J. (1983). Evaluation as a basis for intervention. In D. Peins & R. Ingham (Eds.), *Treatment of stuttering in early childhood*, 128–152. San Diego, CA: College-Hill.

Riley, G., & Riley, J. (1984). A component model for treating stuttering in children. In M. Prins (Ed.), *Contemporary approaches in stuttering therapy*. Boston: Little, Brown.

Riley, G., & Riley, J. (1986). *Oral motor assessment and treatment*. Tigard, OR: C.C. Publications.

Riley, G. D. (1972). A stuttering severity instrument for children and adults. *Journal of Speech and Hearing Disorders*, *37*, 314–321.

Robinson, V. M. (1991). *Humor and the health professions*. Throrfare, NJ: Slack.

Rogers, C. R. (1951). *Client-centered therapy*. Boston: Houghton Mifflin.

Rogers, C. R. (1961). *On becoming a person*. Boston: Houghton Mifflin.

Rogers, C. R. (Ed.). (1967). *The therapeutic relationship and its impact*. Madison: University of Wisconsin Press.

Rogers, C. R. (1980). *A way of being*. Boston: Houghton Mifflin.

Rogers, C. R. (1986). Rogers, Kohut, and Erickson. *Person-Centered Review*, *1*, 125–140.

Rosenbek, J., Messert, B., Collins, M., & Wertz, T. (1978). Stuttering following brain damage. *Brain and Language*, *6*, 82–86.

Rosenheim, E. (1974). Humor in psychotherapy: An interactive experience. *American Journal of Psychotherapy*, *28*, 584–591.

Roth, C. R., Aronson, A. E., & Davis, L. J., Jr. (1989). Clinical studies in psychogenic stuttering of adult onset. *Journal of Speech and Hearing Disorders*, *54*, 634–646.

Rousey, C. G., Arjunan, K. N., & Rousey, C. L. (1986). Successful treatment of stuttering following closed head injury. *Journal of Fluency Disorders*, *11*, 257–261.

Rubin, H. (1986). Postscript: Cognitive therapy. In G. H. Shames & H. Rubin (Eds.), *Stuttering then and now*, 474–486. Columbus, OH: Merrill.

Rubin, H., & Culatta, R. (1971). A point of view about fluency. *ASHA*, *13*, 93–116.

Rudolf, S. R., Manning, W. H., & Sewell, W. R. (1983). The use of self-efficacy scaling in training student clinicians: Implications for working with stutterers. *Journal of Fluency Disorders*, *8*, 55–75.

Runyan, C. M., & Adams, M.R. (1978). Perceptual study of the speech of "successfully therapeutized stutterers." *Journal of Fluency Disorders*, *3*, 25–29.

Runyan, C. M., Bell, J. N., & Prosek, R.A. (1990). Speech naturalness ratings of treated stutterers. *Journal of Speech and Hearing Disorders*, *55*, 434–438.

Runyan, C. M., Hames, P. E., & Proseck, R. A. (1982). A perceptual comparison between paired stimulus and single stimulus methods of presentation of the fluent utterances of stutterers. *Journal of Fluency Disorders*, *7*, 71–77.

Runyan C. M., & Runyan, S. E. (1986). A fluency rules therapy program for young children in the public schools. *Language, Speech, and Hearing Services in Schools, 17,* 276–284.

Rusk, T. (1989). *So you want to change: Helping people help themselves.* Presentation given at the Twelfth Annual Conference for Trainers, Consultants, and other HRD Professionals, sponsored by University Associates (San Diego), San Francisco.

Rustin, L. (1987). The treatment of childhood dysfluency through active parental involvement. In L. Rustin, H. Purser, & H. Rowley (Eds.), *Progress in the treatment of fluency disorders* (pp. 166–180). London: Taylor & Francis.

Rustin, L., & Cook, F. (1995). Parental involvement in the treatment of stuttering. *Language, Speech, and Hearing Services in Schools, 26,* 127–137.

Ryan, B. (1979). Stuttering therapy in a framework of operant conditioning and programmed learning. In H. Gregory (Ed.), *Controversies about stuttering therapy* (pp. 129–174). Baltimore, MD: University Park Press.

Ryan, B. (1980). *Programmed therapy for stuttering children and adults* (3rd ed.), Springfield, IL: Charles C. Thomas.

Ryan, B., & Van Kirk, B. (1974). The establishment, transfer, and maintenance of fluent speech in 50 stutterers using delayed auditory feedback and operant procedures. *Journal of Speech and Hearing Disorders, 39,* 3–10.

Sacco, P. R., Metz, D. E., & Schiavetti, N. (1992). *Speech naturalness of nonstutterers and treated stutterers: Acoustical correlates.* Paper presented to the annual meeting of the American Speech-Language-Hearing Association, San Antonio, TX.

Salamy, J. N., & Sessions, R. B. (1980). Spastic dysphonia. *Journal of Fluency Disorders, 5,* 281–290.

Satcher, D. (1986). Research needs for minority populations. In F. H. Bess, B. S. Clark, & H. R. Mitchel (Eds.), *Concerns for Minority Groups in Communication Disorders,* 89–92. (ASHA Reports, No. 16, ISSN 0569–8553). Rockville, MD: American Speech-Language-Hearing Association.

Schaeffer, M. L., & Shearer, W. M. (1968). A survey of mentally retarded stutterers. *Mental Retardation, 6,* 44–45.

Schiff, J. L. (1975). *Cathexis reader: Transactional analysis treatment of psychosis.* New York: Harper & Row.

Schimel, J. (1978). The function of wit and humor in psychoanalysis. *Journal of the American Academy of Psychoanalysis, 6*(3), 369–379.

Schwartz, H., & Conture, E. (1988). Subgroupings of young stutterers: Preliminary behavioral observations. *Journal of Speech and Hearing Research, 31,* 62–71.

Schwartz, H. D., Zebrowski, P. M., & Conture, E. G. (1990). Behaviors at the outset of stuttering. *Journal of Fluency Disorders, 15,* 77–86.

Scripture, E. W. (1931). *Stuttering, lisping, and correction of the speech of the deaf.* New York: Macmillan.

Shames, G. H., & Florance, C. L. (1980). *Stutter free speech: A goal for therapy.* Columbus, OH: Merrill.

Sheehan, J. (1958). Projective studies of stuttering. *Journal of Speech and Hearing Disorders, 23,* 18–25.

Sheehan, J. (1970). *Stuttering: Research and therapy.* New York: Harper & Row.

Sheehan, J. (1975). Conflict theory and avoidance-reduction therapy. In J. Eisenson (Ed.), *Stuttering, a second symposium,* 97–198. New York: Harper & Row.

Sheehan, J., & Martyn, M. (1966). Spontaneous recovery from stuttering. *Journal of Speech and Hearing Research, 9,* 121–135.

Sheehan, J. G. (1980). Problems in the evaluation of progress and outcome. In W. H. Perkins (Ed.), *Seminars in speech, language and hearing,* 389–401. New York: Thieme-Stratton.

Sheehan, J. G., & Costley, M. S. (1977). A reexamination of the role of heredity in stuttering. *Journal of Speech and Hearing Disorders, 42,* 47–59.

Sheehy, G. (1974). *Passages: Predictable crises of adult life.* New York: Bantam Books.

Shields, D. (1989). *Dead languages.* New York: Knopf.

Shine, Richard E. (1980). *Systematic fluency training for young children.* Tigard, OR: C. C. Publications.

Siegel, G. (1970). Punishment, stuttering and disfluency. *Journal of Speech and Hearing Disorders, 13,* 677–714.

Silverman, E. (1974). Disfluency behavior of elementary-school stutterers and nonstutterers. *Language, Speech, and Hearing Services in Schools, 5,* 32–37.

Silverman, E. (1973). Clustering: A characteristic of preschoolers' speech disfluency. *Journal of Speech and Hearing Research, 16,* 578–583.

Silverman, E., & Zimmer, C. (1982). Demographic characteristics and treatment experiences of women and men who stutter. *Journal of Fluency Disorders, 7,* 273–285.

Silverman, F. H. (1976). Long-term impact of a miniature metronome on stuttering: An interim report. *Perceptual and Motor Skills, 43,* 398.

Silverman, F. H. (1981). Relapse following stuttering therapy. In N. J. Lass (Ed.), *Speech and language, advances in basic research and practice* (Vol. 5), 56–78. New York: Academic Press.

Silverman, F. H. (1988a). Impact of a T-shirt message on stutterer stereotypes. *Journal of Fluency Disorders, 13,* 279–281.

Silverman, F. H. (1988b). The monster study. *Journal of Fluency Disorders, 13,* 225–231.

Silverman, F. H. (1996). *Stuttering and other fluency disorders.* Englewood Cliffs, NJ: Prentice Hall.

Silverman, F. H., & Hummer, K. (1989). Spastic dysphonia: A fluency disorder? *Journal of Fluency Disorders, 14,* 285–291.

Snidecor, J. C. (1947). Why the Indian does not stutter. *Quarterly Journal of Speech, 33,* 493–495.

Sommers, R. K., & Caruso, A. J. (1995). *American Journal of Speech-Language Pathology, 4*(3), 22–28.

Starke, A. (1994). Why do stutterers reject artificial speech? The message incompatibility conflict. Proceedings of the 1984 meeting of the International Fluency Association.

Starkweather, C. W. (1987). *Fluency and stuttering.* Englewood Cliffs, NJ: Prentice-Hall.

Starkweather, C. W. (1992). Response and reaction to Hamre, "Stuttering Prevention I." *Journal of Fluency Disorders, 17,* 43–55.

Starkweather, C. W. (1995). Personal communication, July 8, 1995.

Starkweather, C. W., & Gottwald, S. R. (1990). The demands and capacities model II: Clinical implications. *Journal of Fluency Disorders, 15,* 143–157.

Starkweather, C. W., Gottwald, S. R., & Halfond, M. H. (1990). *Stuttering Prevention: A Clinical Method.* Englewood Cliffs, NJ: Prentice-Hall.

Starkweather, C. W., Hirschmann, P., & Tannenbaum, R. (1976). Latency of vocalization: Stutterers v. nonstutterers. *Journal of Speech and Hearing Research, 19,* 481–492.

Starkweather, C. W., St. Louis, K. O., Blood, G., Peters, T., & Westbrook, J. (1994). American Speech-Language-Hearing Association (1995, March). Guidelines for Practice in Stuttering Treatment. *Asha,* 37 (Suppl. 14, p. 26).

Stetson, R. H. (1951). *Motor Phonetics.* 2nd Ed. Amsterdam: North-Holland.

St. Louis, K. O. (1982). *Transfer and maintenance of fluency in stuttering clients.* Short course presented to the annual meeting of the American Speech-Language-Hearing Association, Toronto, Ontario.

St. Louis, K. O. (1986a). *The atypical stutterer: Principles and practices of rehabilitation.* Orlando, FL: Academic Press.

St. Louis, K. O. (1986b). The problem of the atypical stutterer: An introduction. In K. O. St. Louis (Ed.), *The atypical stutterer: principles and practices of rehabilitation,* 1–8. New York: Academic Press.

St. Louis, K. O., & Durrenberger, C. H. (1992). *Clinician preferences for managing various communication disorders.* Paper presented at the American Speech-Language-Hearing Association Convention, San Antonio, TX.

St. Louis, K. O., & Hinzman, A. R. (1986). Studies of cluttering: Perceptions of cluttering by speech-language pathologists and educators, *Journal of Fluency Disorders, 11,* 131–149.

St. Louis, K. O., & Lass, N. J. (1981). A survey of communicative disorders attitudes toward stuttering. *Journal of Fluency Disorders, 6,* 49–80.

St. Louis, K., & Myers, F. (1995). Clinical management of cluttering. *Language, Speech, and Hearing in Schools, 26,* 187–195.

St. Louis, K., Murray, C., & Ashworth, M. (1991). Coexisting communication disorders in a random sample of school-aged stutterers. *Journal of Fluency Disorders, 16,* 13–23.

St. Louis, K. O., & Rustin, L. (1992). Professional awareness of cluttering. In F. M. Myers & K. O. St. Louis (Eds.), *Cluttering: A clinical perspective,* 23–35. San Diego, CA: Singular Publishing Group, Inc.

St. Louis, K. O., & Westbrook, J. B. (1987). The effectiveness of treatment for stuttering. In L. Rustin, H. Purser, & D. Rowley (Eds.), *Progress in the treatment of fluency disorders*, 235–257. London: Taylor & Francis.

Stetson, H. R. (1951). *Motor phonetics* (2nd ed.). Amsterdam, Holland: North-Holland.

Stocker, B. (1980). *The Stocker Probe technique for diagnosis and treatment of stuttering in young children.* Tulsa, OK: Modern Education Corporation.

Stocker, B., & Gerstman, L. (1983). A comparison of the probe technique and conventional therapy for young stutterers. *Journal of Fluency Disorders, 8,* 331–339.

Stocker, B., & Usprich, C. (1976). Stuttering in young children and level of demand. *Journal of Fluency Disorders, 1,* 116–131.

Sugarman, M. (1980). It's O.K. to stutter: A personal account. *Journal of Fluency Disorders, 5,* 149–157.

Thompson, J. (1983). *Assessment of fluency in school-age children* (resource guide). Danville, IL: Interstate Printers and Publishers.

Tiffany, W. R. (1980). The effects of syllable structure on diadochokinetic and reading rates. *Journal of Speech and Hearing Research, 23,* 894–908.

Tiger, R. J., Irvine, T. L., & Reiss, R. P. (1980). Cluttering as a complex of learning disabilities. *Language, Speech, and Hearing Services in the Schools, 11,* 3–14.

Toscher, M. M., & Rupp, R. R. (1978). A study of the central auditory processes in stutterers using the Synthetic Sentence Identification (SSI) test battery. *Journal of Speech and Hearing Research, 21,* 779–792.

Travis, L. E. (1957). The unspeakable feelings of people with special reference to stuttering. In L. E. Travis (Ed.), *Handbook of speech pathology,* 916–946. New York: Appleton-Century-Crofts.

Travis, L. E. (1971). The unspeakable feelings of people with special reference to stuttering. In L. E. Travis (Ed.). *Handbook of speech pathology and audiology,* 1001–1003. New York: Appleton-Century-Crofts.

Travis, L. E. (1978). Personal communication, July 10, 1978.

Trotter, W. D., & Silverman, F. H. (1973). Experiments with the stutteraid. *Perceptual and Motor Skills, 36,* 1129–1130.

Truax, C. B., & Carkhuff, R. R. (1966). *Toward effective counseling and psychotherapy.* Chicago: Aldine Press.

Tuckman, B. (1965). Developmental sequence in small groups. *Psychological Bulletin, 63,* 384–399.

Tudor, M. (1939). *An experimental study of the effect of evaluative labeling on speech fluency.* Master's thesis, University of Iowa.

Umeda, N. (1975). Vowel duration in American English. *Journal of the Acoustical Society of America, 58,* 434–445.

Valiant, G. E. (1977). *Adaptation to life.* Boston: Little, Brown & Co.

Van Riper, C. (1971). *Speech correction: Principles and methods* (5th ed.). Englewood Cliffs, NJ: Prentice-Hall.

Van Riper, C. (1973). *The treatment of stuttering* (2nd ed.). Englewood Cliffs, NJ: Prentice-Hall.

Van Riper, C. (1974). A handful of nuts. *Western Michigan Journal of Speech*

Therapy, 11 (2), 1–3.

Van Riper, C. (1975). The stutterer's clinician. In Jon Eisenson (Ed.), *Stuttering, a second symposium* (pp. 453–492). NY: Harper & Row.

Van Riper, C. (1977). *Adult Stuttering Therapy.* A series of eight videotapes produced at Western Michigan University, Kalamazoo, MI. Distributed by The Stuttering Foundation of America.

Van Riper, C. (1978). Personal communication. July 1, 1978.

Van Riper, C. (1979). *A career in speech pathology.* Englewood Cliffs, NJ: Prentice-Hall.

Van Riper, C. (1982). *The nature of stuttering* (2nd ed.). Englewood Cliffs, NJ: Prentice-Hall.

Van Riper, C. (1984). Henry Freund: 1896–1982. *Journal of Fluency Disorders, 9,* 93–102.

Van Riper, C. (1990). Final thoughts about stuttering, *Journal of Fluency Disorders, 15,* 317–318.

Van Riper, C. (1992a). Foreword. In F. Florence & K. St. Louis (Eds.), *Cluttering: A clinical perspective,* xii–xix. Leicester, England: Wurr Publications.

Van Riper, C. (1992b). Some ancient history. *Journal of Fluency Disorders, 17,* 25–28.

Waldrop, J., & Exter, T. (1990). What the 1990 census will show. *American Demographics, 12,* 20–30.

Walker, C., & Black, J. (1950). *The intrinsic intensity of oral phrases* (Joint Project Report No. 2). Pensacola, FL: United States Naval School of Aviation Medicine, Naval Air Station.

Wall, M. J. (1980). A comparison of syntax in young stutterers and nonstutterers. *Journal of Fluency Disorders, 5,* 345–352.

Walle, G. (1975). *The prevention of stuttering, part 1.* (film). Memphis, TN: Stuttering Foundation of America.

Watson, J. B. (1988). A comparison of stutterers and nonstutterers affective, cognitive, and behavioral self-reports. *Journal of Speech and Hearing Research, 31,* 377–385.

Webster, E. (1966). Parent counseling by speech pathologists and audiologists. *Journal of Speech and Hearing Disorders, 31,* 331–345.

Webster, E. (1968). Procedures for group counseling in speech, pathology and audiology. *Journal of Speech and Hearing Disorders, 31,* 331–345.

Webster, R. L. (1974). A behavioral analysis of stuttering: Treatment and theory. In *Treatment methods in psychopathology.* New York: Wiley.

Webster, R. L. (1975). *Clinicians' program guide: The precision fluency shaping program.* Roanoke, VA: Communication Development Corp.

Webster, R. L. (1979). Empirical considerations regarding stuttering therapy. In H. H. Gregory (Ed.), *Controversies about stuttering therapy,* 209–239. Baltimore, MD: University Park Press.

Webster, R. L. (1986). Postscript: Stuttering therapy from a technological point of view. In G. H. Shames & H. Rubin (Ed.), *Stuttering then and now,* 407–414. Columbus, OH: Merrill.

Weiss, A. L. (1993). The pragmatic context of children's disfluency. *Seminars in Speech and Language*, *14*, (3) 215–224.

Weiss, A. L., & Zebrowski, P. M. (1992). Disfluencies in the conversation of young children who stutter: Some answers about questions. *Journal of Speech and Hearing Research*, *35*, 1230–1238.

Weiss, D. A. (1964). *Cluttering*. Englewood Cliffs, NJ: Prentice-Hall.

Weiss, D. A. (1967). Similarities and differences between stuttering and cluttering. *Folia Phoniatrica*, *19*, 98–104.

West, R., & Ansberry, M. (1968). *The rehabilitation of speech* (4th ed.). New York: Harper & Row.

White, E. B. (1954/1960) Some remarks on humor. The second tree from the corner. In J. J. Enck, E. T. Forter, and A. Whitley (Eds.), *The comic in theory and practice* (pp. 102–108). New York: Appleton-Century-Crofts.

Williams, D. (1979). A perspective on approaches to stuttering therapy. In H. Gregory (Ed.), *Controversies about stuttering therapy*, 241–268. Baltimore, MD: University Park Press.

Williams, D. (1983). Working with children in the school environment. In J. Fraser Gruss (Ed.), *Stuttering therapy: Transfer and maintenance* (Publication No. 19). Memphis, TN: Stuttering Foundation of America.

Williams, D. (1985). Talking with children who stutter. In J. Fraser (Ed.). *Counseling stutterers* (pp. 35–45). Memphis, TN: Stuttering Foundation of America.

Williams, D., & Silverman, F. (1968). Note concerning articulation of school-age stutterers. *Perceptual and Motor Skills*, *27*, 713–714.

Williams, D. E. (1971). Stuttering therapy for children. In L. E. Travis (Ed.), *Handbook of speech pathology*, 1073–1093. New York: Appleton-Century-Crofts.

Williams, D. E., Silverman, F. H., & Kools, J. A. (1968). Disfluency behavior of elementary school stutterers and nonstutterers: The adaptation effect. *Journal of Speech and Hearing Research*, *11*, 622–630.

Wingate, M. (1959). Calling attention to stuttering. *Journal of Speech and Hearing Research*, *2*, 326–335.

Wingate, M. (1964). A standard definition of stuttering. *Journal of Speech and Hearing Disorders*, *29*, 484–489.

Wingate, M. (1968). Research trends in stuttering. *Voice*, (Journal of the California Speech and Hearing Association), *17*, 2–6.

Wingate, M. E. (1969). Sound and pattern in "artificial" fluency. *Journal of Speech and Hearing Research*, *12*, 677–686.

Wingate, M. (1971). The fear of stuttering. *Journal of the American Speech-Language-Hearing Association*, *13*, 3–5.

Wingate, M. E. (1988). *The structure of stuttering, a psycholinguistic analysis*. New York: Springer-Verlag.

Wolfe, V. I., Ratusnik, D. L., & Feldman, A. (1979). Acoustic and perceptual comparison of chronic and incipient spastic dysphonia. *Laryngoscope*, *89*, 1478–1486.

Woods, C. L., & Williams, D. E. (1976). Traits attributed to stuttering and normally fluent males. *Journal of Speech and Hearing Research, 19,* 267–278.

Woolf, G. (1967). The assessment of stuttering as struggle, avoidance and expectancy. *British Journal of Disorders of Communication, 2,* 158–171.

World Almanac Book of Facts. (1995). Mahwah, NJ: Funk and Wagnalls Corp.

World Health Organization. (1977). *Manual of the international statistical classification of diseases, injuries, and causes of death* (Vol. 1). Geneva, Switzerland: World Health Organization.

Wyatt, G. L. (1969). *Language learning and communication disorders in children.* New York: Free Press.

Yairi, E. (1981). Disfluencies of normally speaking two-year-old children. *Journal of Speech and Hearing Research, 24,* 490–495.

Yairi, E. (1982). Longitudinal studies of disfluencies in two-year-old children. *Journal of Speech and Hearing Research, 25,* 155–160.

Yairi, E. (1983). The onset of stuttering in two- and three-year-old children. *Journal of Speech and Hearing Disorders, 48,* 171–177.

Yairi, E. (1993). Epidemiologic and other considerations in treatment efficacy research with preschool-age children who stutter. *Journal of Fluency Disorders, 18*(2–3), 197–219.

Yairi, E., & Ambrose, N. (1992a). A longitudinal study of stuttering in children: A preliminary report. *Journal of Speech and Hearing Research, 35,* 755–760.

Yairi, E., & Ambrose, N. (1992b). Onset of stuttering in preschool children: Selected factors. *Journal of Speech and Hearing Research, 35,* 782–788.

Yairi, E., Ambrose, N. G., & Niermann, R. (1993). The early months of stuttering: A developmental study. *Journal of Speech and Hearing Research, 36,* 521–528.

Yairi, E., & Clifton, N. F. (1972). Disfluent speech behavior of preschool children, high school seniors and geriatric persons. *Journal of Speech and Hearing Research, 15,* 714–719.

Yairi, E., & Hall, K. D. (1993). Temporal relations within repetitions of preschool children near the onset of stuttering: A preliminary report. *Journal of Communication Disorders, 26,* 231–244.

Yairi, E., & Lewis, B. (1984). Disfluencies at the onset of stuttering. *Journal of Speech and Hearing Research, 27,* 155–159.

Yairi, E., & Williams, D. (1971). Reports of parental attitudes by stuttering and nonstuttering children. *Journal of Speech and Hearing Research, 14,* 596–604.

Yates, A. J. (1963). Delayed auditory feedback. *Psychological Bulletin, 60,* 213–232.

Young, M. A. (1975). Onset, prevalence, and recovery from stuttering. *Journal of Speech and Hearing Disorders, 40,* 49–58.

Zebrowski, P. M., Conture, E. G., & Cudahy, E. A. (1985). Acoustic analysis of young stutterers' fluency: Preliminary observations. *Journal of Fluency*

Disorders, 10, 173–192.

Zemlin, W. R. (1988). *Speech and hearing science: Anatomy and physiology* (3rd ed.). Englewood Cliffs, NJ: Prentice-Hall.

Zenner, A., Ritterman, S., Bowden, S., & Gronhovd, D. (1978). Measurement and comparison of anxiety levels of parents of stuttering, articulatory defective and normal-speaking children. *Journal of Fluency Disorders, 3,* 273–284.

Zimmerman, G. (1980). Stuttering: A disorder of movement. *Journal of Speech and Hearing Research, 23,* 122–136.

Zimmerman, G. (1981). Stuttering: In need of a unifying conceptual framework. *Journal of Speech and Hearing Research, 24,* 25–31.

Name Index

Subject Index